ALLE · ZEIT · WACH · 1842

J. Ragaz I.M. Ariel (Eds.)

High-Risk Breast Cancer

Diagnosis

With 67 Figures and 40 Tables

Springer-Verlag Berlin Heidelberg New York
London Paris Tokyo Hong Kong

Joseph Ragaz, MD, FRCP
Medical Oncology, Cancer Control Agency of British Columbia
600 West 10th Avenue, Vancouver, B.C. V5Z 4E6, Canada

Irving M. Ariel, MD
Foundation for Clinical Research Inc.
80 East End Avenue, New York, NY 10028, USA

ISBN-13: 978-3-642-73720-6 e-ISBN-13: 978-3-642-73718-3
DOI: 10.1007/978-3-642-73718-3

Library of Congress Cataloging-in-Publication Data.
High-risk breast cancer: diagnosis/J. Ragaz, I.M. Ariel (eds.). p. cm. Includes index.
ISBN-13: 978-3-642-73720-6 (U.S.: alk. paper)
1. Breast-Cancer-Diagnosis. I. Ragaz, J. (Joseph), 1945-. II. Ariel, Irving M.
[DNLM: 1. Breast Neoplasms-diagnosis. WP 870 H638]
RC280.B8H54 189 616.99'449075-dc20 DNLM/DLC 89-11333

Softcover reprint of the hardcover 1st edition 1989

Typesetting: Macmillan India Ltd., Bangalore-25, India

2125/3140-543210-Printed on acid-free paper.

Preface

The most meaningful reward to clinicians and researchers is the absence of recurrent malignancy in their patients. While in some patients the disease will be cured by resection alone, in other similarly staged cases the disease will recur despite adequate locoregional and systemic therapies. Hence, risk assessment is a complex issue with many related or unrelated prognostic factors determining outcome. The purpose of this volume is to review some of the most relevant prognostic factors of newly diagnosed breast cancer, focusing on features determining the magnitude of risk. The ultimate value of establishing the significance of each prognostic factor in a given patient will be the resulting ability to plan *individualized* therapies for patients at different risk of recurrence at the time of diagnosis. To secure the maximum benefit for high-risk patients, while avoiding undue toxicity in those with low-risk lesions, a well-integrated analysis of all known prognostic factors will be essential in the early postdiagnostic period. In addition to well-established staging criteria such as axillary nodes, tumor size, receptors, scanning and radiographic examinations, the more sophisticated laboratory techniques, as discussed by several authors herein, will play a crucial role in risk assessment. Most of them, – ploidy determination, oncogenes, tumor markers, monoclonal antibodies, growth factors, etc. – are presently available in only a minority of treatment centers. Their routine use may not only enhance the academic and scientific approach to some fundamental issues of cancer etiology, but also be of practical assistance to clinicians in determining the risk in individual patients at diagnosis. The integration of these risk factors with the conventionally more frequently utilized criteria will greatly refine the assessment of prognosis and overall risk.

This first volume on high-risk breast cancer deals with the diagnosis of the disease. Band and Deschamps review the epidemiological aspects, offering some suggestions for interventional studies of high-risk women without breast cancer. MacKay and Steel, and Fiore and Viola review their and others' exciting data on the significance of oncogenes in breast cancer, while the risk factors assessed by pathological examination are discussed comprehensively by Fisher. The survival benefit associated with screening mammography is brought to our attention by Miller and by Tabar, who place particular emphasis on early detection as the major contribution to cure. Merkel, Hill, McGuire and Shek, Godolphin summarize the significance of estrogen and progesterone receptors, while Hedley and Muss and Kute discuss comprehensively the significance of ploidy and kinetic as determined using flow cytometry. Meyer's chapter clarifies the complex issue of tumor kinetics and summarizes the laboratory techniques of kinetic determination. LeRiche et al. discuss the promising role of fine needle aspiration in the diagnosis and follow-up of breast cancers, while Simpson-Herren offers data indicating that therapeutic maneuvers, including cytoreduction, may lead to profound kinetic alterations in the residual tumor. The exciting role of growth factors in the regulation of proliferation of breast cancer is described by Yee and Lippman. The role of tumor markers, particularly monoclonal antibodies and circulating immune complexes, is reviewed by Mansi and Coombes and by Salinas. Horsman highlights the significance of chromosome aberrations in breast lesions. With more sophisticated laboratory techniques for their visualization, these would probably be found to be present more frequently than is currently realized. Emerman indicates that in vitro culturing of individual lesions at diagnosis may provide great improvement in such an analysis, in addition to enabling testing for sensitivity to therapeutic agents and determination of other tumor characteristics such as oncogenic expression.

We gratefully acknowledge the assistance of all coauthors of this volume. Also, we give special thanks to the following individuals: to Mary Naylor, for devoted secretarial assistance; to David Noble, for skillful editing of the manuscripts and bibliographies; to Springer, for efficient coordination in publication; to Ciba-Geigy Canada, for funding our breast research projects; and to the medical staff of the Cancer Control Agency of British Columbia, for their input and ideas associated with this project.

Spring 1989

J. Ragaz
I. M. Ariel

Contents

List of Contributors *

* The address of the principal author is given on the first page of each contribution.

[1] Page on which contribution begins.

Introduction

High-Risk Breast Cancer: Definition of the Risk

J. Ragaz[1] and I.M. Ariel[2]

[1] Medical Oncology, Cancer Control Agency of British Columbia, 600 West 10th Avenue, Vancouver, B.C. V5Z 4E6, Canada
[2] Pack Medical, B7 East, 36th Street, New York, NY 10016, USA

Introduction

High-risk breast cancer is defined in this volume as a disease with a high probability of dissemination, implying aggressive behavior, presence of micrometastases at diagnosis, resistance to therapy and ultimate recurrence with poor overall survival. This is in contrast to low-risk disease, which is curable in most instances by conventional surgery. The first part of this chapter reviews the known prognostic factors predicting the magnitude of risk. The ultimate value of refined risk assessment may be demonstrated by improvement in planning of therapeutic strategies. Accordingly, different intensities of treatment for different risk subgroups will be suggested, avoiding overtreatment of low-risk cases and undertreatment of high-risk patients.

Risk of Breast Cancer: Background

Evidence is accumulating which indicates that the origin of tumor characteristics can be traced to the genome of the malignant cell [13, 29, 105, 104, 121]. Figure 1 illustrates the primary importance of the genotype, determining all subsequent tumor phenotypic characteristics, including kinetics, stage, grade, receptors, ploidy, and propensity to metastasize. Hence, our first conclusion is the following: The magnitude of risk could be assessed in a more refined way either by a sophisticated integration of all known phenotypic characteristics or, alternatively, by pinpointing the crucial locus in the DNA – either a single gene or an as yet unidentifiable factor X – responsible for the phenotype. Integrated knowledge and quantification of the phenotypic and genotypic characteristics may provide the ultimate risk assessment.

Kinetic Assessment of Risk

Several studies indicate a good correlation between tumor kinetics and outcome, implying a more aggressive behavior in fast-growing tumors [17, 69, 70, 72, 73, 102, 103] (Table 2). The most important data on kinetics have come from studies assessing tumor labeling index [70, 71, 73, 102, 103], or from flow cytometry studies

Ragaz/Ariel (Eds.), High-Risk Breast Cancer

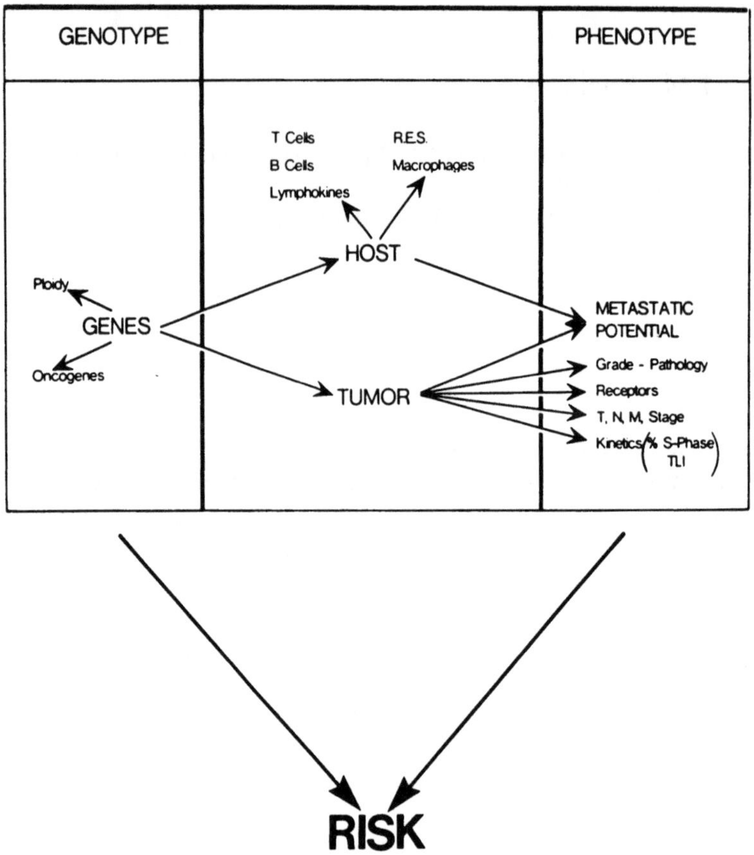

Fig. 1. This illustration shows the contribution of genotype and phenotype to risk determination. It reveals the primary importance of genotype, which influences characteristics not only of the tumor but also of the host. It also indicates the effect of the host on tumor characteristics, the immune surveillance system being the most likely modulating mechanism. *R.E.S.*, resticuloendothelial system

of the proportion of cells in S phase [51, 52, 62, 72, 73]. As discussed by Meyer, Hedley, and Muss and Kute in this volume, actively proliferating tumors, although perhaps better targets for instantaneous cell kill by chemotherapy or radiotherapy, are almost uniformly associated with decreased survival and with other high-risk prognostic factors (Table 2). Figure 2 clarifies several points of this complex association. The level of clinical detection (line d) is the minimum tumor burden permitting clinical or radiological diagnosis. Tumors with a very short doubling time (short cell cycle time, reduced cell death, or both), will grow above the level of clinical detection soon after the malignant transformation of the first cell. Rapidly growing and aggressive tumors (lines a1-a4, mean a) may more frequently emerge before the menopause, although diagnosis at any age is possible (lines a5, a6). Two extreme examples of tumors exhibiting rapid growth are inflammatory breast cancer and, in the lung, oat cell carcinoma. Tumors with longer doubling times

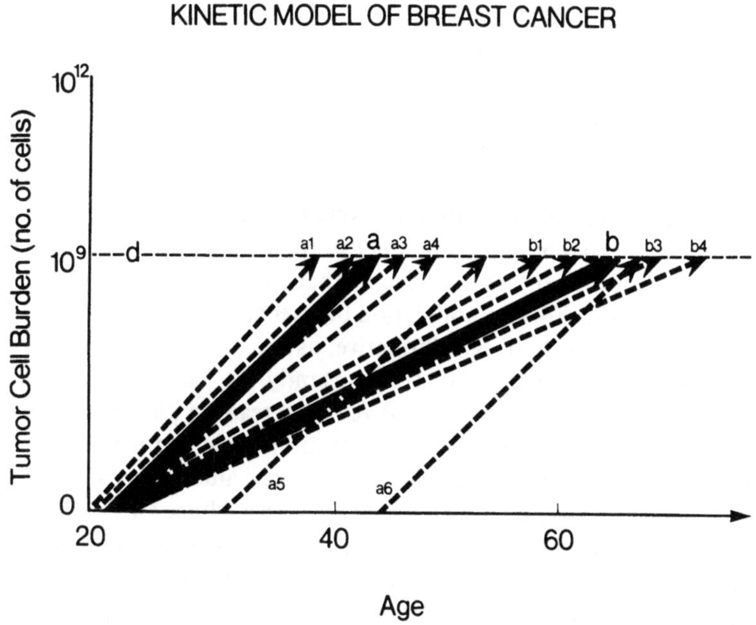

Fig. 2. The time for which the tumor remains subclinical and the slope of tumor development are functions of the rates of tumor stem cell division (intrinsic tumor doubling time), and of cell death (tumor cell necrosis and elimination, loss of metastatic potential, differentiation, etc.). Hence, the intrinsic (genotypic) characteristics of the tumor, and its interaction with the host, may determine not only the time of diagnosis (duration of subclinical period), but also the complex phenotypic characteristics, determining the behavior of the tumor. *Lines a1-a4* (mean *a*): Slopes of tumors with a short subclinical period, usually developing and emerging when the patient is younger. *Lines a5, a6*: Slopes of tumors with a short subclinical period, developing and emerging when the patient is older. *Lines b1-b4* (mean *b*): Slopes of tumors with a long subclinical period, emerging at an older age. *Line d*: Level of clinical detection

(lines b1-b4, mean b) will be diagnosed after a significantly longer subclinical period and may more often emerge after the menopause. Thus, age, the menopause, or any other single prognostic factor may not *alone* determine the behavior of the tumor; rather, the interaction of the tumor's intrinsic genotypic characteristics with the host is decisive (Fig. 1).

Mammography and Risk Assessment

No other interventional technique in breast cancer management has yielded survival gains matching those achieved by screening mammography, as reported by several major screening studies [100, 109, 119]. Elsewhere in this volume, both Tabar and Miller conclude that a substantial survival gain has already resulted from the use of this technique [100, 109, 119]. Several authorities, however, still question the therapeutic benefit of mass screening mammography. Fisher, in his chapter herein, indicates that only up to 10% of patients with large tumors would have been free of disease had their primary tumors been removed when less than 2 cm in size. Had the delay of diagnosis been the main determining factor, he argues, the improvement in disease-free survival should have been much greater. Hence, other factors, rather than the time delay alone, may be responsible for the high risk at diagnosis.

Several questions remain unanswered. Firstly, would earlier detection of the tumors by screening mammography prevent metastatic spread in tumors of *any* degree of aggressiveness? In a given patient, the answer to such a question can be only speculative. For the population of screened women, as argued by Tabar and Miller, the answer is likely affirmative, as the survival gains in screened patients have already been documented. Importantly, the magnitude of the survival gain, particularly for women aged 40-50 years, increases with the duration of follow-up. This was seen by the update of the HIP study, documenting survival benefits of the screened population of younger women only after 8 years follow-up [100]. Of particular importance are results showing that although the overall incidence of breast cancer has not changed as a result of the screening, the proportion accounted for by in situ and stage I disease has risen significantly [100, 109]. Hence, the main value of mass screening has already been established: the proportion of low-risk tumors is increasing, survival gains have been confirmed, and side effects, particularly tumor induction, are not significant.
Several points still require clarification:

1. The extent to which self-examination of the breast and mass education contribute to the survival gains presently attributed to screening mammography.
2. The combination of mammography with other screening diagnostic modalities – imaging techniques with tumor-specific monoclonal antibodies, light scanning assessment, etc.
3. The maximum benefit that can be achieved. Will improvements in equipment and in the interpretative skills of mammographers have further impact on survival? Also, could radiologists outside the centers currently conducting screening trials reproduce the results of their motivated and experienced colleagues?

Considering the rising interest in and improved quality of screening mammography, these points will likely be clarified in the near future.

TNM Staging

Nodes

Axillary Nodes. There is a consensus that involvement of the axillary lymph nodes is the most significant prognostic factor in breast cancer both for disease-free and for overall survival ([33, 36, 48, 49, 85, 98, 106] see also Fisher, this volume). The significance of nodes in most published series is independent of other factors, and a consistently rising negative correlation with survival is seen with an increasing number of affected lymph nodes [75]. Conventional adjuvant chemotherapy regimens will not affect the prognostic importance of lymph nodes, as inferior survival in patients with an increasing number of involved nodes is still seen in adjuvantly treated patients [14, 15, 88]. These data call for more innovative programs for those with high numbers of affected nodes.

Internal Mammary Nodes. The involvement of the internal mammary nodes is associated with inferior outcome both in node-positive and, particularly, in node-negative patients [120]. Internal mammary scintigraphy studies [30, 68], correlating the outcome with the status of these nodes have confirmed these observations. In experienced hands, therefore, this imaging technique could become useful for risk assessment if used more uniformly.

Node-Negative Patients. Node-negative patients survive significantly longer than their node-positive counterparts, yet up to 30% will manifest recurrence at 10- to 15-year follow-up [4, 16, 56, 77].

Most recent studies document the benefit of adjuvant chemotherapy in high-risk subsets of node-negative patients [16, 56]. The question to ask is whether additional risk factors can be identified accurately, so as not to subject the whole group of node-negative patients to adjuvant treatment [93, 94]. The factors so far associated with high risk for relapse in node-negative cases include low yield of estrogen receptor density [28, 111, 117, 118], poor differentiation [89], high thymidine labelling index [72, 73], aneuploidy [28], and invasion of lymph or blood vessels [4, 96]. More recently, involvement of bone marrow in stage 1 patients documented by monoclonal antibodies was correlated with increased rate of recurrence and with subsequent development of bone metastases [20]. These studies indicate that adverse prognostic factors in node-negative patients may increase the risk of recurrence to a level resembling that seen in node-positive cases. Furthermore, patients with involved lymph nodes, but no additional adverse factors may survive longer than high-risk node-negative cases. Therefore, the decision on whether to employ adjuvant chemotherapy should embrace consideration not only of nodal stage but also of the overall risk.

Size

Correlation of Tumor Size and Outcome. Most reports correlate greater tumor size at diagnosis with greater risk of recurrence and shorter duration of survival [32, 49, 60, 75]. Large size has also been repeatedly correlated with high numbers of involved nodes. A review of three large studies showed histological involvement of axillary nodes in 34%, 27%, and 39% of in tumors smaller than 2 cm in diameter, compared with 65%, 49%, and 62% in tumors larger than 5 cm [32, 49, 75]. In a report on one of the largest investigations on tumor size, a positive correlation of T stage with recurrence rate was seen on follow-up for as long as 25 years [60].

How do we interpret data correlating greater tumor size with a higher number of involved axillary nodes? In this regard, several studies are of interest [88]. In our randomized adjuvant study [88], the univariate analysis of 316 patients showed the following prognostic factors to have a significant effect on disease-free survival: number of axillary nodes ($P < 0.0001$), age ($P = 0.0064$), tumor size ($P = 0.022$), and estrogen receptors ($P = 0.03$). In multivariate analysis, when controlling for nodes, only age ($P = 0.0021$) and tumor size ($P = 0.04$) remained significant. When, however, controlling for both nodes and age, tumor size retained only marginal prognostic significance ($P = 0.08$). Similarly, among our 143 node-negative patients, those with T1, T2, and T3 tumors had similar 5-year disease-free survival rates of 75.7%, 76.2%, and 66.7% ($P = > 0.5$).

The next study of importance regarding the association between tumor size and outcome is that by Fracchia et al. [41, 42], who identified a group of patients with large, locally advanced tumors but negative nodes (stages T3-4, N0). They observed a surprisingly good 10-year survival rate of 75.3%, compared with only 15% in patients in the same T categories with positive axillary nodes. Similarly, Arnold and Lesnick [2] reported an unexpectedly good 10-year survival rate of 63% in patients with T3, N0 tumors. These data, therefore, support the observations in other studies [32, 49, 75] that nodal status, rather than size, is of importance. However, more refined analysis of tumor size integrated with nodal status and *all* other prognostic risk factors is needed to determine the *additional* contribution of tumor size to risk of recurrence.

Comments on Large Lesions. There are several possible theoretical explanations for the presence of large tumors, making the association of tumor size and natural history of disease more complex. Firstly, the existence of at least two subtypes of large-size breast cancer lesions is evident. In the first, type A, the diagnostic delay accounts for the advanced tumor stage. The size itself does not necessarily imply aggressiveness. These "neglected" tumors may present as stage III, either operable or categorically inoperable lesions (T3a, b, T4a-c) [49]. In type A tumors, the risk of dissemination will be proportional to the magnitude of the diagnostic delay. An extremely benign subtype of these large tumors has been identified, with consistent, slow locoregional progression but infrequent systemic dissemination [41, 42]. Type A large tumors are usually receptor positive and thus amenable to hormonal treatments, and despite their size a palliative "toilet" mastectomy can frequently achieve long-term control. The other type of large tumor, type B, is typical of rapid systemic dissemination occurring in parallel with locoregional expansion [39]. Extreme examples of type B large lesions are inflammatory breast cancers, and subsets of locally advanced lesions presenting metastatic lesions at diagnosis or soon afterwards. Type B large tumors are usually refractory to hormonal or chemotherapeutic treatments. As discussed earlier in this chapter, widely different intrinsic tumor characteristics, probably at the level of genetic control, are responsible for the great behavioral heterogeneity. In summary, therefore, large size may not always be associated with aggressiveness and reduced survival. Furthermore, it is unlikely that earlier diagnosis will significantly influence the outcome of subtype B large lesions, as aggressive behavior, rapid systemic dissemination, and early transition to resistance are frequent preclinical phenomena. On the other hand, early diagnosis, for instance by screening mammography, assisted by self-examination and general awareness on the part of the patient, may significantly influence the curability of type A large lesions.

Receptor Status

Elsewhere in this volume, Merkel et al., Shek and Godolphin, and Fisher summarize previous studies which indicate a clear correlation of receptors not only with response to hormones, but also with disease-free, overall, and postrecurrence survival [45, 71, 118]. The significance of receptors in risk assessment is enhanced by the appreciation that as a biochemical expression of intact cytosol and nuclear function, their increasing quantity likely correlates with differentiation and reduced aggressiveness. Hence, a higher number of receptors can be considered a biochemical expression of a less aggressive genome, subject to mutational changes within the life of the tumor. The loss of hormonal responses attests to such transitions, echoing observations on somatic mutation in bacteria [66] and in chemotherapy treatments [46]. Several well-confirmed observations correlating the absence of estrogen and progesterone receptors with inferior outcome make receptor status a powerful factor in the global risk [19, 28, 71, 118]. It remains to be seen whether the superiority of progesterone over estrogen receptors as predictors of risk [54, 55] will be reproduced in multivariate analysis using all factors of significance. There is, nevertheless, a smooth transition, from good to poor survival, from groups where both estrogen and progesterone receptors are highly positive to groups where one of them is negative to groups where both are negative [19, 55].

Preliminary data indicate that effective adjuvant chemotherapy may reduce the value of receptors in risk assessment [15]. This may be due to the preferential chemotherapy cell kill effect of receptor-negative clones. Some results, however, indicate a preferential effectiveness of adjuvant chemotherapy in estrogen receptor-positive patients [83]. Further data will be needed to clarify these very important observations.

Pathology

Differentiation: Grade

Both histological and nuclear differentiation can be used for the quantitative expression of risk, because a good correlation of differentiation with lymph node status and outcome has been documented in previous publications [12, 35, 37, 91]. According to several studies, of particular significance is such a correlation in node-negative patients [24, 84, 91, 92]. Of further interest is an association of DNA ploidy, proportion of cells in S-phase (% S-phase), and differentiation. As seen in Tables 1 and 2, aneuploid tumors and, in most series, tumors with high % S-phase were correlated with poor differentiation and also with other adverse prognostic factors [8, 26, 34, 52, 58, 72, 74, 78, 110], including absence of hormone receptors [37], younger age [11, 21, 22, 87, 110], and a high number of axillary nodes [69, 70,

72, 73]. The correlation of nuclear morphometry (a quantitative assessment of nuclear diameter and configuration) with nodal metastases and with the outcome provides further credence for the concept of the association of DNA and tumor behavior [61, 67, 91, 124].

Lymphangitic and Vascular Involvement

In node-negative patients, lymphangitic involvement is seen in up to 15% of cases and is associated with poor outcome ([10, 42, 76, 92-94] see also Fisher, this volume). According to Fisher (this volume); such correlation could not be seen as clearly in patients with positive axillary nodes. In several studies, vascular invasion was clearly identified more often in cases with than without recurrence [10, 91]. According to Rosen, visceral metastases occurred in 67% of patients with, and in 37% without vascular invasion [91]. Most studies agree that the adverse impact of both vascular and lymphangitic involvement is more frequently observed in node-negative patients. This indicates that, in node-positive patients, risk features like lymphangitic and vascular invasion are of lesser importance. Only refined quantitative analysis of each individual risk factor may obviate the additional risk contribution of vessel invasion.

Role of Flow Cytometry in Risk Determination: Ploidy and % S-Phase

The technique of flow cytometry, as discussed by Hedley, Muss and Kute and Meyer in this volume, offers a unique possibility to examine the DNA content and cell-cycle phase of individual cells within the tumor. Such information is yielding insight into the role of DNA in risk determination, and when combined with chromosomal and oncogenic assessment, it will likely enable a more comprehensive understanding of the involvement of DNA in the malignant process. The work of Emerman and of Horsman, as summarized in this volume, indicates that in vitro cultures grown from a given patient may provide more detailed chromosomal and perhaps other DNA information not expressed in the original biopsy sample. Tables 1 and 2 illustrate the various associations of ploidy and % S-phase with outcome and other prognostic factors, and although they do not represent a complete review of the literature, they nevertheless reflect the consensus expressed in most published studies.

Table 1. DNA ploidy and risk. Correlation of ploidy with tumor phenotypic characteristics is indicated by a + or a – sign. The + sign indicates a positive association of ploidy with each individual risk factor as indicated by the statements in parentheses; the – sign a lack of such an association

Survival (worse in aneuploid)		
Overall:		
Harvey et al.	50	+
Atkin and Kay	5	+
Cornelisse et al.: postmenopausal	22	+
Cornelisse et al.: premenopausal	22	–
Hedley et al.: univariate	51, 52	+
Hedley et al.: multivariate	51, 52	–
Kallioniemi et al.	58	–
Auer et al.: FNA	6	+
Dowle et al.	26	+
Opferman et al.	81	–
Owainati et al.	82	–
Klintenberg et al.	59	–
Dressler et al.: stage I	28	+
Coulson et al.	23	+
Kute et al.	62	–
Disease-free:		
Atkin and Kay	5	+
Hedley et al.	51, 52	+
Kute et al.	62	+
Ewers et al.	31	+
Retsky et al.	90	+
Owainati et al.	82	–
Kallioniemi et al.	58	+
Cornelisse et al.: postmenopausal	22	+
Cornelisse et al.: premenopausal	22	–
Dressler et al.: stage I	28	+
Owens stage I	this volume	+
Nodes (more involvement in aneuploid)		
Dowle et al.	26	
Hedley et al.	51, 52	+
Atkin and Kay	5	+
Ewers et al.	31	–
Kute et al.	62	–
Moran et al.	74	–
Klintenberg et al.	59	+
Cornelisse et al >10 nodes positive	22	+
Cornelisse et al $\leqslant 10$ nodes positive	22	–
Fossa et al.	40	+
Jakobsen et al.	57	+
Bedrossian et al.	8	–
Harvey et al.	50	+

Table 1 (continued)

Estrogen/progesterone receptors (lower value in aneuploid)		
Kute et al.	62	+
Hedley et al.	51, 52	+
Klintenberg et al.	59	+
Olszewski et al.	78, 79	+
Kallioniemi et al.	58	+
Bichel et al.	11	+
Abandowitz et al.: premenopausal	1	−
Abandowitz et al.: postmenopausal	1	+
Auer et al.	6	+
Cornelisse et al.	21	+
Jakobsen et al.	57	+
Coulson et al.	23	−
Fossa et al.	40	−
Horsfal et al.	53	−
Raber et al.	87	−
Histological grade (more undifferentiated in aneuploid)		
Dowle et al.	26	+
Hedley et al.	51, 52	+
Kallioniemi et al.	58	+
Thorud et al.	112	+
Moran et al.	74	+
Olszewski et al.	78, 79	+
Bedrossian et al.	8	−
Fossa et al.	40	+
Age (more aneuploid in younger patients)		
Dowle et al.	26	+
Taylor et al.	110	+
Kute et al.	62	−
Kallioniemi et al.	58	−
Abandowitz et al.	1	+
Haag et al.	47	−
Bedrossian et al.	8	−
Fossa et al.	40	−
Hedley et al.	51, 52	−
Tumor size (larger in aneuploid)		
Hedley et al.	51, 52	−
Kute et al.	62	−
Kallioniemi et al.	58	−
Thorud et al.	112	+
Ewers et al.	31	+
Cornelisse et al.: T2 only	21, 22	+
Cornelisse et al.: T1 and T3	21, 22	−
Haag et al.	47	

Table 2. Tumor kinetics (TLI, % S-phase, mitotic index) and risk. Correlation of tumor kinetics with individual risk factors. Tumor kinetics are determined by measurements of the tumor labeling index (TLI) or % S-phase as obtained from flow cytometry. Correlation of kinetics with tumor phenotypic characteristics is indicated by a + or a − sign. The + sign indicates a positive association of kinetics with each individual risk factor as indicated by the statements in parentheses, the − sign a lack of such an association

***Survival* (*lower in tumors with increased kinetics*)**		
Overall:	References	
Meyer et al.	72, 73	+
Silvestrini et al.: stage I	102, 103	+
Tubiana et al.	114, 115	+
Hedley et al.	51, 52	−
McDivitt et al.	69, 70	+
Disease-free		
Meyer et al.: local recurrence	71, 72	+
Meyer et al.: distant recurrence	71, 72	−
Silvestrini et al.: stage I	102, 103	+
Tubiana et al.	114	+
Klintenberg et al.	59	+
Kallioniemi et al.	58	+
Coulson et al.	23	+
Hedley et al.: univariate	51, 52	+
Hedley et al.: multivariate	51, 52	−
Kute et al.	62	−
McDivitt et al.	69, 70	+
Dressler et al.	28	+
Clark and McGuire	19	+
Owens	this volume	+
***Estrogen/progesterone receptors* (*increased kinetics in lower values*)**		
Gentilli et al.	44	+
Meyer et al.		+
Kute et al.	62	+
Olszewski et al.	78, 79	+
Bedrossian et al.	8	+
Dressler et al.	28	+
McDivitt et al.	69, 70	+
Hedley et al.	51, 52	−
Klintenberg et al.	59	+
Kallioniemi et al.	58	+
Strauss et al.	108	+
Bertuzzi et al.	9	+
***Tumor grade* (*increased kinetics in undifferentiated tumors*)**		
Hedley et al.	51, 52	−
Kallioniemi et al.	58	+
Meyer et al.	72, 73	+

Table 2 (*continued*)

***Tumor grade* (increased kinetics in undifferentiated tumors)**		
Moran et al.	74	+
Taylor et al.	110	+
***Ploidy* (increased kinetics in aneuploid)**		
Coulson et al.	23	+
Kute et al.	62	+
Kallioniemi et al.	58	+
Meyer et al.	72, 73	+
Frankfurt et al.	43	+
Hedley et al.	51, 52	+
Haag et al.	47	+
Bedrossian et al.	8	−
Fossa et al.	40	+
Dressler et al.	28	+
Olszewski et al.	78, 79	+
***Age* (increased kinetics in younger patients)**		
Abandowitz et al.	1	+
Kute et al.	62	−
Meyer et al.	72, 73	+
Bedrossian et al.	8	−
Gentilli et al.	44	+
Bertuzzi et al.	9	+
Silvestrini et al.	102, 103	+
***Tumor size* (increased kinetics in larger tumors)**		
Kute et al.	62	−
Meyer et al.	72, 73	+
Bedrossian et al.	8	+
Gentilli et al.	44	+
Tubiana et al.	114	+
Hedley et al.	51, 52	−
Silvestrini et al.	102, 103	+

Growth Factors

As growth factors influence cell division and tumor growth in vitro, their quantitative or qualitative assessment in a clinical setting may correlate with the kinetic and perhaps also with the metastatic potential of a given tumor. As discussed by Yee and Lippman in this volume, an association of tumor growth with several growth factors has been recently documented by many laboratories [63, 64, 107, 113, 116, 123]. Receptors for most growth factors have been identified, and early data show that their binding with monoclonal antibodies interrupts the signal pathway of a measured growth factor. Hence, information not only on growth factors, but also on their receptors, and ultimately on their genes, will be needed for the final assessment of this complex interaction [18, 25, 107, 113].

It has been suggested recently that hormones may also act partially through the stimulation of the production of growth factor proteins, which, in paracrine or autocrine fashion, mediate growth stimulation [3, 63, 64]. Estrogens enhance activity of transforming growth factor alpha (TGF-alpha, a known mitogen), while tamoxifen increases levels of transforming growth factor beta (TGF-beta, a suppressor of cell division in breast cancer cell lines). Also, TGF-alpha is thought to act via epidermal growth factor (EGF) receptor, believed to be a product of the newly identified c-erb/her/neu oncogene [27, 97]. Hence, a sensitive interplay among hormones, growth factors, their genes, and between the stimulatory and inhibitory growth factors may determine the overall tumor growth potential. Of great interest are recent data showing TGF-alpha activity in benign epithelium, as determined in samples obtained from reduction mammoplasty [7]. Even in benign tissue, however, TGF-alpha RNA was expressed more in the rapidly proliferating breast epithelial cell line but not in the organoid cell line, rendering TGF-alpha a marker for increased growth also in benign epithelium. With regard to the association of tamoxifen and increasing levels of TGF-beta, (suppression of cell division) there are data showing increased expression of an epithelial membrane antigen upon TGF-beta stimulation, a marker of differentiated non-malignant epithelial cells [122]. Such observations substantiate a possible role of TGF-beta, and indirectly also tamoxifen, in the induction of differentiation [122].

Concerning the rising significance of growth factors in the clinical setting, several recent studies of EGF are of importance: Fitzpatrick et al. [38], studying a subset of human breast cancer tumors, observed expression of EGF but not estrogen receptors, and postulated that for some breast cancer patients, EGF rather than estrogen is the main growth regulator. Perez et al. [86] confirmed the presence of EGF receptors in 50% of human breast cancer samples, with an inverse relationship of EGF receptors and estrogen receptors. Therefore, EGF may have a very important regulatory role in the growth of breast cancer. This intriguing association was confirmed by Sainsbury et al. [95] in a study correlating EGF receptors, estrogen receptors, and survival in 135 breast cancer patients. Multivariate analysis, their data showed EGF receptors to be the most significant prognostic factor for node-negative patients and the second most important prognostic factor for node-positive patients.

Most recent reports have shown that methods utilizing immunohistochemistry and immunohybridization may permit intracellular visualization of growth factors, with great promise for diagnosis of human cancer [63]. Also, experiments documenting a decrease of tumor growth after interruption of TGF-alpha receptors by a polyclonal antibody indicate a promising role of growth factors in therapy [3].

Several intriguing questions arise: Could growth factors not only mediate the growth of established tumors, but also initiate the transformation of benign into malignant cells? Sherwin et al. documented TGF-alpha in the urine of 18/22 patients with disseminated cancer, but not in the normal controls [101]. In an established malignancy, could the ongoing process of mutations alter the balance of stimulatory and inhibitory growth factors, rendering the tumor more aggressive? Could any kinetic alterations, including initial tumor growth, or subsequent growth fluctuations, also be mediated systemically by growth factors?

Whether examination of growth factors, their receptors, and DNA will be of assistance in diagnosis and therapy [18] remains to be seen, but the coming few years will likely see growth factors in a position of extreme importance in the clinical setting.

Oncogenes and Breast Cancer

There is increasing evidence for an association of malignancy with several groups of oncogenes or their products [13, 65, 104, 105]. MacKay and Steel (this volume) discuss the significance of genetic factors in breast cancer. They also outline the methodology for genetic analysis, indicating its enormous complexity, yet tempting one to make correlations between oncogenes, restriction fragment length polymorphism, and cancer. Fiore and Viola present clinically available data associating the protein product of the H-*ras* oncogene and the aggressiveness of breast cancer. The data correlating the magnitude of oncogenic expression with the aggressiveness of the disease are reminiscent of the elegant work of Seeger et al. (99), who reported the association of an increased expression of N-*myc* oncogene with a reduction of disease-free survival in patients with neuroblastoma. Similar clinical data on breast cancer come from Slamon and colleagues [104, 105]. In their work, the overexpression of *her/neu* oncogene was associated with significantly inferior disease-free and overall survival, independent in a multivariate analysis from nodes and from estrogen and progesterone receptors. Repeated analysis with an updated follow-up at 53 months confirmed the findings and the significance of *her/neu* oncogene in predicting relapse and shorter overall survival in node-positive, but not node-negative patients [104].

The ongoing debate on the connection between oncogenes and outcome must be interpreted with caution because of several factors. Firstly, most laboratories differ greatly in the magnitude of the problems they experience with the DNA technology. Also, insufficient numbers of patients have been studied so far. Nevertheless, the very fact that some association is found between genetic loci and tumor behavior is of extreme importance. It not only indicates that genetic phenomena may be responsible for the initial tumor transformation, but also indicates that regulatory genetic control can be assessed and quantitated at diagnosis. The potential significance of such an assessment in the clinical setting can be appreciated more clearly in light of the fact that of more than 40 known oncogenes, only a few have so far been submitted to rigorous clinical testing. Also, it is not unrealistic, considering the rate of progress in genetic research over the last few years, to predict that probes for other as yet unidentified oncogenes and other genetic loci will likely be developed.

What can oncogenic research offer clinicians in terms of risk assessment? Firstly, the increasing availability and standardization of laboratory techniques may make oncogenes, pending confirmation of their significance in cancer follow-up, a part of the routine risk assessment at the time of diagnosis. Secondly, their impact may be greatly increased if a battery of oncogenes, rather than a single one, can be obtained from the patient and assessed in conjunction with other prognostic factors. Such an approach will likely yield further insight into the association between genetic influences and overall phenotypic risk characteristics, and the overall risk will be assessed more accurately.

Conclusion

This volume provides solid evidence that increasing numbers of individual phenotypic tumor characteristics correlating with the outcome of breast cancer are being identified and, hence, can be used at diagnosis for risk assessment. The important point may be not only the magnitude of the risk predicted by these various characteristics *individually*, but their additional contribution when controlling for several of the most important risk factors in combination. For example, knowing the nodal status, tumor size, and receptor status, do we have to have information about ploidy, oncogenes, differentiation, etc.? The ultimate improvement in risk assessment will lie in the identification of one or several crucial factors rendering other risk factors unnecessary for prediction of outcome. Identification of such a single factor may be sufficient to determine the risk, and ultimately to indicate different intensities of treatment for different risk subgroups. Until then, however, the contributions of all individual phenotypic characteristics toward the risk of recurrence, as determined from multivariate analysis, are considered important. The main value of such an approach is to offer curative treatment to most patients while improving the therapeutic ratio. Undertreatment of high-risk patients and overtreatment of low-risk patients may thus be minimized.

Acknowledgements. The authors would like to thank the following individuals for their assistance: Dr. Martin Pollock, for input into the section on growth factors; Mary Naylor, for help in preparing the manuscript; David Noble, for editorial comments; John Spinelli, for critical analysis of the figures, tables, and conclusions.

References

1. Abandowitz HM, Oow KT, Hardy D et al. (1987) Relationship between flow cytometric parameters, steroid receptors and menopausal status in breast cancer. Oncology 4: 24-29
2. Arnold DJ, Lesnick G (1979) Survival following mastectomy for stage III breast cancer. Am J Surg 137: 362–366
3. Arteaga CL, Osborne CK (1988) Blockade of the epidermal growth factor (EGF) receptor inhibits transforming growth factor alpha (TGF alpha)-induced but not estrogen-induced growth of hormone-dependent human breast cancer. Proc Am, Assoc Cancer Res 29: 238
4. Atiba J, Coppin C, Ragaz J et al. (1988) Clinical significance of lymphatic, vascular or neural invasion in node negative breast cancer. Proc Am Soc Clin Oncol 7: 12
5. Atkin NB, Kay R (1979) Prognostic significance of model DNA value and other factors in malignant tumors, based on 1465 cases. Br J Cancer 40: 210-221

6. Auer G, Ericksson E, Azavedo E et al. (1984) Prognostic significance of nuclear DNA content in mammary adenocarcinoma in human. Cancer Res 44: 394-396
7. Bates SE, Valverius EM, Stampfer M et al. (1988) Transforming growth factor alpha (TGF alpha) production by proliferating normal breast epithelial cells. Proc Am Assoc Cancer Res 29: 52
8. Bedrossian CWM, Raber M, Barlogie B (1981) Flow cytometry and cytomorphology in primary resectable breast cancer. Anal Cytol 3: 112-116
9. Bertuzzi A, Diadone MG, DiFronzo G et al. (1981) Relationship among estrogen receptors, proliferative activity and menopausal status in breast cancer. Breast Cancer Res Treat 1: 253-262
10. Bettelheim R, Penman HG, Thornton-Jones H et al. (1984) Prognostic significance of peritumoral vascular invasion in breast cancer. Br J Cancer 50: 771-777
11. Bichel P, Paulsen HS, Andersen J. (1982) Estrogen receptor content and ploidy of human mammary carcinomas. Cancer 50: 1771-1774
12. Bloom HJG, Richardson WW (1957) Histological grading and prognosis in breast cancer. A study of 1049 cases, of which 359 have been followed 15 years. Br J Cancer 11: 359
13. Bishop JM (1986) Oncogenes. Sci Am 246 (3): 80-92
14. Bonadonna G, Valagussa P, Rossi A et al. (1979) CMF adjuvant chemotherapy in operable breast cancer. In: Jones SE, Salmon SE (eds) Adjuvant therapy of cancer. II. Grune and Stratton, New York, pp 227-237
15. Bonadonna G, Valagussa P, Rossi A. Multimodal therapy with CMF in resectable breast cancer with positive axillary nodes. The Milan Institute experience. In: Salmon SE, Jones SE (eds) Adjuvant therapy of cancer. III. Grune and Stratton, New York, pp 435-445
16. Bonadonna G, Valagussa P, Zambetti M et al. (1987) Milan adjuvant trials for stage I, II breast cancer. In: Salmon SE (ed) Adjuvant therapy of cancer V. Grune and Stratton, New York, pp 211-221
17. Boyd NF, Meakin JW, Hayward JL et al. (1981) Clinical estimation of the growth rate of breast cancer. Cancer 48: 1037-1042
18. Carpenter J, Stoscheck CH, Preston YA et al. (1983) Antibodies to the epidermal growth factor receptor block. The biological effects of sarcoma growth factor. Proc Natl Acad Sci USA 80: 5627-5630
19. Clark GM, McGuire WL (1988) Steroid receptors and other prognostic factors in primary breast cancer. Semin Oncol 15: 20-25
20. Coombes RC, Berger U, Mansi J et al. (1986) Prognostic significance of micrometastases in bone marrow in patients with primary breast cancer. NCI Monogr 1: 51-53
21. Cornelisse CJ, De Koning HR, Moolenaar AJ et al. (1984) Image and flow cytometry analysis of DNA content in breast cancer. Relation to estrogen receptor content and lymph node involvement. Anal Quant Cytol 6: 9
22. Cornelisse CJ, Velde CJH, Caspers RJC et al. (1987) DNA ploidy and survival in breast cancer patients. Cytometry 8: 225-234
23. Coulson PB, Thornthwaite JT, Woolley TW et al. (1984) Prognostic indicators including DNA histogram type, receptor content, and staging related to human breast cancer patients' survival. Cancer Res 44: 4187-4196
24. Dawson PJ, Ferguson DJ, Karrison T (1982) The pathologic findings of breast cancer in patients surviving 25 years after radical mastectomy. Cancer 50: 2131-2138

25. Dickson RB, Kasid A, Huff KK et al. (1987) Activation of growth factors' secretion in tumorogenic state of breast cancer induced by 17 beta estradiol or V-HA ras oncogene. Proc Natl Acad Sci USA 84: 837-841
26. Dowle CS, Owainati A, Riobirns A et al. (1987) Prognostic significance of the DNA content of human breast cancer. Br J Surg 74: 133-136
27. Downward J, Yarden Y, Mayes E et al. (1984) Close similarity of epidermal growth factor receptor and V-ERB oncogene protein sequences. Nature 307: 521-527
28. Dressler L, Clark G, Owens M et al. (1987) DNA flow cytometry predicts for relapse in node negative breast cancer patients. Proc Am Soc Clin Oncol 6: 57
29. Duesberg PH (1983) Retroviral transforming genes in normal cells. Nature 304: 219-226
30. Ege JN (1978) Internal mammary lymphoscintography: a rational adjunct to the staging and management of breast carcinoma. Clin Radiol 29: 453
31. Ewers SP, Langstrom E, Baldetorp B et al. (1984) Flow cytometry DNA analysis in primary breast carcinomas and clinical pathological correlations. Cytometry 5: 408-419
32. Fisher B, Slack NH, Bross IDJ et al. (1969) Cancer of the breast: size of neoplasm and prognosis. Cancer 24: 1071-1080
33. Fisher B, Slack NH, Katrych D et al. (1975) 10 year follow-up results of patients with carcinoma of the breast in a cooperative clinical trial evaluating surgical adjuvant chemotherapy. Surg Gynecol Obstet 140: 528-534
34. Fisher B, Redmond C, Fisher ER (1986) Systemic adjuvant therapy in treatment of primary operable breast cancer: National Surgical Adjuvant Breast and Bowel Project experience. NCI Monogr 1: 35-45
35. Fisher ER (1986) Prognostic and therapeutic significance of pathologic features of breast cancer. NCI Monogr 1: 29-35
36. Fisher ER, Gregorio RM, Fisher B (1975) The pathology of invasive breast cancer. Cancer 36: 1-85
37. Fisher ER, Osborne CK, McGuire WL et al. (1981) Correlation of primary breast cancer histopathology and estrogen receptor content. Breast Cancer Res Treat 1: 37-41
38. Fitzpatrick SL, Brightwell J, Wittliff JL (1984) Epidermal growth factor finding by breast tumor biopsies and relationship to estrogen receptor and progesterone receptor levels. Cancer Res 44: 3448-3453
39. Folkman J, Klagsprun M (1987) Angiogenic factors. Science 235: 442-447
40. Fossa SD, Thorud E, Shoaib MC et al. (1984) DNA flow cytometry in primary breast carcinoma. Acta Pathol Microbiol Immunol Scand [A] 92: 475-480
41. Fracchia AA, Evans JF, Eisenberg BL (1980) Stage III carcinoma of the breast. A detailed analysis. Ann Surg 192: 705-710
42. Fracchia AA, Rosen PP, Ashikari R (1980) Primary carcinoma of the breast without axillary lymph node metastases. Surg Gynecol Obstet 151: 375
43. Frankfurt OS, Greco WR, Slocum HK et al. (1984) Proliferative characteristics of primary and metastatic human solid tumors by DNA flow cytometry. Cytometry 5: 629-635
44. Gentili C, Sanfilippo O, Silvestrini R (1981) Cell proliferation in relation to clinical features and relapse in breast cancers. Cancer 48: 974-979
45. Godolphin W, Elwood JM, Spinelli JJ (1981) Estrogen receptor quantification and staging as complementary prognostic indicators in breast cancer: a study of 583 patients. Eur J Cancer Clin Oncol 28: 677-683
46. Goldie JH, Coldman AJ (1979) A mathematical model for relating the drug sensitivity of tumors to the spontaneous mutation rate. Cancer Treat Rep 63: 1727-1733
47. Haag D, Goerttler K, Tschahargane C (1984) The proliferative index (PI) of human breast cancer as obtained by flow cytometry. Pathol Res Pract 178: 315-322

48. Haagensen CD (1977) Treatment of curable carcinoma of the breast. Int J Radiat Oncol Biol Phys 2: 975-980
49. Haagensen CD (1986) Diseases of the breast, 3rd edn. Saunders, Philadelphia, p 656
50. Harvey J, DeKlerk N, Berryman I et al. (1987) Nuclear DNA content and prognosis in human breast cancer. Static cytophotometric study. Breast Cancer Res Treat 9: 101-109
51. Hedley DW, Friedlander ML, Taylor IW (1985) Application of DNA flow cytometry to paraffin-embedded archival material for the study of aneuploidy and its clinical significance. Cytometry 6: 327-333
52. Hedley DW, Rugg CA, Gelber RD (1987) Association of DNA index and S-phase fraction with prognosis of node positive early breast cancer. Cancer Res 47: 4729-4735
53. Horsfall DJ, Tilley WD, Orell SR et al. (1986) Relationship between ploidy and steroid hormone receptors in primary invasive breast cancer. Br J Cancer 53: 23-28
54. Horwitz KB (1988) The central role of progesterone receptors and progestational agents in the management and treatment of breast cancer. Semin Oncol 15: 14-19
55. Horwitz KB, Wei LL, Sedlack SM et al. (1985) Progestine action and progesterone receptor structure in human breast cancer: a review. Recent Prog Horm Res 41: 249-316
56. Jakesz R, Kolb R, Reiner G et al. (1985) Effects of adjuvant chemotherapy in stage I and II breast cancer is dependent on tumor differentiation and estrogen receptor status. Proc Am Soc Clin Oncol 4: 69
57. Jakobsen A, Skovgaard-Poulsen H, Lindegaard ME et al. (1984) Ploidy level of human breast carcinoma. Acta Radiol Oncol 23: 103-107
58. Kallioniemi OP, Hietanen T, Mattila J et al. (1987) Aneuploid DNA content and a high S-phase fraction of tumor cells are related to poor prognosis in patients with primary breast cancer. Eur J Cancer Clin Oncol 23: 277-282
59. Klintenberg C, Stal O, Nordenskjold B et al. (1986) Proliferative index, cytosol estrogen receptor and axillary node status as prognostic predictors in human mammary carcinoma. Breast Cancer Res Treat [Suppl] 7: 99-106
60. Koscielny S, Tubiana M, Le MG et al. (1984) Breast cancer: relationship between the size of the primary tumor and the probability of metastatic dissemination. Br J Cancer 49: 709-715
61. Kuenen-Boumeester V, Hop WCJ, Blonk DI et al. (1984) Prognostic scoring using cytomorphometry and lymph node status of patients with breast carcinoma. Eur J Cancer Clin Oncol 20: 337
62. Kute TE, Muss HP, Hopkins M et al. (1985) Relationship of flow cytometry results of clinical and steroid receptor status in human breast cancer. Breast Cancer Res Treat 6: 113-121
63. Lippman ME, Dickson RB, Bates S (1986) Autocrine and paracrine growth regulation of human breast cancer. Breast Cancer Res Treat 7: 59-70
64. Lippman ME, Huff KK, Jakesz R et al. (1986) Estrogens regulate production of specific growth factors in hormone dependent human breast cancer. Ann NY Acad Sci 464: 11-16
65. Lundy J, Grimson R, Mishriki Y et al. (1986) Elevated ras oncogene expression correlates with lymph node metastases in breast cancer patients. J Clin Oncol 4: 1321-1325
66. Luria SE, Delbruck M (1943) Mutations of bacteria from virus sensitivity to virus resistance. Genetics 491
67. Maehle BO, Thoresen S, Skjaerven R et al. (1982) Mean nuclear area and histological grade of axillary node tumor in breast cancer: relation to prognosis. Br J Cancer 46: 95-100
68. Manji MF (1982) Internal mammary lymphoscintigraphy in breast carcinoma: possible significance in relation to current treatment. J Can Assoc Radiol 33: 10-14

69. McDivitt RW, Stone KR, Meyer JS (1984) A method for dissociation of viable human breast cancer cells that produces flow cytometric kinetic information similar to that obtained by thymidine labeling. Cancer Res 44: 2628-2633
70. McDivitt RW, Stone KR, Craig RB et al. (1986) A proposed classification of breast cancer based on kinetic information derived from a comparison of risk factors in 168 primary operable breast cancers. Cancer 57: 269-276
71. McGuire WL (1986) Prognostic factors in primary breast cancer. In: Bulbrook RD (ed), Cancer surveys – advances and prospects in clinical, epidemiological and laboratory oncology, vol 5. Oxford University Press, Oxford, pp 527-536
72. Meyer JS, Friedman E, McCrate M et al. (1983) Prediction of early course of breast carcinoma by thymidine labelling. Cancer 51: 1879-1886
73. Meyer JS, Prey MU, Babcock DS et al. (1986) Breast carcinoma cell kinetics, morphology, stage and host characteristics. A thymidine labelling study. Lab Invest 54: 41-51
74. Moran RE, Black MM, Alpert L et al. (1984) Correlation of cell cytokinetics, hormone receptors, histopathology, and nodal status in human breast cancer. Cancer 54: 1586-1590
75. Nemoto T, Vanna J, Bedwani RN et al. (1980) Management and survival of female breast cancer: results of a national survey by the American College of Surgeons. Cancer 45: 2917-2924
76. Nime F, Rosen PP, Thaler H et al. (1977) Prognostic significance of tumor emboli in intramammary lymphatics in patients with mammary carcinoma. Am J Surg Pathol 1: 25
77. Nissen-Meyer R, Host H, Kjellgren K et al. (1986) Perioperative adjuvant chemotherapy of breast cancer: the Scandinavian experience. In: Ragaz J, Band PR, Goldie JH (eds) Preoperative (neoadjuvant) chemotherapy. Springer, Berlin Heidelberg New York, pp 95-103
78. Olszewski W, Darzynkiewicz Z, Rosen PP et al. (1981) Flow cytometry of breast carcinoma. I. Relation of DNA ploidy level to histology and estrogen receptor. Cancer 48: 980-984
79. Olszewski W, Darzynkiewicz Z, Rosen PP et al. (1981) Flow cytometry of breast carcinoma. II. Relation of tumor cell cycle distribution to histology and estrogen receptor. Cancer 48: 985-988
80. Olszewski W, Darzynkiewicz Z, Rosen PP et al. (1982) Flow cytometry of breast carcinoma. III. Possible altered kinetics in axillary lymph node metastases. Anal Quantit Cytol 4: 275-278
81. Opfermann M, Brugal G, Vassilakos P. (1987) Significance of ploidy balance and proliferation index. Cytometry 8: 217-224
82. Owainati AAR, Robins RA, Hinton C et al. (1987) Tumor aneuploidy, prognostic parameters and survival in primary breast cancer. Br J Cancer 55: 449-454
83. Padmanabhan N, Howell A, Rubens RD (1986) Mechanism of action of adjuvant chemotherapy in early breast cancer. Lancet II: 411-414
84. Parl FF, Dupont WD (1982) A retrospective cohort study of histologic risk factors in breast cancer patients. Cancer 50: 2410-2416
85. Payne WS, Taylor WF, Khonsari S et al. (1970) Surgical treatment of breast cancer: trends and factors affecting survival. Arch Surg 101: 105-113
86. Perez R, Betsholtz C, Westermark B et al. (1987) A frequent expression of growth factors for mesenchymal cells in human mammary carcinoma cell lines. Cancer Res 47: 3425-3429

87. Raber MN, Barlogie B, Latreille J et al. (1982) Ploidy, proliferative activity and estrogen receptor content in human breast cancer. Cytometry 3: 36-41
88. Ragaz J, Jackson S, Wilson K et al. (1988) Randomized study of locoregional radiotherapy and ovarian ablation in premenopausal patients with breast cancer treated with adjuvant chemotherapy. Proc Am Soc Clin Oncol 7: 12
89. Rank F, Dombernowski P, Jespersen NCB et al. (1987) Histologic malignancy grading of invasive ductal breast cancer. A regression analysis of prognostic factors in low risk carcinomas from 9 multicentre trials. Cancer 60: 1299-1305
90. Retsky MW, Swartzendruber DE, Wardell RH (1985) Predicting the disease free survival of breast cancer patients using DNA index and a stochastic numerical model of breast cancer growth. International Conference on analytical cytometry 11: Hilton Head, Abstract 343
91. Rosen PP (1983) Tumor emboli in intramammary lymphatics in breast carcinoma: pathologic criteria for diagnosis and clinical significance. Pathol Annu 18 (2): 215
92. Rosen PP (1987) The pathology of breast carcinoma. In: Harris JR, Hellman S, Henderson IC, Kinne DW (eds) Breast diseases. Lippincott, Philadelphia, pp 147-210
93. Rosen PP, Saigo PE, Braun DW et al. (1981) Predictors of recurrence in stage I (T1 N0 M0) breast carcinoma. Ann Surg 193: 15-25
94. Roses DF, Bell DA, Flotte TJ et al. (1982) Pathologic predictors of recurrence in stage I (T1 N0 M0) breast cancer. Am J Clin Pathol 78: 817
95. Sanisbury JRC, Farndon JR, Needham GK (1987) Epidermal growth factor receptor status as predictor of early recurrence of death from breast cancer. Lancet I: 1398-1402
96. Sampat MB, Sirsat MV, Gangadharan P (1977) Prognostic significance of blood vessel invasion in carcinoma of the breast in women. J Surg Oncol 9: 623-632
97. Schlessinger J (1986) Regulation of cell growth by the EGF receptor. In: Kahn P, Graf T (eds) Oncogenes and growth control. Springer, Berlin Heidelberg, New York, pp 77-84
98. Schottenfeld D, Nash AG, Robbins GF et al. (1976) Ten-year results of the treatment of primary operable breast carcinoma. Cancer 38: 1001-1007
99. Seeger RC, Brodeur GM, Sather H et al. (1985) Association of multiple copies of the N-MYC oncogene with rapid progression of neuroblastomas. N Engl J Med 313: 1111-1116
100. Shapiro S (1986) Final results of the breast cancer screening randomized trial: the Health Insurance Plan (HIP) of Greater New York study. UICC workshop on screening for breast cancer, Helsinki
101. Sherwin SA, Twardzik DR, Bohn WH et al. (1983) High molecular weight transforming growth factor activity in the urine of patients with disseminated cancer. Cancer Res 43: 403-407
102. Silvestrini RS, Diadone MG, Gasparini G (1985) Cell kinetics as a prognostic marker in node negative breast cancer. Cancer 56: 1982-1987
103. Silvestrini RS, Diadone MG, DiFronzo G et al. (1986) Prognostic implication of labelling index versus estrogen receptors and tumor size in node negative breast cancer. Breast Cancer Res Treat 7: 161-169
104. Slamon DJ, Clark DJ (1988) Amplification of C-ERB-2 and aggressive human breast tumors? Science 240: 1795-1798
105. Slamon DJ, Clark GM, Wong SG et al. (1987) Human breast cancer: correlation of relapse and survival with amplification of the HER-2/NEU oncogene. Science 235: 177-182
106. Spratt JS, Donegan WL (eds) (1971) Carcinoma of the breast. Saunders, Philadelphia, p 136
107. Stiles CD (1985) The biological role of oncogenes – insights from platelet-derived growth factor: Rhodes memorial award lecture. Cancer Res 45: 5215-5218

108. Strauss MJ, Moran R, Muller RE et al. (1982) Estrogen receptor heterogeneity and the relationship between estrogen receptor and the thymidine labelling index in human breast cancer. Oncology 39: 197-200
109. Tabar L, Fagerberg CJG, Gad A. (1985) Reduction in mortality from breast cancer after mass screening with mammography: randomized trial from the Breast Screening Group of the Swedish National Board of Health and Welfare. Lancet 1: 829-832.
110. Taylor IW, Musgrove EA, Friedlander ML et al. (1983) The influence of age on the DNA ploidy levels of breast tumors. Eur J Cancer Clin Oncol 19: 623-628
111. Thorpe SM, Rose C, Rasmussen BB et al. (1987) Prognostic value of steroid hormone receptors: multivariate analysis of systemically untreated patients with node negative primary breast cancer. Cancer Res 47: 6126-6133
112. Thorud E, Fossa SD, Vaage S et al. (1986) Flow cytometric DNA pattern in relation to clinical and histopathologic characteristics. Cancer 57: 808-811
113. Todaro GJ, Frylling C, De Larco JE (1980) Transforming growth factors produced by certain human tumor cells: polypeptides that interact with human EgR receptors. Proc Natl Acad Sci USA 77: 5258-5262
114. Tubiana M, Chauvel P, Ranaud A et al. (1975) Vitesse de croissants et histoire naturelle du cancer du sein. Bull Cancer 62: 341-358
115. Tubiana M, Pejovic MH, Chavaudra N et al. (1984) The long-term prognostic significance of the thymidine labelling index in breast cancer. Int J Cancer 33: 441-445
116. Ullrich A, Coussens L, Hayflick JS et al. (1984) Human epidermal growth factor receptor cDNA sequence and aberrant expression of the amplified gene in A431 epidermoid carcinoma cells. Nature 309: 418-425
117. Valagussa P, Bonadonna G, Veronesi U (1978) Patterns of relapse and survival following radical mastectomy. Cancer 41: 1170-1178
118. Valagussa P, DiFronzo G, Bignami P et al. (1981) Prognostic importance of estrogen receptors to select node negative patients for adjuvant chemotherapy. In: Salmon SE, Jones SE (eds) Adjuvant therapy of cancer. III. Grune and Stratton, Orlando, pp 329-335
119. Verbeek ALM, Hendriks JHCL, Holland R (1984) Reduction of breast cancer through mass screening with modern mammography: first results of the Nijmegen project, 1975-1981. Lancet 1: 1222-1224
120. Veronesi U, Scascinelli N, Greco M et al. (1985) Prognosis of breast cancer patients after mastectomy and dissection of internal mammary nodes. Ann Surg 202: 702-707
121. Viola MV, Fromowitz S, Oravez S et al. (1985) Ras oncogene p 21 expression is increased in pre-malignant lesions and high grade bladder carcinomas. J Exp Med 161: 1213-1218
122. Walker-Jones, Valverius EM, Stauffer MS et al. (1988) Transforming growth factor beta stimulates expression of milk fat globule protein in normal and oncogene-transformed human mammary epithelial cells. Proc Am Assoc Cancer Res 29: 249
123. Yarden Y, Harari I, Schlessinger J (1985) Purification of an active EgR receptor kinase with monoclonal anti-receptor antibodies. J Biol Chem 260: 315-319
124. Zajdela A, De Lariva LS, Ghossein NA (1979) The relation of prognosis to the nuclear diameter of breast cancer cells obtained by cytological aspiration. Acta Cytol 23: 75

Epidemiology

Breast Cancer Risk and Chemoprevention

P.R. Band, A.J. Coldman, and M. Deschamps*

Division of Epidemiology, Biometry and Occupational Oncology, Cancer Control Agency of British Columbia, 600 West 10th Avenue, Vancouver, B.C. V5Z 4E6, Canada

Introduction

The purpose of this chapter is to discuss the potential role of retinoids in breast cancer chemoprevention. Chemoprevention may be defined as the use of natural substances and their synthetic analogs or of other chemicals to reduce the likelihood of cancer development. For epithelial cancers, which account for the majority of human malignancies, chemoprevention consists of intervention measures taken during the development of the neoplastic process up to the stage of in situ carcinoma. Excellent reviews [8, 32, 50] have discussed this topic since the concept and the term were introduced a decade ago [73]. However, the question of dose of chemopreventive agents in relation to the stages of tumor formation has not been adequately addressed. This issue will be specifically considered from a clinical perspective based on an overview of experimental, epidemiologic, and clinical evidence.

Before doing so, however, it is first necessary to consider the risk factors associated with breast cancer, the contribution of epidemiology in assessing the probability of a woman to develop breast cancer, and its important function in the selection of a high risk target population for chemoprevention trial. Our intention is not to give an exhaustive review of the voluminous literature pertaining to breast cancer epidemiology, but rather to exemplify how epidemiologic information may be integrated with chemoprevention strategies.

Breast Cancer Risk Factors

Epidemiologic studies have pointed to a number of breast cancer risk factors which will be briefly summarized. The reader is referred to reviews on the subject for detailed information [31, 39, 53].

* Fellow of the National Health and Research Development Program, Health and Welfare, Canada.

Ragaz/Ariel (Eds.), High-Risk Breast Cancer

Age

Age represents the most important breast cancer risk factor. In western countries, the incidence rate of breast cancer steeply increases between the ages of 20 and 40, reaches a plateau between the ages of 40 and 45, and increases thereafter, but at a much slower rate [86]. About 85% of all breast cancer cases are detected in women over the age of 40; of these, 67% are diagnosed after the age of 50 years. Less than 1.5% of the cases occur in women under the age of 30 years [49]. In Japan and other Asian countries, breast cancer incidence rates also increase to a premenopausal plateau, but progressively decline thereafter [86].

Age at Menarche

An early age at menarche is associated with a higher risk of breast cancer. Women whose menarche occurred before the age of 12 have about a twofold increase in relative risk (RR) compared with those whose menstruations began after that age [39]. Establishment of regular menstrual cycles within 1 year of menarche is an associated risk factor [53]; the combination of early menarche and rapid onset of regular menstrual cycles further increases (RR = 3.7) the risk of breast cancer.

Age at First Pregnancy

An early age at first pregnancy exerts a protective effect against breast cancer development, but only a full-term pregnancy provides this protection [29]. A late age at first pregnancy and nulliparity carry a three- and twofold risk of breast cancer respectively. Although an early age at first birth appears to be a strong factor in reducing breast cancer risk, parity may also have an independent protective effect [83].

Age at Menopause

Women who become menopausal after the age of 45 years have a twofold breast cancer risk compared with those whose menopause occurred earlier [84]. A protective effect of an artificial menopause has been reported by several investigators; women with a bilateral oophorectomy performed before the age of 35 years have about one-third the breast cancer risk of those experiencing a natural menopause between the ages of 45 and 54 years [52, 84].

Family History of Breast Cancer

Many studies have indicated that women having a first-degree relative with breast cancer have a two- to threefold increased risk of developing the disease [51, 82].

This risk is greatly influenced by the laterality of the disease and the menopausal status of the relative at the time of diagnosis, being greater for premenopausal rather than postmenopausal, for bilateral rather than unilateral, and greatest when the disease is both premenopausal and bilateral [2].

Personal History of Benign Breast Diseases

Benign breast diseases (BBD) consist of a variety of distinct histologic entities which have only recently been considered for their potential relation to breast cancer. Page and co-workers, examining the different histologic types of BBD, established that atypical lobular hyperplasia carried the greatest risk for the development of breast cancer, with no increased risk associated with nonproliferative lesions [65].These findings were subsequently corroborated in cohort studies of women with BBD [22, 37, 62, 66].

It was also demonstrated that the breast cancer risk associated with the different histologic subtypes of BBD was strongly affected by nonhistologic risk factors. Age at first birth, nulliparity, and breast size were found to increase the risk of breast cancer in women with atypical hyperplasia, but had little effect in women without proliferative disease [23].

Recently, the Cancer Committee of the College of American Pathologists further helped to clarify the cancer risks associated with the histologic types of BBD. It was concluded that only women with BBD characterized by moderate and severe hyperplasia with atypia (RR = 5) and without atypia (RR = 2) had an increased risk of breast cancer compared with women with nonbiopsied BBD [15].

Mammography

Mammography was first used by Wolfe to identify breast parenchymal changes indicative of breast cancer risks [93]. This author reported that women with mammographic patterns characterized by prominent ducts (P2) or "dysplasia" (Dy) involving greater than 25% of the breast parenchyma were at an increased risk of developing breast cancer. Other investigators have since provided confirmatory evidence for an association between these mammographic patterns and breast cancer risks [9, 11, 76, 80]. Of substantial interest is the positive correlation reported by Wellings between mammographic Dy patterns and atypical ductal hyperplasia [88].

Other

A positive relationship has been observed for postmenopausal women between obesity and risk of developing breast cancer [18, 77]. Whether this effect is related to high caloric intake, low energy expenditure, or increased consumption of specific nutrients such as dietary fat [42, 60] remains, however, to be clarified. No definite association with breast cancer has been demonstrated for oral contraceptive use [13] or for estrogen replacement therapy [77].

Risk Assessment and Selection of a High Risk Target Population

Relative Risk and Probability of Disease

Knowledge of breast cancer risk factors has mainly been derived from epidemiologic case-control studies. In this design, which involves the comparison of risk factors among women with and without breast cancer, results are usually expressed in terms of relative risks of developing the disease between women exposed to (or having) and not exposed to (or not having) these risk factors. For example, RR = 2 for a given factor signifies a twofold increased risk of developing breast cancer in women exposed compared with those not exposed to this factor. Although RRs are of great interest for indicating possible etiologic factors, they do not by themselves enable one to define target populations for intervention trials. To do this requires information on the individual's probability of developing the disease over the duration of the study. This probability is equal to the incidence rate of disease in a group in which each individual has the same risk factors. As an example, let us consider a hypothetical group of women (group I), all with identical breast cancer risk factors, whose yearly breast cancer incidence is 1000 cases per 100 000. In this situation, we would estimate that an individual having the same risk factors as the group would have a 0.01 probability (1000/100 000) of developing breast cancer in 1 year. Now consider a second group of women (group II), again homogeneous in known risk factors for breast cancer, in whom we wish to estimate the probability that an individual will develop breast cancer in 1 year. If we know RR of disease between groups II and I, for instance RR = 5, then we may estimate the incidence rate of disease in group II as

$$\begin{aligned}\text{Incidence rate in group II} &= \text{RR} \times \text{incidence rate of group I}\\ &= 5000 \text{ per } 100\,000 \text{ women per year}\end{aligned}$$

Thus, the probability that a woman with the same risk factors as those in group II will develop breast cancer is 0.05 (5000/100 000) in 1 year. Based on the preceding, it becomes a simple matter to estimate the probability that an individual will develop a disease as long as the incidence rate for one group and the risk of that individual in relation to the group are known.

Probability of Disease for Combinations of Risk Factors

Given the many known risk factors for breast cancer and the possible combinations of these factors, many groups of women with differing risk of developing breast cancer may be defined. In epidemiologic studies one wishes to estimate the effect of a single risk factor in the presence of a variety of risk factor combinations. In this situation the difficulty is solved by applying statistical models (e.g., binary logistic regression) to the data where it is assumed that RR for multiple factors is the joint product of RR for each factor. For example, if RR for a personal history of BBD and for a family history of breast cancer are 2 and 3 respectively, then RR for both factors is 6 (2×3). Based on this model, RR for any combinations of risk factors may be computed if RR for each factor is known. Care should be exercised, however, to use RR estimates derived from studies which consider the same factors one intends to select, since this will reduce the likelihood of confounding. Using this statistical model, the probability that a woman will develop breast cancer can be estimated if the following information is available: (a) the woman's risk factors; (b) RR for each of these factors; (c) the distribution of these risk factors in a group for which the incidence rate of breast cancer is known.

In planning breast cancer chemoprevention trials, the objective is to identify which combinations of risk factors result in a minimum specified probability of disease over the duration of the study. Information on RR for each factor may be obtained from case-control studies of breast cancer in populations similar to the one from which participants in the chemoprevention trial are to be selected. To calculate the probability of disease, incidence rates from a population-based cancer registry may be used if information is also available on the distribution of breast cancer risk factors in a representative sample of the population.

The calculations required to estimate the probability of disease for various combinations of risk factors may be expressed as follows: let R_i represent RR for a particular combination of risk factors, R_p the mean breast cancer RR for the general population (obtained from the sample), and I_p the incidence rate of breast cancer in the general population. If I_i is the incidence rate of breast cancer for the combination of risk factors of interest, then

$$I_i = \frac{R_i}{R_p} I_p$$

Given the correspondence between incidence and probability of disease, it is a simple matter to calculate the probability of disease for various combinations of risk factors.

Selection of Participants for Chemoprevention

The method discussed to estimate the probability of disease for various combinations of risk factors may be used to identify, in a given population, subjects eligible for a chemoprevention trial. This approach will be illustrated with data from British Columbia. In the following example, the incidence rates of breast cancer were taken from the British Columbia provincial tumor registry and the distribution of risk factors in the general population was obtained from a recent case-control study of breast cancer in British Columbia [33]. Six known breast cancer risk factors will be considered: age; family history of breast cancer; personal history of clinical BBD; age at menarche; age at first birth; age at menopause. Only women aged 55 years or above were considered in order to identify menopausal age accurately. These risk factors were chosen because their distribution was available in our series. Clearly, any other factors could be included provided their RRs and distributions are known.

The distribution and RRs for the selected factors and the mean RRs are shown in Table 1. RRs were assigned on the basis of values obtained from a recent review [39]. As indicated previously, each individual's overall RR may be estimated by taking the product of RR for each factor; the results of this calculation are given under the last heading in Table 1. As can be seen, considerable variation in risk exists, with a mean RR = 6.53 for the entire sample.

When planning a randomized chemoprevention trial for breast cancer, sample size is of critical concern. As an example, let us consider a two-arm trial in which one is a placebo arm, and the hypothesized reduction in breast cancer risk due to chemoprevention is 50%. For a group with a 2% probability of developing breast cancer over a fixed time interval then, for a significance level of 0.05 and a power of 0.80, approximately 2500 participants would be required in each arm. A similar trial in a group with a 5% probability of breast cancer over the study period would need 1000 subjects per arm.

The information in Table 1 and the knowledge of the general population incidence rates of breast cancer may be used to estimate what combinations of risk factors result in individuals having the probability of breast cancer specified for the trial. Examples of such calculations are given in Table 2. Estimates of the proportion of the general population that have the required probability of disease development may also be derived from these calculations. For example, Table 2 indicates that, for a chemoprevention trial in a group of women aged 60 years with a mean probability of breast cancer of 5% over a 5-year period, approximately 2% of the general population of women of that age will be eligible to participate. It is important to notice that the calculations in Table 2 analyze the probability of developing breast cancer across all subjects. A group with a mean risk of 2% does not imply that the risk of an individual member of the group is exactly 2% as it may be either lower or higher than the group average. If for each participant a risk of at least 2% is needed, the calculation can be repeated incorporating this requirement. However, a smaller number of cases will be eligible for such a study.

Chemoprevention

Carcinogenesis is a complex multistep process evolving over a prolonged period of time, which has been characterized into the stages of initiation, promotion, and progression [5, 24]. Initiation results in hereditary and irreversible cellular genetic damage induced by carcinogens. Promotion leads to clonal expansion of the initiated cells and to a variety of phenotypic changes which may become irreversible over time [87]. The poorly understood process of progression encompasses the subsequent development of precursor lesions and cancer.

When considering chemopreventive strategies at least two phases of the neoplastic process must be distinguished conceptually. First, the initiation and early reversible promotion phase; second, the later more autonomous phase of tumor development. We suggest that these distinctions are of crucial importance as the

Table 1. Distribution of breast cancer risk factors of 441 women aged 55 years or over in British Columbia

Risk factor	Relative risk	Women with indicated risk factor Number	Percent
1. Family history of breast cancer in a first-degree relative			
None	1.0	426	96
Unilateral postmenopausal	1.2	2	1
Unilateral premenopausal	1.8	9	2
Bilateral postmenopausal	4.0	2	1
Bilateral premenopausal	8.8	2	1
Mean	1.07		
2. Personal history of benign breast disease			
No	1.0	353	80
Yes	2.0	88	20
Mean	1.20		
3. Age at menarche (years)			
18 and over	0.3	6	1
12-17	1.0	393	89
<12	2.0	42	10
Mean	1.08		
4. Age at first birth (years)			
<20	1.0	45	10
20-24	1.3	151	34
25-29	1.8	112	25
30-35	2.2	61	14
36 and over	3.0	10	2
Nulliparous	2.0	62	14
Mean	2.89		
5. Age at menopause (years)			
<35	1.0	10	2
35-44	1.7	36	8
45-54	2.5	252	57
55 and over	4.0	143	32
Mean	2.89		
6. Overall relative risk[a]			
<5	3.37	168	38
5-9.99	6.40	205	46
10-14.99	11.58	49	11
15 and greater	21.87	19	4
Mean	6.53		

[a] Obtained from the product of the individual risk factors selected.

Table 2. Estimated proportion of women in the general population eligible for participation in a chemoprevention trial as a function of study duration, age of participants and specified probability of breast cancer development over the study period

Age of study entrant	Study duration (years)	Probability of cancer over study duration (%)	Required relative risk compared to population average	Percent eligible
55	5	2	7.3	27
55	5	5	22.0	1
55	10	5	9.0	15
60	5	2	7.0	34
60	5	5	17.6	2
60	10	5	8.9	19
65	5	2	7.0	34
65	5	5	16.2	2
65	10	5	8.1	21

effective dose of chemopreventive agents may differ, depending on the stage of tumor development. Failure to take these considerations into account could result in negative or inconclusive chemoprevention trials. This discussion focuses on retinoids (vitamin A and its synthetic analogs) since these substances have been the most thoroughly studied for their chemopreventive properties in vitro and in vivo, and are currently undergoing intensive clinical trial [17]. For simplicity the term retinoids will be used in this chapter for both vitamin A and its derivatives unless otherwise specified.

Anticarcinogenic Action of Retinoids

Retinoids suppress, in vitro, the process of malignant transformation [12, 30, 59, 81], restore contact inhibition and anchorage-dependent growth to transformed cells [20, 21], and inhibit or reverse the hyperplastic and metaplastic changes produced by carcinogens in organ cultures of various organs, including the mammary gland [16, 19, 45, 46, 48]. In vivo, many studies have similarly shown that retinoids inhibit the process of carcinogenesis in many organs [6, 7, 70, 74], notably in the mammary gland [28, 54-58, 79, 89, 90].

Although not fully elucidated, the mechanism by which retinoids exert their anticarcinogenic action appears to be mainly related to their antipromotion effect [6, 85] and to their role in controlling cellular proliferation [25, 61, 91] and differentiation.

Of particular significance is the ability of vitamin A and retinoids to enhance differentiation of putative premalignant lesions [46, 48] and of fully transformed malignant cells [10, 75]. These effects imply a role of vitamin A in the control of gene expression involved in cell differentiation [72], possibly through a direct interaction with nuclear DNA mediated by specific intracellular retinoid-binding proteins [38]. Retinoic acid-binding proteins have been documented in human breast dysplastic and neoplastic cells [36, 44].

Distinction Between Maintenance of Normal Cellular Differentiation and Chemoprevention

Vitamin A is essential for the maintenance of normal epithelial differentiation. Vitamin A deficiency leads in many tissues to squamous cell metaplasia [92], morphologically similar to changes induced by chemical carcinogens [47], and to an increased susceptibility to tumor formation [14, 26, 64, 69]. Of special interest are the observations that this increased susceptibility is prevented by normal or moderately increased dietary levels of vitamin A, with no added protective effect provided by high levels of this substance in the diet [14, 26, 64, 69]. In parallel, a number of independent epidemiologic studies have shown an inverse correlation between the frequent consumption of food rich in vitamin A and/or provitamin A (β-carotene) and cancer risk [43, 68]. These studies, which substantiate experimental data, indicate that adequate or moderately increased dietary levels of vitamin A and/or its provitamin, exert a protective effect against cancer development in humans. Taken together, the experimental and epidemiologic evidence point to the effectiveness of maintenance levels of vitamin A, and/or provitamin A, in inhibiting the initiation and/or reversible promotion processes. As preneoplastic lesions develop, however, it is clear that this protective effect has been overwhelmed.

In vitro studies aimed at reversing established precursor lesions induced by chemical carcinogens have either required high doses of vitamin A [46] or shown a dose-dependent [48] or a time-dependent effect, with decreasing effectiveness related to delayed retinoid administration [54]. In experimental animal systems pharmacologic doses of retinoids have generally been necessary to inhibit tumor development [16, 28, 78]. Retinoids given in the postinitiation phase of the carcinogenesis process have also shown a dose-dependent inhibition of preneoplastic and malignant lesions [7, 61, 74, 78], and a progressive loss of chemopreventive potential associated with delayed retinoid treatment [54]. Furthermore, whereas low nontoxic doses of retinoids are effective in inducing differentiation of malignant cells in vitro [10, 75], high toxic doses have been required to produce similar changes in vivo [75].

In humans, retinoids have shown promising chemopreventive activity in a variety of premalignant conditions [27, 34, 40], in patients with high risk BBD [4], and in preventing tumor recurrence [1, 67]. These clinical trials, which generally used a single dosage schedule, have required the administration of pharmacologic doses of retinoids invariably associated with toxicity except in one study [27]. Since dose-response effects were not evaluated, it is impossible to conclude whether lower nontoxic doses would have been active. However, a reduction in retinoid dosage has been correlated with a decreased therapeutic activity [41, 67], and in a large chemoprevention trial in patients with premalignant esophageal lesions, doses of vitamin A of about two to three times the recommended daily allowance have been shown to be ineffective [63].

It would thus appear that the effective doses of retinoids depend on the timing of their administration in relation to the stage of cancer development. Considering the protective effect of early and long-term administration of maintenance levels of vitamin A and/or β-carotene against cancer formation, it would seem justified to recommend an adequate dietary intake of food rich in these substances as a potential means to reduce cancer incidence in the general population.

In the more advanced stages of tumor development, particularly in the presence of premalignant lesions, maintenance levels of vitamin A or equivalent doses of retinoids are likely to be ineffective and pharmacologic treatment with these compounds is needed. Since currently used retinoids produce dose-limiting side effects [1, 3, 8], a certain degree of toxicity will be difficult to avoid and will need to be accepted until new synthetic compounds with improved therapeutic indices become clinically available.

Discussion

The efficacy of retinoids against mammary gland tumor development has been amply documented experimentally, setting the stage for chemoprevention trials in high risk women. However, several problems confront the planning of chemoprevention trials of breast cancer. First, in comparison with smoking as a risk for lung cancer, the individual risk factors for breast cancer are generally weak. Consequently, selection of participants needs to be based on combinations of risk factors satisfying the minimum level of risk required by the trial. Setting a high risk level reduces the number of study participants required, but also reduces the number of eligible candidates in the population. Hence, specification of the risk level for participant selection is critically dependent on the knowledge of the distribution of risk factors in the population where the study is contemplated. It is likely that the high risk mammographic patterns will play an increasing role in the selection of women for intervention trials, in situations where the population distribution of these patterns is known.

Second, whereas chemoprevention-induced reversal of premalignant lesions of the cervix could readily be noted by repeated cytologic, tests observing similar changes in the breast would be difficult. Thus, the potential efficacy of an agent for breast cancer chemoprevention must be inferred from evidence of activity in animal mammary tumor models and possibly, in humans, from reversal of dysplasia observed in sites other than the breast.

Retinoids and chemopreventive agents in general ought to be investigated in a manner analogous to that of chemotherapeutic drugs. Thus, phase I pharmacologic and toxicologic studies should be undertaken to determine pharmacokinetic parameters, maximum tolerated dose, toxicity, and the time course pattern of the reversibility of side effects. Prior to considering large intervention trials, phase II studies need to be carried out in patients having well-defined precursor lesions such as dysplastic oral leukoplakia, cervical dysplasia, or actinic keratosis, with particular attention to dose-response effect. In this respect, the dose-intensity approach recently suggested for the investigation of chemotherapeutic drugs [35] appears equally appropriate to phase II studies aimed at establishing the dose-response curves of chemopreventive agents. Careful monitoring of the lesions would enable one to determine the dose range at which regressions are observed, the degree and duration of regression, as well as an eventual enhancement effect [71]. Furthermore, such studies would enable one to select the least toxic effective chemopreventive dose for intervention trials in high risk populations, which could then be undertaken based on evidence of activity.

References

1. Alfthan O, Tarkkanen J, Grohn P, Heinonen E, Pyrhonen S, Saila K (1983) Tigason (etretinate) in prevention of recurrence of superficial bladder tumors. A double-blind clinical trial. Eur Urol 9: 6-9
2. Anderson DE (1974) Genetic study of breast cancer: identification of a high risk group. Cancer 34: 1090-1097
3. Band PR, Besner JG, Leclaire R, Girard C, Diorio G, Deschamps M, Gelinas M, Larochelle D (1982) Phase I study of 13-*cis*-retinoic acid toxicity. Cancer Treat Rep 66: 1759-1761
4. Band PR, Deschamps M, Falardeau M, Ladouceur J, Coté J (1984) Treatment of benign breast disease with vitamin A. Prev Med 13: 549-554
5. Berenblum I (1982) Sequential aspects of chemical carcinogenesis: skin. In: Becker FF (ed) Cancer, vol 1. Plenum, New York, pp 451-484
6. Bollag W (1972) Prophylaxis of chemically induced benign and malignant epithelial tumors by vitamin A acid (retinoic acid). Eur J Cancer 8: 689-693
7. Bollag W (1974) Therapeutic effects of an aromatic retinoic acid analog on chemically induced skin papillomas and carcinomas of mice. Eur J Cancer 10: 731-737
8. Bollag W (1983) Vitamin A and retinoids: from nutrition to pharmacotherapy in dermatology and oncology. Lancet i: 860-863
9. Boyd NF, O'Sullivan B, Campbell JE, Fishell E, Simon I, Cooke G, Germanson T (1982) Mammographic signs as risk factors for breast cancer. Br J Cancer 45: 185-193
10. Breitman TR, Selonick SE, Collins SJ (1980) Induction of differentiation of the human promyelocytic leukemia cell line (HL-60) by retinoic acid. Proc Natl Acad Sci USA 77: 2936-2940
11. Brisson J, Merletti F, Sandowsky NL, Twaddle JA, Morrison AS, Cole P (1982) Mammographic features of the breast and breast cancer risk. Am J Epidemiol 115: 428-437
12. Chatterjee M, Banerjee MR (1982) Influence of hormones on *N*-(4-hydroxyphenyl)-retinamide inhibition of 7,12-dimethylbenz(*a*)anthracene transformation of mammary cells in organ culture. Cancer Lett 16: 239-245
13. Clavel F, Benhamou E, Sitruk-Ware R, Mauvais-Jarvis P, Flamant R (1985) Breast cancer and oral contraceptive: a review. Contraception 6: 553-569
14. Cohen SM, Wittenberg JF, Bryan GT (1976) Effect of avitaminosis A and hypervitaminosis A on urinary bladder carcinogenicity of *N*-[4-(5-nitro-2-furyl)-2-thiazolyl] formamide. Cancer Res 36: 2334-2339
15. Consensus meeting (1986) Is "fibrocystic disease" of the breast precancerous. Arch Pathol Lab Med 110: 171-173

16. Crocker JJ, Sanders LL (1970) Influence of vitamin A and 3,7-dimethyl-2,6-octadienal (citral) on the effect of benzo(*a*)pyrene on the hamster trachea in organ culture. Cancer Res 30: 1312-1318.
17. De Wys WD, Greenwald P (1983) Clinical trials: a recent emphasis in the prevention program of the National Cancer Institute. Semin Oncol 10: 360-364
18. deWaard F, Baanders-van Helewijn EA (1974) A prospective study in general practice on breast cancer risk in postmenopausal women. Int J Cancer 14: 153-160
19. Dickens MS, Custer RP, Sorof S (1979) Retinoid prevents mammary gland transformation by carcinogenic hydrocarbons in whole organ culture. Proc Natl Acad Sci USA 76: 5891-5895
20. Dion LD, Blalock JE, Gilford GE (1977) Vitamin A-induced density dependent inhibition of L-cell proliferation. J Natl Cancer Inst 58: 795-801
21. Dion LD, Blalock JE, Gilford GE (1978) Retinoic acid and the restoration of anchorage dependent growth to transformed mammalian cells. Exp Cell Res 117: 15-22
22. Dupont WD, Page DL (1985) Risk factors for breast cancer in women with proliferative breast disease. New Engl J Med 312: 146-151
23. Dupont WD, Page DL (1987) Breast cancer risk associated with proliferative disease, age at first birth, and a family history of breast cancer. Am J Epidemiol 125: 769-779
24. Farber E (1984) The multi-step nature of cancer development. Cancer Res 44: 4217-4223
25. Fraker LD, Halter SA, Forbes JT (1984) Growth inhibition by retinol of a human breast carcinoma cell line in vitro and in athymic mice. Cancer Res 44: 5757-5763
26. Fujimaki Y (1926) Formation of gastric carcinoma in albino rats fed on deficient diets. J Cancer Res 10: 469-477
27. Gouveia J, Hercend T, Lemaigre G, Mathé G, Gros F, Santelli G, Homasson JP, Angebault M, Lededente A, Parrot R, Gaillard JP, Bonniot JP, Marsac J, Pretet S (1982) Degree of bronchial metaplasia in heavy smokers and its regression after treatment with a retinoid. Lancet i: 710-712
28. Grubbs CJ, Moon RC, Sporn MB, Newton DL (1977) Inhibition of mammary cancer by retinyl methyl ether. Cancer Res 37: 599-602
29. Hadjimichael OC, Boyle CA, Meigs JW (1986) Abortion before first live birth and risk of breast cancer. Br J Cancer 53: 281-284
30. Harisiadis L, Miller RC, Hall EJ, Borek C (1978) A vitamin A analogue inhibits radiation induced oncogenic transformation. Nature 274: 486-487
31. Henderson BC, Pike MC, Ross RK (1984) Epidemiology and risk factors. In: Bonadonna G (ed) Breast cancer: diagnosis and management. Wiley, Toronto, pp 15-33
32. Hill DL, Grubbs CJ (1982) Retinoids as chemopreventive and anticancer agents in intact animals (review). Anticancer Res 2: 111-124
33. Hislop TG, Coldman AJ, Elwood JM, Skippen DH, Kan L (1986) Relationship between risk factors for breast cancer and hormonal status. Int J Epidemiol 15: 469-476
34. Hong WK, Endicott J, Itri LM, Doos W, Batsakis JG, Bell R, Fofonoff S, Byers R, Atkinson EN, Vaughan C, Toth BB, Kramer A, Dimery IW, Skipper P, Strong S (1986) 13-*cis*-Retinoic acid in the treatment of oral leukoplakia. N Engl J Med 315: 1501-1546
35. Hryniuk W, Bush H (1984) The importance of dose intensity in chemotherapy of metastatic breast cancer. J Clin Oncol 2: 1281-1288
36. Huber PR, Geyer E, Kung W, Matter A, Torhorst J, Eppenberger U (1978) Retinoic acid-binding protein in human breast cancer and dysplasia. J Natl Cancer Inst 61: 1375-1378
37. Hutchinson WB, Thomas DB, Hamlin WB, Roth GJ, Peterson AV, Williams B (1980) Risk of breast cancer in women with benign disease. J Natl Cancer Inst 65: 13-20

38. Jetten AR, Jetten MER (1979) Possible role of retinoic acid and binding protein in retinoid stimulation of embryonal carcinoma cell differentiation. Nature 278: 180-182
39. Kelsey JL, Hildreth NE (1983) Breast and gynecologic cancer epidemiology. CRC, Boca Raton, pp 5-50
40. Kerndrup G, Bendix-Hansen K, Pedersen B, Ellegaard J, Hokland P (1986) Primary myelodysplastic syndrome: treatment of 6 patients with 13-*cis*-retinoic acid. Scand J Haematol 36 (Suppl 45): 128-132
41. Koch HF (1978) Biochemical treatment of precancerous oral lesions: the effectiveness of various analogues of retinoic acid. J Maxillofac Surg 6: 59-63
42. Kolonel LN, Nomura AM, Hinds MW, Hirohata T, Hankin JH, Lee J (1983) Role of diet in cancer incidence in Hawaii. Cancer Res 43: 2397s-2402s
43. Kummet T, Moon TE, Meyskens FL (1983) Vitamin A: evidence for its preventive role in human cancer. Nutr Cancer 5: 96-106
44. Kung WM, Geyer E, Eppenberger U, Huber PR (1980) Quantitative estimation of cellular retinoic acid-binding protein activity in normal, dysplastic and neoplastic human breast tissue. Cancer Res 40: 4265-4269
45. Lane BP, Miller SL (1976) Effects of vitamin A on carcinogen induced changes in tracheal epithelial organ cultures (Abstract). Proc Am Assoc Cancer Res 17: 211
46. Lasnitzki I (1955) The influence of A hypervitaminosis on the effect of 20-methylcholanthrene on mouse prostate glands grown in vitro. Br J Cancer 9: 434-441
47. Lasnitzki I (1962) Hypovitaminosis A in the mouse prostate gland cultured in defined medium. Exp Cell Res 28: 40-51
48. Lasnitzki I (1976) Reversal of methylcholanthrene-induced changes in mouse prostates in vitro by retinoic acid and its analogues. Br J Cancer 34: 239-248
49. Leis HP (1978) Epidemiology of breast cancer: identification of high risk women. In: Gallagher HS, Lois HP, Snyderman RK, Urban JA (eds) The breast. Mosby, St Louis, pp 37-48
50. Lotan R (1980) Effects of vitamin A and its analogs (retinoids) on normal and neoplastic cells. Biochim Biophys Acta 605: 33-91
51. Macklin MT (1959) Comparison of the number of breast cancer deaths observed in relatives of breast cancer patients, and the number expected on the basis of mortality rate. J Natl Cancer Inst 22: 927-951
52. MacMahon B, Feinleib M (1960) Breast cancer in relation to nursing and menopausal history. J Natl Cancer Inst 24: 733-753
53. MacMahon B, Cole P, Brown J (1972) Etiology of human breast cancer: a review. J Natl Cancer Inst 50: 21-42
54. McCormick DL, Moon RC (1982) Influence of delayed administration of retinyl acetate on mammary carcinogenesis. Cancer Res 42: 2639-2643
55. McCormick DL, Moon RC (1986) Retinoid-tamoxifen interaction in mammary cancer chemoprevention. Carcinogenesis 7: 193-196
56. McCormick DL, Burns FJ, Albert RE (1980) Inhibition of rat mammary carcinogenesis by short dietary exposure to retinyl acetate. Cancer Res 40: 1140-1143
57. McCormick DL, Sowell ZL, Thompson CA, Moon RC (1983) Inhibition by retinoid and ovariectomy of additional malignancies in rats following surgical removal of the first mammary cancer. Cancer 51: 594-599
58. Mehta RG, Cerny WL, Moon RC (1983) Retinoids inhibit prolactin-induced development of the mammary gland in vitro. Carcinogenesis 4: 23-36
59. Merriman RL, Bertram JS (1979) Reversible inhibition by retinoids of 3-methylcholanthrene-induced neoplastic transformation in C3H/10T 1/2 clone 8 cells. Cancer Res 39: 1661-1666

60. Miller AB (1986) Dietary fat and the epidemiology of breast cancer. Prog Clin Biol Res 222: 17-32
61. Moon RC, Thompson HJ, Becci PJ, Grubbs CJ, Gander RJ, Newton DL, Smith JM, Phillips SL, Henderson WR, Mullen LT, Brown CC, Sporn MB (1979) *N*-(4-Hydroxyphenyl) retinamide, a new retinoid for prevention of breast cancer in the rat. Cancer Res 39: 1339-1346
62. Moskowitz M, Gartside P, Wirman JA, McLaughlin C (1980) Proliferative disorders of the breast as risk factors for breast cancer in a self-selected screened population: pathologic markers. Radiology 134: 289-291
63. Munoz N, Bang LJ, Day NE, Yan WE, Yun ZC, Correa P, Wahrendorf J, Crespi M, Ji ZH, Lin LG, Fang ZS, O'Conor GT, Thurnham DI, Grassi A, Quan LY, Yao LJ, Bosch X (1985) No effect of riboflavine, retinol, and zinc on prevalence of precancerous lesions of oesophagus. Randomized double-blind intervention study in high risk population of China. Lancet ii: 111-114
64. Nettesheim P, Snyder C, Kim JCS (1979) Vitamin A and the susceptibility of respiratory tract tissues to carcinogenic insult. Environ Health Perspect 29: 89-93
65. Page DL, Zanderswaag RV, Rogers LW, Williams LT, Walker WE, Hartmann WH (1978) Relation between component parts of fibrocystic disease complex and breast cancer. J Natl Cancer Inst 61: 1055-1063
66. Page DL, Dupont WD, Rogers LW, Rados MS (1985) Atypical hyperplastic lesions of the female breast: a long-term follow-up study. Cancer 55: 2698-2708
67. Peck GL, Gross EG, Butkus D, DiGiovanna JJ (1982) Chemoprevention of basal cell carcinoma with isotretinoin. J Am Acad Dermatol 6: 815-823
68. Peto R, Doll R, Buckley JD, Sporn MB (1981) Can dietary β-carotene materially reduce human cancer rates? Nature 290: 201-208
69. Rogers AE, Herndon BJ, Newberne PM (1973) Vitamin A and dimethylhydrazine-induced colon carcinoma in the rat. Cancer Res 33: 1003-1009
70. Saffiotti U, Montesano R, Sellakumar AR, Borg SA (1967) Experimental cancer of the lung. Inhibition by vitamin A of the induction of tracheobronchial squamous metaplasia and squamous cell tumors. Cancer 20: 857-864
71. Shroder EW, Black PH (1980) Retinoids: tumor preventers or tumor enhancers? J Natl Cancer Inst 65: 671-674
72. Sporn MB, Roberts AB (1983) Role of retinoids in differentiation and carcinogenesis. Cancer Res 43: 3034-3040
73. Sporn MB, Dunlop NM, Newton DL, Smith JM (1976) Prevention of chemical carcinogenesis by vitamin A and its synthetic analogs. Fed Proc 35: 1332-1338
74. Sporn MB, Squire RA, Brown CC, Smith JM, Wenk ML, Springer S (1977) 13-*cis*-Retinoic acid: inhibition of bladder carcinogenesis in the rat. Science 195: 487-489
75. Strickland S, Sawey MJ (1980) Studies on the effect of retinoids on the differentiation of teratocarcinoma stem cells in vitro and in vivo. Dev Biol 78: 76-85
76. Tabar L, Dean PB (1982) Mammographic parenchymal patterns: risk indicator for breast cancer? JAMA 247: 185-189
77. Thomas DB, Chu J (1986) Nutritional and endocrine factors in reproductive organ cancers: opportunities for primary prevention. J Chronic Dis 39: 1031-1050
78. Thompson HJ, Becci PJ, Grubbs CJ, Shealy YF, Stanek EJ, Brown CC, Sporn MB, Moon RC (1981) Inhibition of urinary bladder cancer by *N*-(ethyl)-all-*trans*-retinamide and *N*-(2-hydroxyethyl)-all-*trans*-retinamide in rats and mice. Cancer Res 41: 933-936
79. Thompson HJ, Meeker LD, Tagliaferro AR, Becci PJ (1982) Effect of retinyl acetate on the occurrence of ovarian hormone-responsive and -nonresponsive mammary cancers in the rat. Cancer Res 42: 903-905

80. Threatt B, Norbeck JM, Ullman N, Kummer R, Roselle P (1980) Association between mammographic parenchymal pattern classification and incidence of breast cancer. Cancer 45: 2550-2556
81. Todaro GJ, De Larco JE, Sporn MB (1978) Retinoids block phenotypic cell transformation produced by sarcoma growth factor. Nature 276: 272-274
82. Tokuhata GK (1969) Morbidity and mortality among offspring of breast cancer mothers. Am J Epidemiol 89: 139-153
83. Trapido EJ (1983) Age at first birth, parity and breast cancer risk. Cancer 51: 946-948
84. Trichopoulos D, MacMahon B, Cole P (1972) Menopause and breast cancer risk. J Natl Cancer Inst 48: 605-613
85. Verma AK, Boutwell RK (1977) Vitamin A acid (retinoic acid), a potent inhibitor of 12-*O*-tetradecanoyl-phorbol-13-acetate-induced ornithine decarboxylase activity in mouse epidermis. Cancer Res 37: 2196-2201
86. Waterhouse J, Muir C, Correa P, Powell J (eds) (1976) Cancer incidence in five continents, vol 3. IARC, Lyon (IARC scientific publication no 15)
87. Weinstein IB, Yamasaki H, Wigler M, Lee L-S, Fisher PB, Jeffrey A, Grunberger D (1979) Molecular and cellular events associated with the action of initiating carcinogens and tumor promoters. In: Griffin AC, Shaw CR (eds) Carcinogens: identification and mechanisms. Raven, New York, pp 399-418
88. Wellings SR, Wolfe JN (1978) Correlative studies of the histological and radiologic appearance of the breast parenchyma. Radiology 129: 299-306
89. Welsch CW, Brown CK, Goodrich-Smith M, Chiusano J, Moon RC (1980) Synergistic effect of chronic prolactin suppression and retinoid treatment in the prophylaxis of *N*-methyl-*N*-nitrosourea-induced mammary tumorigenesis in female Sprague-Dawley rats. Cancer Res 40: 3095-3098
90. Welsch CW, De Hoog JV, Scieszka KM, Aylsworth CF (1984) Retinoid feeding, hormone inhibition, and/or immune stimulation and the progression of *N*-methyl-*N*-nitrosourea-induced rat mammary carcinoma: suppression by retinoids of peptide hormone-induced tumor cell proliferation in vivo and in vitro. Cancer Res 44: 166-171
91. Wetherall NT, Taylor CM (1986) The effects of retinoid treatment and antiestrogens on the growth of T47D human breast cancer cells. Eur J Cancer Clin Oncol 22: 53-59
92. Wolbach SB, Howe PR (1925) Tissue changes following deprivation of fat soluble A vitamin. J Exp Med 42: 753-777
93. Wolfe JN (1976) Risk for breast cancer development determined by mammographic parenchymal pattern. Cancer 37: 2486-2492

Oncogenes

Genetic Aspects of Human Breast Cancer

J. MacKay and M. Steel

Department of Clinical Surgery, Edinburgh University Medical School and
MRC Department of Human Genetics, Edinburgh, Scotland, Great Britain

Risk Factors in General

In common with many neoplasms, the incidence of breast cancer increases with age [24]. It is slightly higher in socioeconomic classes I and II [52] and in North American and European women compared with African and Asian women [127]. The behaviour of the ovary appears to play a central role in the aetiology of breast cancer; several studies showing that early age of menarche (below 14 years) and late age of menopause, increase the risk [20, 107, 12, 119]. The effects of pregnancy are less clear; childbearing appears protective if the first child is born before the mother reaches the age of 30, although bearing more than five children increases the risk [12, 26, 125, 76, 1]. Alterations of the hormonal environment, as in prolonged use of oral contraceptives or postmenopausal oestrogens, do not appear to affect the risk in most recent studies, but this remains a controversial issue [12, 51, 122, 123, 124, 98, 78]. Artificial menopause, for example by oophorectomy, is reported to be protective; the earlier it is performed the greater the reduction in risk [69, 33].

Past medical history is of particular importance in the assessment of risk. A previous diagnosis of cancer in one breast significantly increases the likelihood of developing a second primary tumour in the other [66, 110]. Many studies have suggested that a history of benign breast disease, particularly if a biopsy was performed, increases risk [25, 77, 48] although this has been disputed [12, 18] and certainly the pathological findings in the biopsy are not predictive [78]. A history of primary cancer in the ovary or endometrium has also been reported to increase the chance of subsequent breast cancer [75, 92].

Many other factors, such as body mass, have been shown to be related to very small increases in risk [65, 61], but the strongest predictive factor so far identified and the one which we will now examine in more detail, is a positive family history of breast cancer.

Family History

The occurrence of families containing a large number of individuals affected by breast cancer has been recognised for many centuries. The first detailed report was published in 1866 by the French surgeon Paul Broca [13] who ascertained the

Ragaz/Ariel (Eds.), High-Risk Breast Cancer

cause of death in 38 individuals through five generations of his wife's family. Of the 24 women in that family, 10 died of breast cancer and several more individuals died from other malignancies. Both Broca and his contemporary Sir James Paget [84, 63] expressed concern that multiple instances of such a common disease might appear in a small number of families by coincidence, but, using the available data on cancer mortality rates in the normal population, they concluded that a tendency to develop breast cancer could indeed be inherited.

Advances in statistics, epidemiology and genetics allowed more rigorous examination of these initial observations in the first half of the twentieth century. Several groups attempted to compare the mortality from breast cancer in a population of patients with one or more affected relatives and in a normal control population [49, 132, 4, 52, 70]. These studies highlighted the importance of pathological verification of malignancy, of assessing the incidence of malignancies other than breast cancer and of using large numbers of families plus reliable data on cancer incidence and mortality in the general population. Overall, they showed that there was a twofold increase in breast cancer incidence in the close female relatives of breast cancer patients. Underreporting of disease by control subjects was recognised as a significant problem which remains hard to surmount. Further analysis of data collected in the course of these studies hinted at the possibility of there being two separate types of breast cancer, sporadic and hereditary, and suggested that several features were commoner in one type than the other.

The important characteristics of familial breast cancer in a number of countries have been defined by H.T. Lynch and colleagues [71]:

1. Significantly early age of onset
2. Excess of bilaterality
3. Excess of multiple primaries at various sites
4. Vertical transmission (mother to daughter)
5. Impaired survival when compared with sporadic forms.

Applying these criteria, he estimates that 5% of *all* breast cancer is familial, but 11.5% of patients with breast cancer diagnosed before the age of 50 have a familial form of the disease. Anderson [5, 6] adopted a somewhat different approach, dividing his cases into subgroups and identifying the groups in which the risk was increased beyond the two- or threefold level observed in the earlier studies. The relative risk to first-degree female relatives of patients with premenopausal breast cancer was 3.1, while no increase in risk was observed among relatives of postmenopausal patients. If the patient had bilateral breast cancer the risk to first-degree female relatives was increased fivefold. If both conditions applied (i.e. the patient was premenopausal *and* had bilateral disease), the risk to first-degree relatives was increased ninefold. Furthermore, the relatives of patients with bilateral disease were at a ninefold times greater risk of developing bilateral disease themselves as compared with relatives of patients with unilateral disease.

The importance of age and of bilaterality have been confirmed in other studies [7, 17] and so, despite one dissenting report from a large Swedish study in which the effects of family history, age of onset and bilaterality were rather weak [2], we are now in a position to identify a group of women who are at significantly higher risk of developing breast cancer than the general population, who are likely to be more aware of (and concerned about) their susceptibility to the disease [50], and who therefore require detailed and accurate counselling about that risk [83]. By combining complex statistical analyses and laboratory investigation it is possible to define more precisely the genetic component in what is acknowledged to be a disease of multifactorial aetiology.

Segregation Analysis

In some "classical" genetic disorders, inspection of the pedigrees of a few affected families will reveal the mode of transmission (autosomal or sex-linked, dominant or recessive). However, in the vast majority of diseases, where the genetic component is less clear cut, a more comprehensive statistical analysis is required. Segregation analysis is the name given to the process of determining the probable mode of transmission of a trait, from an observed distribution of phenotypes in a pedigree or a number of pedigrees.

The procedure involves calculating how well the observed distribution of phenotypes fits various hypotheses and can thus establish the validity of some of these hypotheses, though it may not prove conclusively that a trait *is* transmitted genetically. The larger the families examined, the more affected individuals in each family; the larger the total number of families, the better will be the data and the more secure the final conclusions.

Several statistical advances, such as maximum likelihood scoring, the concept of multifactorial inheritance, the "mixed model" and a sampling correction to allow for the manner in which the pedigrees have been ascertained and relatives added [29, 30, 80, 27, 60, 81], have all been incorporated into a segregation analysis performed on 200 Danish families with breast cancer [131].

The observed distribution of breast cancer in these families was compatible with transmission of a single autosomal gene with dominant expression, the frequency of the abnormal (disease) allele being 0.7%, and the penetrance varying with age. According to that model, by age 80, a female heterozygous for the abnormal allele would have a 57% chance of developing breast cancer. For cancers presenting before age 30, 88% of affected females would be carriers of the disease gene whereas for the total population (presentation up to age 80), only 13% of affected females would carry the gene, the other 87% having developed "sporadic" breast cancer.

Several similar analyses have been performed on another large family with breast cancer and all agree that an autosomal dominant gene with incomplete penetrance is the most likely mode of transmission [35, 44, 36]. Increasing the complexity of a segregation analysis may well improve the accuracy of estimates of gene frequency and penetrance, but it cannot give any indication as to what gene is involved and where in the human genome it may be.

The Principles of Linkage Analysis

The most practical approach to locating the gene for susceptibility to breast cancer is by the technique of linkage analysis, based on the segregation of defined genetic markers in affected and unaffected family members [133]. The human genome is composed of genes arranged in a linear fashion along the 23 pairs of chromosomes. Genes which are close together on the same chromosome tend to be transmitted together, i.e. to segregate nonindependently. Genes on different chromosomes segregate independently so that every possible combination of alleles appears with equal frequency in the gametes, as illustrated by Fig. 1. The disease gene is *D* (normal allele *d*) and the marker gene alleles are represented by *T* and *t*.

If the disease gene and the marker gene are physically very close together, they will be transmitted together, so that the gametes formed are either *DT* or *dt* as shown in Fig. 2. This departure from independent segregation is termed "linkage", with *D* and *T* being very tightly linked in the example shown. If *D* and *T* are slightly further apart on the chromosome, the two genes may well be transmitted together, but because they can segregate by crossing over and recombination at meiosis, a few gametes with genotypes *Dt* or *dT* will appear, as illustrated in Fig. 3. These gametes are known as recombinants and the proportion of recombinant gametes in the total pool is the recombinant fraction. The further apart the two genes are, the more likely it is that recombination will occur, until eventually the two genes will appear to be segregating independently as all four possible genotypes will be represented equally, giving a recombinant fraction of 50%, as illustrated in Fig. 4.

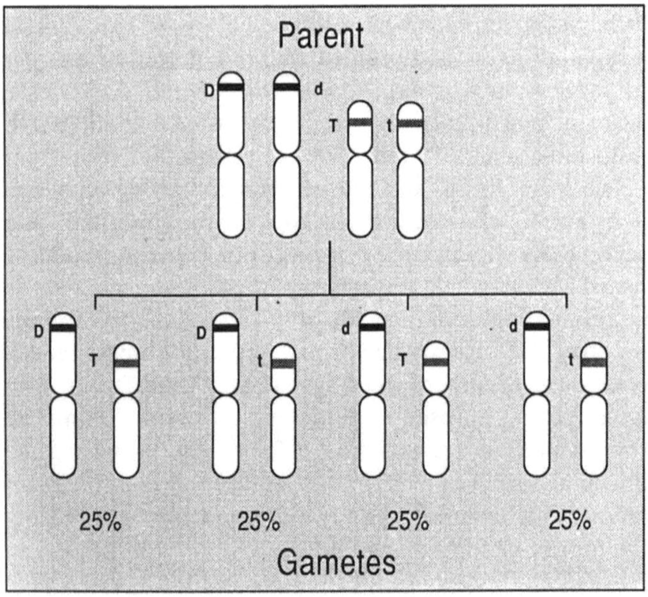

Fig. 1. Independent assortment of alleles at meiosis for a disease locus (alleles *D* and *d*) and a marker locus (alleles *T* and *t*) on different chromosomes. (After [133])

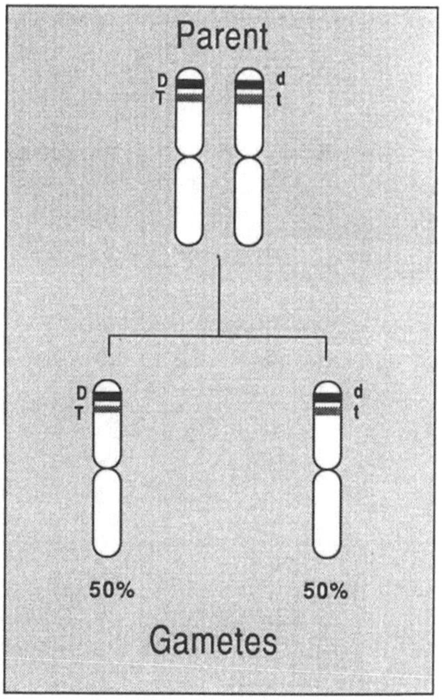

Fig. 2. Absence of independent assortment of alleles at meiosis for disease and marker loci very close together on the same chromosome (tight linkage). (After [133])

The markers used in linkage analysis must be polymorphic (i.e. more than one allelic form found in the population), and ideally the chromosomal location should be known. After identifying which allelic forms of the marker are present in every individual (both affected and unaffected) in a family, it is possible to calculate *a* the probability of the observed distribution occurring by chance if there is no linkage between the marker gene and the disease, and *b* the probabilities of such a pattern appearing if there is linkage at different recombination fractions. The logarithm of b/a, known as the "lod" (logarithm of odds) score, is calculated for various recombinant fractions [79]. To attain statistical significance it is usually necessary to combine data from several families, and the lod scores from each family for each recombination fraction can be added together. A lod score greater than $+3$ is usually taken as demonstrating significant linkage, but obviously the more families examined, the greater the confidence one can place in the lod score.

King, Go and colleagues [53, 38] used segregation analysis to identify ten families showing genetic transmission of the breast cancer trait and performed linkage analysis with 21 independent polymorphic markers. They suggested that in seven families there was significant linkage between an autosomal dominant gene for susceptibility to breast cancer and the enzyme glutamate-pyruvate transaminase (GPT), the gene which is located on chromosome 16 [73]. They reported a lod score of $+1.95$, at a recombination fraction of zero and accepted that such a result should be viewed with caution. When a larger number of families was examined, it was conclusively shown that there was no linkage between GPT and susceptibility to breast cancer [74].

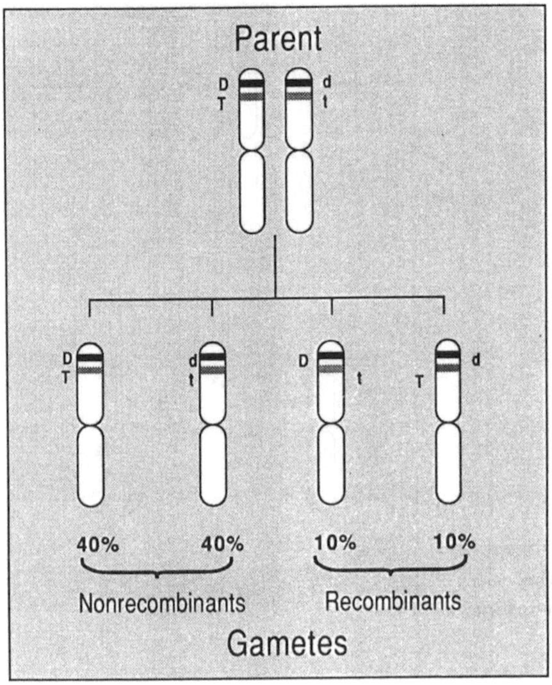

Fig. 3. Disease and marker loci nearby on the same chromosome showing linkage. The recombination fraction is 20%. (After [133])

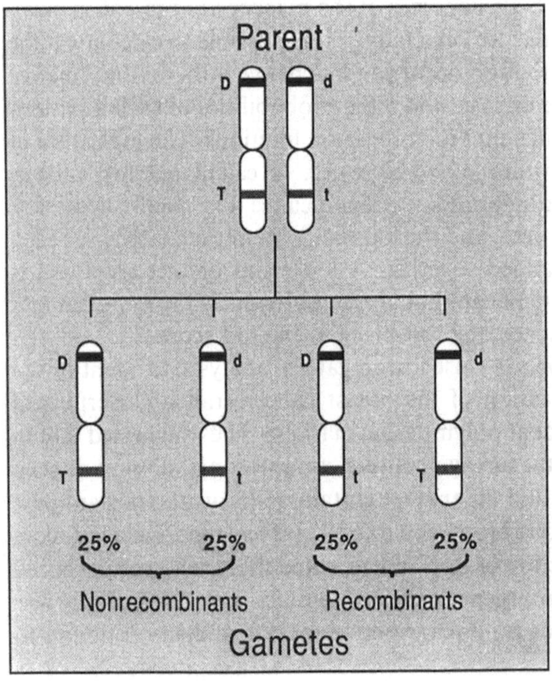

Fig. 4. Disease and marker loci far apart on the same chromosome mimic independent assortment and linkage cannot be detected. The recombination fraction is 50%. (After [133])

Confusion sometimes arises between the terms " linkage" and "association" in the context of genetics. As explained, linkage between two DNA sequences means that they are physically close together in the genome. Hence if *one* is polymorphic, so that inheritance of the different alleles can be traced within a family, it can be used to "tag" the other sequence. It does not follow that the *same* allelic forms of the two sequences are linked in all cases. For example, in the case illustrated in Fig. 2 a single chromosome carried *D* and *T* in tight linkage so that *T* would serve as a marker for *D* in this family. In another family, however, the relevant chromosome might carry the alleles *D* and *t* in which case the marker for *D* would be *t*. In other words, there is no functional relationship between the gene with alleles *Dd* and that with alleles *Tt*. The important practical consequence is that even if strong linkage is established between these genes, there is no purpose in screening a population, say for carriers of the *t* allele, since one could not predict which of the individuals so identified would also carry *D*. That type of prediction is valid only *within* each family.

"Association", however, is quite a different matter. The term implies that a particular *allele* of a given gene is overrepeated among the total population of patients with a particular genetic disorder. There are, for example, over 100 diseases associated with individual alleles of the major histocompatibility system [118]. *HLA-B27* and ankylosing spondylitis, or *DR4* and rheumatoid arthritis are well-known instances. These associations hold across family boundaries (though, interestingly, they may not apply in all racial groups) and can therefore be useful in population screening. Association in this sense may come about because the disease arose through a single mutation event affecting a gene so close to the "marker" sequence that the disease and marker alleles have never become separated throughout the succeeding generations. This so-called founder effect implies that all the affected individuals in a population are actually related through they may not be aware of it. An equally likely mechanism, however, is a *causal* relationship between the marker allele and the disease itself. In other words, individuals with the *HLA* type *B27* are at risk from ankylosing spondylitis not because an "*ank-spond*" gene lies close to the *HLA* complex on the short arm of chromosome 6, but because the *B27* gene product is actually involved in the aetiology of the disease.

Returning to the problem of genetic susceptibility to breast cancer, the search for linkage, in the strict sense, simply means extension of the approach used by King, Go and their colleagues, namely the analysis of large numbers of randomly chosen polymorphic markers in families with multiple cases of premenopausal disease. An alternative approach would be to try to identify "candidate" genes suspected, for one reason or another, of possible involvement in breast cancer. The gene encoding the oestrogen receptor might be an obvious choice as would a number of oncogenes (see later). Until recently, the shortage of useful genetic polymorphisms has restricted both of these approaches, but the situation has been transformed by the discovery of DNA restriction fragment length poymorphisms and other advances in molecular biology discussed in the next section.

Basic Molecular Biology

The total human gene complement is stored and transmitted in the form of deoxyribonucleic acid. DNA is a double-stranded helix. Each strand is composed of a string of sugar and phosphate molecules forming the backbone, with a series of bases protruding. In DNA there are four possible bases, adenine, guanine, thymidine and cytosine, and in native double-stranded DNA, A must be opposite T, and G opposite C. The genetic information coded by the order of bases in the DNA is transcribed into RNA, and RNA is then translated into protein. Because of the requirements for complementary base pairing (A-T and G-C) a single strand of DNA uniquely defines its complementary strand of DNA or RNA.

Under appropriate conditions of pH, temperature and ionic strength, single-stranded DNA or RNA fragments will stick to (or "hybridise" with) complementary single strands of DNA. The stability of the double-stranded complex ("hybrid") depends upon the degree of complementarity between the two nucleic acid strands. By increasing the pH or temperature or altering the ionic strength, hybridisation conditions can be made more stringent until only strands that are perfectly matched at every base pair will remain as hybrids. This property is exploited in the technique of gene probing.

DNA is extracted from cells by well-defined chemical procedures involving phenol extraction and ethanol precipitation, stripped of contaminating RNA and protein and then must be cleaved into fragments of manageable size. This is most conveniently achieved by digestion with restriction enzymes, large numbers of which have become commercially available over the past 10 years. Each of these enzymes, isolated from bacteria and fungi, recognises a specific base sequence in double-stranded DNA and cuts the strands at that point [94].

The fragments thus produced can be separated by electrophoresis in an agarose gel. The shorter fragments will move faster through the gel and so will travel further away from the origin in a given time than large heavier fragments [108].

It is much easier to work with DNA on a solid support than in a gel and therefore the DNA is transferred onto either nitrocellulose paper or a nylon membrane by a method first described by Dr. E.M. Southern [106]. This maintains the spatial relationship between the DNA fragments generated by the gel electrophoresis. After "denaturing" the DNA with NaOH, to separate the two strands, the gel is placed on a piece of filter paper, supported by a glass plate, with both ends dipping into a concentrated salt solution. The membrane is placed on top of the gel and pressed down onto it with a heavy weight. The salt moves down its concentration gradient, carrying the DNA from the gel to the membrane, and the weight assists by gradually compressing the gel, forcing the DNA out. After this overnight "blotting" procedure, the membrane is exposed to ultraviolet light for 2-5 min. This links the single-stranded DNA to the membrane by covalent bonds. A similar blotting technique can also be applied to RNA transfer [117].

The next step is to create a labelled DNA or RNA probe (i.e. millions of identical copies of a particular base sequence). The probes themselves are obtained by cloning the required piece of DNA as an insert in a virus-like vector which will grow in a bacterial host, usually *Escherichia coli*. The commonest method of labelling a

DNA probe is "nick translation" [93]; a segment of double-stranded DNA is incubated with a mixture of three unlabelled nucleotides plus one nucleotide containing radioactive ^{32}P atoms. The enzymes DNAse and DNA polymerase I are added. The DNAse introduces breaks ("nicks") at random in one DNA strand and the DNA polymerase moves along that strand cutting out nucleotides and then replacing them, using the other strand as a template. In the course of this repair phase, ^{32}P-labelled nucleotides are introduced into the DNA. Other methods have been used to label DNA and RNA probes to a higher specific activity with ^{32}P and the use of nonradioactive labels has also been explored [45].

The membrane, bearing the imprint of the original DNA gel fragments, is immersed in a complex hybridisation solution containing the labelled probe, shaken overnight at 68°C and then washed to remove unhybridised probe. If stringent washing conditions are used, the probe will hybridise only to those fragments of DNA on the filter to which it is exactly complementary. After autoradiographic exposure (1-10 days at −70°C), one or more discrete bands appear on the film. These bands correspond to the DNA fragments on the membrane to which the probe has hybridised and the size of these fragments can be determined from the positions of the bands (Fig. 5).

At least 90% of the DNA in a human cell does not encode any protein product, i.e. does not consist of "genes". While this material is not necessarily devoid of function, it is evidently much more tolerant of variation in base sequence than the genes themselves. Hence, within the species there is much more polymorphism of the nontranslated DNA than of the genes. One aspect of this polymorphism is the gain or loss of restriction enzyme cleavage sites, the positions of which can vary considerably from one individual to another. Thus, when DNA is cleaved with a restriction enzyme and the Southern blot probed with a particular labelled sequence, the size of fragment bearing the complementary sequence is quite likely to show some variation within the population. This "restriction fragment length polymorphism" (RFLP) provides an enormous pool of genetic markers since the positions of restriction sites are still sufficiently stable for the DNA fragment lengths to behave as alleles obeying the simple laws of Mendelian inheritance. "Anonymous" DNA probes recognising sequences that are not necessarily parts of structural genes, now represent a major resource in human gene mapping and genetic analysis. They may be used simply to increase the pool of "random" polymorphisms for the conventional "shotgun" approach to linkage studies or they may serve to provide polymorphic markers for adjacent candidate genes. The latter application, ironically, tends to blur the distinction just made (at some length!) between "linkage" and "association" for the candidate gene and by definition, will be causally related to the disorder (implying "association"). Nevertheless, when the allelic forms of that gene are identified on the basis of RFLP rather than by the putative mutation directly responsible for the disease, then any observed correlation between a *particular allele* and disease susceptibility will apply only within an individual family, i.e. we are dealing with true "linkage". Of course, in such an event, the logical course would be to analyse the implicated gene in sufficient detail to permit direct identification of the crucial DNA lesion which would, in turn, provide a basis for population (as distinct from family-based) screening.

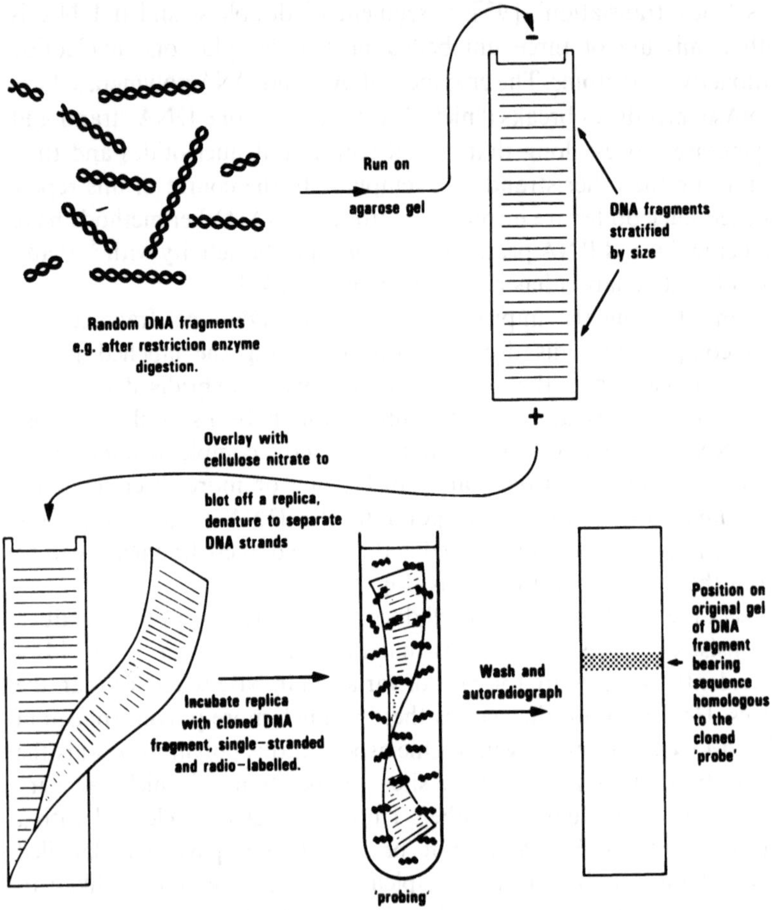

Fig. 5. Southern blotting. [108]

An Outline of Oncogenes

Identification of genes likely to be of importance in the aetiology of human cancer has resulted from three main experimental approaches: investigation of tumour-producing viruses; transfection of human tumourigenic DNA into immortalised cell lines; and direct comparisons of malignant and nonmalignant tissue at the molecular level.

The first clues came from an understanding of the structures of oncogenic retroviruses. The genetic material of these viruses is RNA, but once inside an infected cell, the RNA is copied into DNA which then integrates into the chromosomal DNA of the host. Later it may be transcribed and translated by the host cell's replication system, unleashing a second generation of virus. The viruses can be divided into two broad groups, depending on the rapidity with which they produce tumours. Slowly transforming viruses contain three genes; *gag* which codes for specific antigens mainly located at the core of the virus, *pol*, which codes for reverse transcriptase and *env*, which codes for the envelope protein. The acutely transforming viruses contain another gene, termed an "oncogene", specific to each virus and directly responsible for induction of malignancy in infected cells [10].

Analysis of the nucleotide sequences of retroviral oncogenes revealed that they were very similar to sequences (proto-oncogenes) found in the genome of higher organisms, including humans [109, 8]. It is virtually certain that the acutely transforming viruses arose by recombination between nononcogenic or slowly transforming viruses and the cellular proto-oncogenes. At least 22 viral oncogenes have been identified so far [9].

The second productive experimental approach has been direct DNA transfection/transformation. DNA from human tumours or tumour cell lines is precipitated onto the surface of cells in culture by calcium phosphate. A small proportion of the DNA enters the cells and an even smaller fraction becomes integrated into the genome in a random fashion. Cells "transformed" by this technique exhibit uncontrolled proliferation and form distinct colonies, which can be isolated and cloned up [103]. When injected into immunologically compromised animals, such as nude or neonatally thymectomised and irradiated mice, these transformed cells produce tumours, suggesting that a segment of DNA responsible for producing the original human tumour, has been integrated into the cell's genome [58, 86]. These oncogenes can then be identified by comparing extracted DNA from the transformed cells and from the original cell line.

Eleven new cellular oncogenes, without viral counterparts, have been identified by this technique [9]. Among the few oncogenes identified by both transfection and viral studies are members of the *ras* gene family which will be considered more fully in the next section.

One of the main limitations of DNA transfection studies is that the target cells used, usually 3T3 or C127 mouse fibroblasts, though subject to some normal growth controls, are immortal. They therefore represent an intermediate stage between the normal and full-blown malignant states. Cotransfection of at least two different oncogenes, for example, Ha-*ras* and c-*m̄yc*, is generally required to achieve tumourigenic transformation of normal cells [62]. This observation strengthens the theory that carcinogenesis is a multistage process, but raises the question of what changes have already taken place in immortal cell lines commonly used as targets for transfection assays and hence what (restricted) range of new oncogenic events they may be capable of detecting.

Chromosome Analysis

The alterations in genetic material that are required to induce malignant change are far beyond the limits of resolution by direct visualisation of stained chromosomes. Nevertheless, they may come about in the course of major (visible) structural rearrangements. The easiest neoplastic cells to examine in this fashion come from haematological malignancies. Several well-defined chromosomal abnormalities have been found consistently in various types of leukaemia and lymphoma [97]. By concentrating on regions of the genome involved in specific chromosome aberrations, molecular biologists have identified three novel oncogenes [43, 120, 121] and have achieved greater understanding of the mechanisms involved in cellular oncogene activation. It is much harder to obtain good chromosome preparations from solid tumours, but some progress has been made. There are, for example, reports of recurring deletions in the short arm of chromosome 3 in small cell lung cancer and in renal carcinoma [128, 134]. The possibility of localising a genetic lesion in breast cancer by a similar approach is therefore not to be discounted.

By combining the three experimental approaches already outlined, around 40 DNA sequences in the human genome have been classed as proto-oncogenes [9]. These proto-oncogenes may be activated to become oncogenic by changes either in their structure or in regulatory elements. A specific alteration in the nucleotide sequence (a point mutation) activates the *ras* gene family, resulting in the production of an abnormal protein product [90]. In chronic myeloid leukaemia, translocation between portions of chromosomes 9 and 22 results in the juxtaposition of two oncogenes, leading to the production of a hybrid mRNA and a hybrid protein product [43]. Translocation of another oncogene, c-*myc*, from chromosome 8 to chromosome 14 in Burkitt's lymphoma results in dysregulation of c-*myc*, leading to a continued expression of the normal gene [54, 64, 113], which is usually switched off as the cell differentiates [22, 40]. Overproduction of a normal protein product can also result from an increase in the copy number of an oncogene [102].

Harvey *ras*

In the context of breast and other human cancers, one of the most intensively studied oncogenes is Harvey *ras* (c-Ha-*ras*). The proto-oncogene was first identified as the sequence which, on transfection from a human bladder cancer cell line, was capable of transforming mouse 3T3 fibroblasts into tumourigenic cells [103, 39]. Its similarity to the *ras* oncogene of the Harvey rat sarcoma virus was quickly established and the human gene has been mapped to the short arm of chromosome 11 [72]. Analysis of the nucleotide sequence has shown that the Harvey *ras* proto-oncogene becomes tumourigenic by a point mutation in either the 12th or the 61st codon [90, 100]. There are two other closely related proto-oncogenes: Kirsten *ras* (K-*ras*) on chromosome 12 and N-*ras* on chromosome 1, coding for almost identical proteins of 189 amino acids, known as p21 [14, 112]. By analysis of DNA fragments on Southern blots, alterations involving *ras* sequences have been identified in about 10% of the commonest forms of human solid tumours [88] and in up to 80% of chemically induced rat mammary tumours [111]. A Harvey *ras* gene mutuation has also been found in a cell line derived from a carcinosarcoma of the breast, but not in normal breast cells of the same patient [57].

Abnormally high levels of the normal protein p21, induced by increasing the rate of transcription or the number of copies of the normal Harvey *ras* proto-oncogene, will transfrom 3T3 cells in culture [85, 89]. Primary human breast tumours have significantly higher levels of p21 than normal mammary tissue [46, 82, 129] and alterations in structure or regulation of the Harvey *ras* gene are of importance in the aetiology or progression of breat cancer.

Near the Harvey *ras* gene lies an untranslated region made up of a variable number of repeated DNA subunits [14]. Digestion with the restriction enzyme Bam HI generates a fragment bearing Ha-*ras* plus the untranslated subunits. Since they vary in number, the fragment length is variable, i.e. this is an example of RFLP. There are four common alleles in the normal population, (named A_1, A_2, A_3, A_4) and a number of very much rarer alleles. In 1985 Krontiris et al. [59] reported that among patients with a variety of solid or haematopoietic malgnacies there were significantly more rare alleles than in a control population. Since the alleles can be identified in any tissue, including white blood cells, if this report could be confirmed it would offer a real possibility of identifying a blood-borne marker for high risk of developing cancer.

Furthermore, it suggests that information about a gene involved in familial breast cancer might be obtained from direct analysis of a large series of unselected tumours, rather than concentrating only on patients with multiple affected first-degree relatives, bilateral disease and early age of onset. Though this may seem paradoxical, there are precedents which may prove to be highly relevant. The hereditary form of retinoblastoma is associated with an inherited deletion of part of chromosome 13 and there is evidence that the same region of the genome has become abnormal in tumour tissue from sporadic (i.e. nonhereditary) cases [16]. More recently, the gene for familial adenomatous polyposis (an autosomal dominant condition leading to multiple colon cancers if not treated by early colectomy) has been mapped to the long arm of chromosome 5 and a lesion of the same chromosome arm has been recognised in tumour material from a substantial proportion of sporadic large bowel cancers [11, 105].

Harvey *ras* Alleles in Primary Breast Cancer

The differences in restriction fragment length for the four common Harvey *ras* alleles are considerable and it is therefore relatively simple to separate them. Rare alleles however, tend to be much closer in size to their common counterparts. This is illustrated by the autoradiograph in Fig. 6.

We have determined the frequency of the different Ha-*ras* Bam HI restriction fragments in tumour tissue from a series of 100 female patients with breast cancer prior to treatment in the Department of Clinical Surgery, Edinburgh University Medical School, and in 100 placentae (to act as a control panel representative of the local Edinburgh population). Table 1 shows the relative frequencies of the alleles in these two groups.

There is no significant difference between breast cancer patients and controls in respect of any alleles (rare or common). This large series therefore contradicts the findings of Krontiris and the subsequent report from Lidereau and colleagues [68] which related specifically to breast cancer. Negative findings, however, have emerged from similar studies in myelodysplasia [115], lung cancer [47] and melanoma [37].

In the course of this study we noted that in several of the heterozygous tumours the autoradiographic band representing one allele was darker than the other

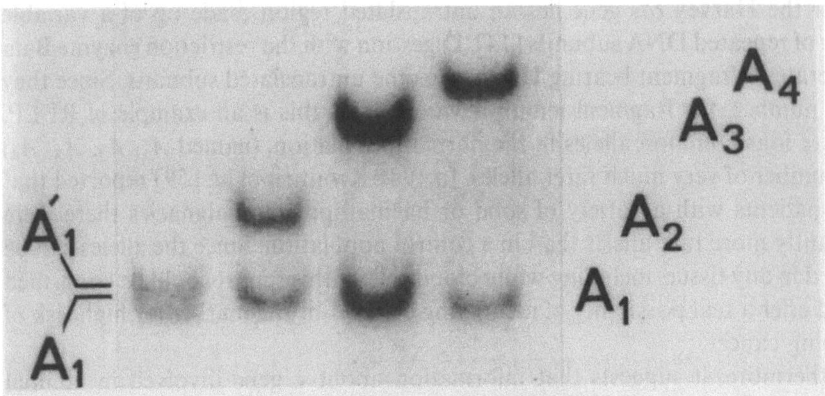

Fig. 6. Alleles of c-Ha-*ras* (Bam HI digests). The left-hand track of this Southern blot contains a "doublet" of allele A_1 and the rare variant A'_1

Table 1. Relative frequencies of Harvey *ras* alleles in breast cancer patients and a control group

	100 Breast cancer patients		100 Placentae	
	Number	(%)	Number	(%)
A_1	122	61	135	67.5
A_2	26	13	27	13.5
A_3	26	13	19	9.5
A_4	21	10.5	15	7.5
A'_1	5	2.5	4	2.0
	200		200	

(Fig. 7). A possible explanation is that the tumour cells have lost one allele and the fainter band results from contamination of the tumour sample by normal white blood cells. This interpretation was supported by comparing tumour DNA and white blood cell DNA from the same patient (Fig. 8). Since a tumour with minimal white blood cell infiltration might appear homozygous, we have examined white blood cell DNA from most of the patients with apparently homozygous tumours and have identified four who are constitutionally heterozygous. The current status of this investigation is set out in Table 2. The 100 tumours therefore fall into three groups: (a) 52 with no allele loss; (b) 13 with loss of one allele; and (c) 35 which await definition, of which 27 are constitutionally homozygous.

As seen in Table 3, loss of Harvey *ras* allele is significantly correlated ($P < 0.05$) with poverty of oestrogen receptor protein, which is known to indicate a poor prognosis [21, 78, 130].

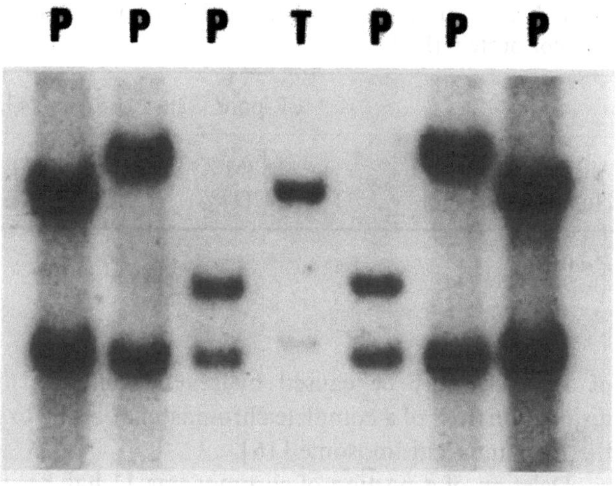

Fig. 7

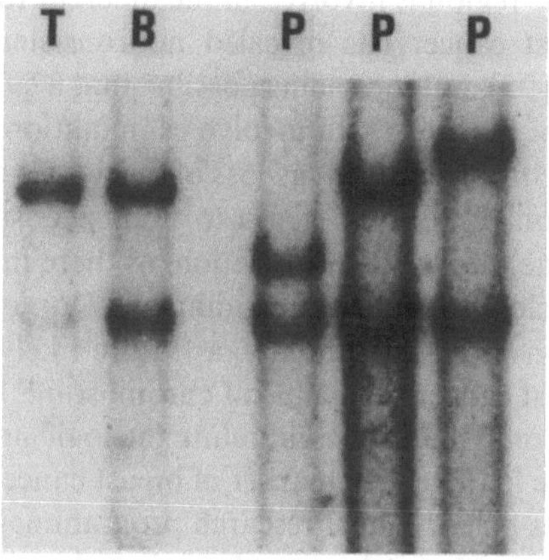

Fig. 8

Table 2. Restriction fragment length polymorphisms (RFLP) in DNA from breast Tumours and white blood cells (WBC)

100 Tumours characterised for Harvey *ras* alleles	
61 Heterozygous	*39 Apparently homozygous*
9 Allelic bands of different density	31 WBC DNA examined
52 Allelic bands of equal density	4 Heterozygous
	27 Homozygous

We are currently evaluating the correlation between allelic loss of Ha-*ras* and other prognostic factors, such as tumour size, progesterone receptor levels and axillary lymph node involvement [99], to clarify the suggestion that loss of a Harvey *ras* allele is a marker for a more aggressive tumour behaviour [3, 114]. Loss

Table 3. Loss of Harvey *ras* allele and poverty of oestrogen receptor protein (ER)

	ER-poor (22)	ER-rich (43)
Allelic loss (13)	8 (61%)	5 (39%)
No allelic loss (52)	14 (27%)	38 (73%)

$P < 0.02$.

of an allele may be caused by several different mechanisms, including non-disjunction (loss of a complete chromosome), alone or followed by reduplication of the remaining chromosome [16].

Deletion of a portion of chromosome 11 has been reported in Wilms' tumour [55, 31, 91], hepatoblastoma [56], hepatocellular carcinoma [96] and transitional cell carcinoma of the bladder [32] although it has yet to be established whether precisely the same region is involved in the different tumours. Cytogenetic analysis of primary breast cancer has revealed no consistent loss of large portions of chromosome 11 [95], but it remains possible that a submicroscopic deletion exists. The next phase of the study will involve examination of other polymorphic genes known to be on chromosome 11, as loss of one whole copy of the chromosome will result in reduction of all these genes to homozygosity. This strategy could also enable us to define the size of any deletion, as there may turn out to be a region of chromosome 11 close to (but not including) the Harvey *ras* gene that is deleted in a higher proportion of breast tumours, a feature likely to be of importance in the aetiology of breast cancer. A change of chromosome 11, but not of the Harvey *ras* gene, would be ironic since it would refute the logic underlying the choice of c-Ha-*ras* as a candidate for a genetic marker of breast cancer susceptibility. Nevertheless serendipity has its place in most research programmes and it is not to be despised.

A note of caution must be sounded when drawing conclusions from genetic lesions found in tumour tissue. Biochemical and cytogenetic evidence has been available for many years to show that malignant cells tend to accumulate multiple aberrations in their DNA, including gene deletions [87, 99]. It is unlikely that all – or even many – of them contribute to the malignant state. Refinements in molecular biology have confirmed and extended these findings [116]. It will therefore be necessary to scan the rest of the genome of breast cancer cells before concluding that a deletion in the vicinity of c-Ha-*ras* is significantly associated with the disease.

The Future

In addition to the Harvey *ras* gene, several other oncogenes have been studied in primary breast cancer. The *erb*-B_2 gene, mapping to the long arm of chromosome 17 [19, 34] codes for a protein similar to epidermal growth factor [101], and is amplified in 30% of primary breast tumours. Amplification of this gene is a prediction of both disease-free interval and overall survival and has a greater prognostic value than oestrogen receptor status [104].

Amplification of another oncogene, c-*myc* on chromosome 8 has been reported in 30% of primary breast tumours [28], but this is not significantly linked to disease progression. A rare restriction fragment bearing the c-*mos* locus (on chromosome 8) has been identified in a small number of patients with breast cancer [67], but in the absence of a formal linkage analysis, the significance of this finding remains unclear.

In addition to the known oncogenes, one of the genes likely to be of interest in breast cancer is the recently cloned gene for the oestrogen receptor protein [42]. A high level of oestrogen receptor protein in a breast tumour is a good prognostic sign [130]. The gene coding for the oestrogen receptor protein maps to chromosome 6 [126, 41] and there is extensive homology between it and the *erb*-A oncogene of the avian erythroblastosis virus [23]. The identification of any rearrangement or amplification of this gene in primary and metastatic breast cancer would be important and the recent finding of an RFLP with the enzyme PVU II, [15] will allow a linkage analysis of families with a high incidence of breast cancer.

In conclusion, it is clear that the techniques of molecular biology can contribute to a better understanding of the aetiology and progression of breast cancer in two ways. Identification of alterations in the genetic material that contribute to progression from a normal breast epithelium cell to a malignant cell is fairly well advanced. However, the search for a genetic marker for high risk of developing breast cancer will gather momentum as more and more polymorphic DNA markers become available. If successful, it will represent a major breakthrough in the targeting of expensive screening techniques to those women who are most likely to benefit.

Acknowledgments. The authors are indebted to their colleagues in the Department of Clinical Surgery, Edinburgh University Medical School and in the Medical Research Council Clinical and Population Cytogenetics Unit, for their many contributions to the work described in this chapter. In particular we wish to thank Dr. Anthony Hawkins, Dr. Peter Middleton, Dr. John Clayton and Mrs. P Elder. James Mackay holds a Margaret and Annie Mackenzie Scholarship from the Edinburgh University Faculty of Medicine.

References

1. Adami HO, Rimsten A, Stenkvist B, Vegeluis J (1978) Reproductive history and risk of breast cancer. A case control study in an unselected Swedish population. Cancer 41: 747-757
2. Adami HO, Hansen J, Jung B, Rimsten A (1981) Characteristics of familial breast cancer in Sweden. Absence of relation to age and unilateral versus bilateral disease. Cancer 48: 1688-1695
3. Ali IU, Lidereau R, Theillet C, Calahan R (1987) Reduction to homozygosity of genes on chromosome 11 in human breast neoplasia. Science 238: 185-188
4. Anderson VE, Goodman HO, Reed SC (1958) Variables related to human breast cancer. University of Minnesota Press, Minneapolis

5. Anderson DE (1971) Some characteristics of familial breast cancer. Cancer 28: 1500-1504
6. Anderson DE (1972) A genetic study of human breast cancer. J Natl Cancer Inst 48: 1029-1034
7. Bain C, Speizer FE, Rosner B, Belanger C, Hennekens CH (1980) Family history of breast cancer as a risk indicator for the disease. Am J Epidemiol 11: 301-308
8. Bishop JM (1981) Enemies within: the genesis of retrovirus oncogenes. Cell 23: 5-6
9. Bishop JM (1983) Cellular oncogenes and retroviruses. Annu Rev Biochem 52: 301-354
10. Bister K, Duesberg PH (1982) Genetic structure and transforming genes of avian retroviruses. Adv Viral Oncol 1: 3-42
11. Bodmer WF, Binley CJ, Bodmer J, Bussey HJR, Ellis A, Gorman P, Lucibello FC, Murday VA, Rider SH, Scambler P, Sheer D, Solomon E, Spurr NK (1987) Localisation of the gene for familial adenomatous polyposis on chromosome 5. Nature 328: 614-616
12. Brinton LA, Williams RR, Hoover RN, Stegens NL, Feinleib M, Fraumeni JF Jr (1979) Breast cancer risk factors among screening program participants. J Natl Cancer Inst 62: 37-43
13. Broca PP (1866) Traite des tumeurs. Asselin, Paris
14. Capon DJ, Chen EY, Levison AD, Seeburg PH, Goeddel DV (1983) Complete nucleotide sequences of the T24 human bladder carcinoma oncogene and its normal homologue. Nature 302: 33-37
15. Castagnoli A, Maestri I, Bernardi F, Del Senno L (1987) PVU II RFLP inside the human estrogen receptor gene. Nucleic Acids Res 15: 866
16. Cavenee WK, Dryja TP, Phillips RA (1983) Expression of recessive alleles by chromosomal mechanisms in retinoblastoma. Nature 305: 779-784
17. Chaudray MA, Millis RR, Bulbrook RD, Hayward JL (1985) Family history and bilateral primary breast cancer. Breast cancer Res Treat 5: 201-205
18. Chetty U, Wang CC, Forrest APM, Roberts MM (1980) Benign breast disease and cancer. Br J Surg 67: 789-790
19. Coussens L, Yang-Feng TL, Liao YC, Chen E, Gray A, McGrath J, Seeburg PH, Libermann TA, Schlessinger J, Francke U et al. (1985) Tyrosine kinase receptor with extensive homology to EGF receptor shares chromosomal location with new oncogene. Science 230: 1132-1139
20. Craig TJ, Comstock JW, Geiser PB (1974) Epidemiologic comparison of breast cancer patients with early and late onset of malignancy and general population controls. J Natl Cancer Inst 53: 1577-1582
21. Croton R, Cooke T, Holt S, George WD Nicolson R, Griffiths K (1981) Oestrogen receptors and survival in early breast cancer. Br Med J 283: 1289-1291
22. Curran T (1984) Induction of c-*fos* gene and protein by growth factors precedes activation of c-*myc*. Nature 312: 716-720
23. Debuire B, Henry C, Bernissa M, Biserte G, Claverie JM, Saule S, Martin P, Stehelin D (1984) Sequencing the *erb*A gene of avian erythroblastosis virus reveals a new type of oncogene. Science 224: 1456-1459
24. Doll R (1975) The epidemiology of cancers of the breast and reproductive system. Scott Med J 20: 305-315
25. Donnelly PK, Baker KW, Carney JA, O'Fallon WM (1975) Benign breast lesions and subsequent breast carcinoma in Rochester, Minnesota. Mayo Clin Proc 50: 650-656
26. Duffy SW, Roberts MM, Elton RA (1983) Risk factors for breast cancer: relevance to screening. J Epidemiol Community Health 37: 127-131

27. Elston RC and Sobel E (1979) Sampling considerations in the gathering and analysis of pedigree data. Am J Hum Genet 31: 62-69
28. Escot C, Theillet C, Lidereau R, Spyratos F, Champeme MH, Gest J, Callahan R (1986) Genetic alteration of the c-*myc* proto-oncogene (MYC) in human primary breast carcinomas. Proc Natl Acad Sci USA 83: 4834-4838
29. Falconer DS (1965) The inheritance of liability to certain diseases, estimated from the incidence among relatives. Ann Hum Genet 29: 51-76
30. Falconer DS (1967) The inheritance of liability to diseases with variable age of onset, with particular reference to diabetes mellitus. Ann Hum Genet 31: 1-20
31. Fearon ER, Vogelstein B, Feinberg AP (1984) Somatic deletion and duplication of genes on chromosome 11 in Wilms' tumor. Nature 309: 176-178
32. Fearon ER, Feinberg AP, Hamilton SH, Vogelstein B (1985) Loss of genes on the short arm of chromosome 11 in bladder cancer. Nature 318: 377-380
33. Feinleib M (1968) Breast cancer and artificial menopause: a cohort study. J Natl Cancer Inst 41: 315-329
34. Fukushiga S-I, Matsubara K-I, Yoshida M, Sasaki M, Suzuki T, Semba K, Toyoshima K, Yamamoto T (1986) Localisation of a novel v-*erb* B-related gene c-*erb*B-2, on human chromosome 17 and its amplification in a gastric cancer cell line. Mol cell Biol 6: 955-958
35. Gardner EJ, Stephens FE (1950) Breast cancer in one family group. Am J Hum Genet 2: 30-40
36. Gardner E (1980) Prevention and cure for hereditary cancers. In: Cairns (ed) Cancer incidence in defined populations, Banbury Rep no. 4. Cold Spring Harbor Lab, Cold Spring Harbor, pp 365-378
37. Gerhard D, Dracopoli NC, Bale SJ, Houghton AN, Watkins P, Payne CE, Greene MH, Housman DE (1987) Evidence against Ha-*ras*-1 involvement in sporadic and familial melanoma. Nature 325: 73-75
38. Go RCP, King M-C, Bailey-Wilson J, Elston RC, Lynch HT (1983) Genetic epidemiology of breast cancer and associated cancers in high risk families. I. Segregation analysis. J Natl Cancer Inst 71: 455-461
39. Goldfarb M, Shimzu K, Perucho M, Wigler M (1982) Isolation and preliminary characterization of a human transforming gene from T24 bladder carcinoma cells. Nature 296: 404-409
40. Gonda TJ, Metcalf D (1984) Expression of *myb*, *myc* and *fos* proto-oncogenes during the differentiation of a murine myeloid leukaemia. Nature 310: 249-251
41. Gosden JR, Middleton PG, Rout D (1986) Localisation of the human oestrogen receptor gene to chromosome 6q 24-27 by in-situ hybridisation. Cytogenet Cell Genet 43: 218-220
42. Green S, Walter P, Kumar V, Krust A, Bornert JM, Argos P, Chambon P (1986) Human oestrogen receptor cDNA: sequence, expression and homology to V. *erb*-A. Nature 320: 134-139
43. Groffen J, Stephenson JR, Heisterkamp N (1984) Philadelphia chromosomal breakpoints are clustered within a limited region, *bcr* on chromosome 22. Cell 36: 93-99
44. Hill JR, Carmelli D, Gardner EJ, Skonick M (1978) Likelihood analysis of breast cancer predisposition in a Mormon pedigree. In: Morton NE, Chung CS (eds) Genetic epidemiology. Academic, New York, pp 304-310
45. Hames BD, Higgins SJ (eds) (1985) Nucleic acid hybridisation: a practical approach. IRL Press, Oxford

46. Hand PH, Thor A, Wunderlich D, Muraro R, Caruso A, Scholm J (1984) Monoclonal antibodies of predefined specificity detect activated *ras* gene expression in human mammary and colon carcinomas. Proc Natl Acad Sci USA 81: 5227-5231
47. Heighway J, Thatcher N, Cerny T, Hasleton PS (1986) Genetic predisposition to human lung cancer. Br J Cancer 53: 453-457
48. Hutchinson WB, Thomas DB, Hamlin WB, Roth GJ, Peterson AV, Williams B (1980) Risk of breast cancer in women with benign breast disease. J Natl Cancer Inst 65: 13-20.
49. Jacobsen O (1946) Heredity in Breast Cancer. Lewis, London, pp 1-306
50. Kelly PT (1890) Counselling needs of women with a maternal history of breast cancer. Patient Counselling and Health Education 2: 118-124
51. Kelsey JL, Holford TR, White C, Mayer ES, Kilty SE Acheson RM (1978) Oral contraceptives and breast disease. An epidemiological study. Am J Epidemiol 107: 236-244
52. Kelsey J (1979) A review of the epidemiology of human breast cancer: epidemiological reviews. Przegl Epidemiol 1: 74-109
53. King M-C, Go RCP, Lynch HT, Elston RC, Terasaki PI, Petrakis NL, Rodgers GC, Lattanzio D, Bailey-Wilson J (1983) Genetic epidemiology of breast cancer and associated cancers in high risk families. II. Linkage analysis. J Natl Cancer Inst 71: 463-467
54. Klein G (1981) The role of gene dosage and genetic transpositions in carcinogenesis. Nature 294: 313-318
55. Koufos A, Hansen MF, Lampkin BC, Workman ML, Copeland NG, Jenkins NA, Cavenee WK (1984) Loss of alleles at loci on human chromosome 11 during genesis of Wilms' tumor. Nature 309: 170-172
56. Koufos A, Harsen MF, Copeland NG, Jenkins NA, Lampkin BC, Cavenee WK (1985) Loss of heterozygosity in three embryonal tumours suggests a common pathogenetic mechanism. Nature 316: 330-334
57. Kraus MH, Yuasa Y, Aaronson SA (1984) A position 12-activated H-*ras* oncogene in all HS 578T mammary carcinosarcoma cells but not normal mammary cells of the same patient. Proc Natl Acad Sci USA 81: 5384-5388
58. Krontiris TG, Cooper GM (1981) Transfroming activity of human tumor DNAs. Proc Natl Acad Sci USA 78: 1181-1184
59. Krontiris TG, Nancy A, Di Martina NA, Colb M, Parkinson DR (1985) Unique allelic restriction fragments of the human Ha-*ras* locus in leukocyte and tumour DNAs of cancer patients. Nature 313: 369-374
60. Lalouel JM, Morton NE (1981) Complex segregation analysis with pointers. Hum Hered 31: 312-321
61. Lancet (editorial) (1982) Obesity – the cancer connection. Lancet 1: 1223
62. Land H, Parada LF, Weinberg RA (1983) Tumorigenic conversion of primary embryo fibroblasts requires at least two cooperating oncogenes. Nature 304: 596-602
63. Lane-Clayton JE (1926) A further report on cancer of the breast, with special reference to its associated antecedent conditions. Rep Minist Health no 32 London
64. Leder P, Battey J, Lenoir G, Moulding C, Murphy W, Potter H, Stewart T, Taub R (1983) Translocations among antibody genes in human cancer. Science 222: 765-771
65. Lew EA, Garfinkel L (1979) Variations in mortality by weight among 750000 men and women. J Chronic Dis 32: 563-576
66. Lewison EF, Neto AS (1971) Bilateral breast cancer at the Johns Hopkins Hospital. Cancer 34: 1090-1097
67. Lidereau R, Matlieu-Mahul D, Theillet C, Renaud M, Mauchauffe M, Gest J, Larsen CJ (1985) Presence of an allelic Eco Rl restriction fragment of the c-*mos* locus in

leukocyte and tumor cell DNAs of breast cancer patients. Proc Natl Acad Sci USA 82: 7068-7070
68. Lidereau R, Chantal E, Theillet C (1986) High frequency of rare alleles of the human c-Ha-*ras*-1 proto-oncogene in breast cancer patients. J Natl Cancer Inst 77: 697-701
69. Lilienfeld AM (1956) The relationship of cancer of the female breast to artificial menopause and mental status. Cancer 9: 927-934
70. Lynch HT, Guirgis HA (1981) Genetics and breast cancer. Van Nostrand Reinhold, New York, p 253
71. Lynch HT, Albano WA, Heieck JJ, Mulcahey GM, Lynch JF, Layton MA, Danes BS (1984) Genetics, biomarkers and control of breast cancer: a review. Cancer Genet Cytogenet 13: 43-92
72. McBride OW, Swan DC, Santos E (1982) Localisation of the normal allele of T24 human bladder carcinoma oncogene to chromosome 11. Nature 300: 773-774
73. McKusick VA (1982) The human gene map. Clin Gen 22: 360-391
74. McLellan T, Cannon LA, Bishop DT, Skolnick MH (1984) The cumulative lod score between a breast cancer susceptibility locus and GPT is 3.86. Cytogenet Cell Genet 37: 536-537
75. MacMahon B, Austin JH (1969) Association of carcinomas of the breast and corpus uteri. Cancer 23: 275-280
76. MacMahon B, Cole P, Lowe CR, Mirra AP, Ravhihar B, Salber EJ, Valaoras VG, Yuasa S (1970) Age at first birth and breast cancer risk. Bull WHO 43: 209-221
77. Monson RR, Yen S, MacMahon B (1976) Chronic mastitis and carcinoma of the breast. Lancet 1: 224-226
78. Moore DH, Moore DUT and Moore CT (1983) Breast carcinoma etiological factors. Adv Cancer Res 40: 189-253
79. Morton NE (1955) Sequential tests for the detection of linkage. Am J Hum Genet 7: 277-318
80 Morton NE, MacLean CJ (1974) Analysis of family resemblance. III. Complex segregation of quantitative traits. Am J Hum Genet 26: 489-503
81. Morton NE, Rao DC, Lanouel JM (1983) Methods in genetic epidemiology. Karger, New York
82. Ohuchi N, Thor A, Page DL, Haran Hand P, Halter SA, Schlom J (1986) Expression of the 21 000 molecular weight *ras* protein in a spectrum of benign and malignant human mammary tissue. Cancer Res 46: 2511-2519
83. Ottman R, Pike MC, King MC, Henderson BE (1983) Practical guide for estimating risk for familial breast cancer. Lancet 2: 556-558
84. Paget J (1853) Lectures on surgical pathology, vol 2. Longman, Brown, Green and Longmans, London
85. Paroda LF, Tabin CJ, Shih C, Weinberg RA (1982) Human EJ bladder carcinoma oncogene is homologue of Harvey sarcoma virus *ras* gene. Nature 297: 474-478
86. Porteous DJ, Morten JEN, Foster ME, Cranston G, Weir-Thompson E, Busuttil A, Bostock CJ, Steel CM (1986) H-*ras* 1 selected chromosome mediated transformants vary in phenotype in vitro and tumorigenic potential in vivo. Int J Cancer 38: 603-612
87. Povey S, Jeremiah S, Arthur E, Steel M, Klein G (1980) Differences in genetic stability between cell lines from patients with and without lymphoreticular malignancies. Ann Hum Genet 44: 119-133
88. Pulciani S, Santos E, Lauver AU, Lang LK, Aaronson SH, Barbacid M (1982) Oncogenes in solid human tumours. Nature 300: 539-542
89. Pulciani S, Santos E, Lang LK, Sorrentino V, Barbacid M (1985) *Ras* gene amplification and malignant transformation. Mol Cell Biol 5: 2836-2841

90. Reddy EP, Reynolds RK, Santos E, Barbacid M (1982) A point mutation is responsible for the acquisition of transforming properties by the T24 human bladder carcinoma oncogene. Nature 300: 149-152
91. Reeve AE, Housiaux PJ, Gardner RJ, Chewings WE, Grindley RM, Millow LJ (1984) Loss of a Harvey *ras* allele in sporadic Wilms' tumor. Nature 309: 174-176
92. Reimer RR, Hoover R, Fraumeni JF, Young RC (1978) Second primary neoplasms following ovarian cancer. J Natl Cancer Inst 61: 1195-1197
93. Rigby PWJ, Dieckmann M, Rhodes C, Berg P (1977) Labelling DNA to high specific activity in vitro by nick translation with DNA polymerase I. J Mol Biol 113: 237-251
94. Roberts RJ (1983) Restriction and modification enzymes and their recognition sequences. Nucleic Acids Res 11: 135-167
95. Rodgers CS, Hill SM, Hulten M (1984) Cytogenetic analysis in human breast carcinoma. I. Nine cases in the diploid range investigated using direct preparations. Cancer Genet Cytogenet 13: 95-120
96. Rogler CE, Shermanm, Su CY, Shafritz DA, Summers J, Shows TB, Henderson A, Kew M (1985) Deletion in chromosome 11p associated with a hepatitis B integration site in hepatocellular carcinoma. Science 230: 319-322
97. Rowley JD (1982) Identification of the constant chromosome regions involved in human hematologic malignant disease. Science 216: 749-751
98. Royal College of General Practitioners (1981) Breast cancer and oral contraceptives: findings in Royal College of General Practitioners study. Br Med J 282: 2089-2093
99. Sandberg AA (1980) The chromosomes in human cancer and leukaemia. Elsevier, New York
100. Santos E, Reddy EP, Puciani S, Feldmann RJ, Barbacid M (1983) Spontaneous activation of a human proto-oncogene. Proc Natl Acad Sci USA 15: 4697-4683
101. Schechter AL, Stern DF, Vaidyanathan L, Decker SJ, Drebin JA, Greene MI, Weinberg RA (1984) The new oncogenes: an *erb*-B-related gene encoding a 185 000-H_r tumour antigen. Nature 312: 513-516
102. Semba K, Kamata N, Toyoshima K, Yamamoto T (1985) A v-*erb* B-related proto-oncogene c-*erb* B-2, is distinct from the c-*erb* B-1/epidermal growth factor-receptor gene and is amplified in a human salivary gland adenocarcinoma. Proc Natl Acad Sci USA 82: 6497-6501
103. Shih C Weinberg RA (1982) Isolation of a transforming sequence from a human bladder carcinoma cell line. Cell 29: 161-169
104. Slamon DJ, Clark GM, Wong SG, Wendy J, Levin, Ullrich A, McGuire WL (1987) Human breast cancer: correlation of relapse and survival with amplification of the HER-2 *neu* oncogene. Science 325: 177-182
105. Solomon E, Voss R, Hall V, Bodmer WF, Jass JR, Jeffreys AJ, Lucibello FC, Patel I, Rider SH (1987) Chromosome 5 allele loss in human colorectal carcinomas. Nature 328: 616-619
106. Southern EM (1975) Detection of specific sequences among DNA fragments separated by gel electrophoresis. J Mol Biol 98: 503-517
107. Staszewski J (1971) Age at menarche and breast cancer. J Natal Cancer Inst 47: 935-940
108. Steel CM (1984) DNA in medicine: the tools. I and II. Lancet 2: 908, 911, 966-968
109. Stehelin D, Varmus HE, Bishop JM, Vogt PK (1976) DNA related to the transforming gene(s) of avian sarcoma viruses is present in normal avian DNA. Nature 260: 170-173
110. Storm HH, Jensen OM (1986) Risk of contralateral breast cancer in Denmark 1943-80. Br J Cancer 54: 483-492

111. Sukumar S, Notano V, Martin-Zanca, Barbacid M (1983) Induction of mammary carcinomas in rats by nitrosomethylurea involves malignant activation of H-*ras*-1 locus by single point mutations. Nature 306: 658-661
112. Taparowsky E, Shmizu K, Goldfarb M (1983) Structure and activation of the human N-*ras* gene. Cell 34: 581-586
113. Taub R, Moulding C, Battey J, Murphy W, Vasicek T, Lenoir GM, Leder P (1984) Activation and somatic mutation of the translocated c-*myc* gene in Burkitt lymphoma cells. Cell 36: 339-348
114. Theillet C, Rosette Lidereau R, Escot C (1986) Loss of a c-H-*ras*-1 allele and aggressive human primary breast carcinomas. Cancer Res 46: 4776-4781
115. Thein SL, Oscier DG, Flint J, Wainscoat JS (1986) Ha-*ras* hyper-variable alleles in myelodysplasia. Nature 321: 84-85
116. Thein SL, Jeffreys AJ, Govi HC, Catler F, Flint J, O'Connor NTJ, Weatherall DJ, Wainscot JS (1987) Detection of somatic changes in human cancer DNA by DNA fingerprint analysis. Br J Cancer 55: 353-356
117. Thomas PS (1980) Hybridisation of denatured RNA and small DNA fragments transferred to nitrocellulose. Proc Natl Acad Sci USA 77: 5201-5205
118. Tiwari JL, Terasaki PI (1985) HLA and disease associations. Springer, Berlin Heidelberg New York Tokyo
119. Trichopoulos D, MacMahon B, Cole P (1972) Menopause and breast cancer risk. J Natl Cancer Inst 48: 605-613
120. Tsujimoto Y, Yunis J, Onorato-Showe L, Erikson J, Nowell PC, Croce CM (1984) Molecular cloning of the chromosomal breakpoint of B-cell lymphomas and leukaemias with the *t*(11,14) chromosome translocation. Science 224: 1403-1406
121. Tsujimoto Y, Cossman J, Jaffe E, Croce CM (1985) Involvement of the *bcl*-2 gene in human follicular lymphoma. Science 228: 1440-1443
122. Vessey MP, Doll R, Jones K, McPherson K, Yeates D (1979) An epidemiological study of oral contraceptives and breast cancer. Br Med J 1: 1755-1758
123. Vessey MP, McPherson K, Doll R (1981) Breast cancer and oral contraceptives: findings in Oxford – Family Planning Association Contraceptive Study. Br. Med J 282: 2093-2094
124. Vessey MP, McPherson K, Yeates D, Doll R (1982) Oral contraceptive use and abortion before first term pregnancy in relation to breast cancer risk. Br J Cancer 45: 327-331
125. Wainwright JM (1931) A comparison of conditions associated with breast cancer in Great Britain and America. Am J Cancer 15: 2610-2614
126. Walter P, Green S, Greene G, Krust A, Bornert JM, Jeitsch JM, Staub A, Jensen E, Scrace G, Waterfield M et al. (1985) Cloning of the human estrogen receptor cDNA. Proc Natl Acad Sci USA 82: 7889-7893
127. Waterhouse J, Shanmugarathnam K, Muir C, Powell J (eds) (1976) Cancer incidence in five continents, vol III. IARC, Lyon
128. Whang-Peng J, Bunn PA Jr, Kao-Shan CS, Lee EC, Carney DN, Gazdar A, Minna JD (1982) A nonrandom chromosomal abnormality, in human small cell lung cancer. Cancer Genet Cytogenet 2: 119-134
129. Whittaker JL, Walker RA, Varley JM (1986) Differential expression of cellular oncogenes in benign and malignant human breast tissue. Int J Cancer 38: 651-655
130. Williams MR, Todd JH, Ellis IO, Dowle CS, Haybittle JL, Elston CW, Nicholson RI, Griffiths K, Blamey RW (1987) Oestrogen receptors in primary and advanced breast cancer. An eight-year review of 704 cases. Br J Cancer 55: 67-73
131. Williams WR, Anderson DE (1984) Genetic epidemiology of breast cancer: segregation analysis of 200 Danish pedigrees. Genet Epidemiol 1: 7-20

132. Woolf CM (1955) Investigations on genetic aspects of carcinoma of the stomach and breast. Bull Public Health 2: 265-349
133. Yates JRW, Connor JM (1986) Genetic linkage. Br J Hosp Med 36: 133-136
134. Zbar B, Brauch H, Talmadae C, Linehan M (1987) Loss of alleles of loci on the short arm of chromosome 3 in renal cell carcinoma. Nature 1: 721-724

Significance of Oncogenes in Breast Cancer: Review

J. Fiore and M.V. Viola

Oncology Division, Department of Medicine, Health Sciences Centre, P-17, 080,
State University of New York at Stonybrook, New York, NY 11794-8174, USA

Introduction

Proto-oncogenes are a restricted set of cellular genes that are frequent targets for mutational alterations in human cancer. Many of these genes were originally identified because they had nucleotide sequence similarity with transforming genes found in acutely transforming retroviruses. The viral oncogene (v-*onc*) was derived from its cellular homolog (c-*onc*) by genetic recombination and in the process of insertion into the viral genome acquired structural alterations. The detailed comparison of the structure of the viral oncogene as compared with the cellular proto-oncogene has provided critical information on the nature of the mutations obligatory for changing a normal protein into one with transforming ability.

There have been more than 30 cellular proto-oncogenes identified, and there is a rapidly growing literature which indicates that proto-oncogene products are important in normal cell growth and development, including cell proliferation. For example, the proto-oncogene c-*sis* appears to be the platelet-derived growth factor [57]. A series of oncogenes (c-*erb*-B, *neu*, c-*fms*, c-*kit*) belong to a family of plasma membrane receptors having tyrosine-specific protein kinase activity. Oncogenes c-*erb*-B and c-*fms* are the epidermal growth factor receptor and colony-stimulating factor 1 receptor respectively; for the remaining proto-oncogene protein "receptors", the ligand has not yet been identified [11, 44]. An additional group of proto-oncogene products localize to the inner surface of the plasma membrane (e.g:, c-*ras*, c-*src*), and appear to transduce signals generated from specific ligand-membrane receptor interactions. The structural and biochemical similarities between the *ras* gene product and another class of signal transducers, the G-proteins, is discussed later in this chapter. Finally, a poorly understood group of proto-oncogene proteins localize to the nucleus (e.g., c-*myc*, c-*fos*, c-*erb*-A). Oncogene c-*erb*-A is the nuclear protein receptor for thyroid hormone and functions as a transcriptional activator [41]. Both c-*fos* and c-*myc* gene products are increased following a number of membrane signals (including those generated by epidermal growth factor) and in turn appear capable of inducing increased transcription of a series of genes. Also, it has been proposed that c-*myc* is intimately involved in the regulation of the cell cycle and is functionally involved in DNA synthesis [50].

Analysis of the structure and organization of viral oncogenes and proto-oncogenes in human tumors has identified those mutations capable of converting a

Ragaz/Ariel (Eds.), High-Risk Breast Cancer

normal gene involved in growth control into an oncogene. The structural changes fall into a number of distinct classes.

Point Mutations

Specific bases of the *ras* gene resulting in amino acid substitutions which alter the function of the p21 molecule are discussed later in this chapter. These mutations are found both in human cancers [5] and in the viral *ras* genes. Point mutations may also alter regulatory sequences in proto-oncogenes and result in deregulation of tightly controlled genes. For example, point mutations at the 3′ end of the noncoding exon 1 of the c-*myc* gene result in the removal of a block to transcriptional elongation, resulting in an alteration of transcriptional control of c-*myc*. Mutations in this region of c-*myc* are frequently found in Burkitt's lymphoma [36].

Gene Truncation

The removal of COOH terminal or NH_2 terminal regions from proto-oncogene-encoded proteins has been found to "activate" proto-oncogenes of the tyrosine kinase type. Loss of the extracellular ligand-binding domain (NH_2 terminal) has been found in v-*kit* and v-*erb*-B [11, 59]. In those instances, loss of the ligand-binding domain of membrane receptor proto-oncogenes may lead to constitutive, unregulated tyrosine kinase activity.

Truncation of the COOH terminal region of tyrosine kinase-type proto-oncogenes has been found in v-*fms*, v-*src*, and v-*kit*. In v-*src*, this mutation removes a regulatory autophosphorylation site which activates the transforming ability of the molecule [25]. Although the mutational activation of c-*src* has been studied in considerable detail, experimentally, an activating mutation of this proto-oncogene has not yet been detected in a human tumor.

Gene Amplification

Alterations in the level of expression or inappropriate expression of specific proto-oncogenes may activate their transforming potential. This is particularly true of the *myc* family of cellular proto-oncogenes, where multiple molecular mechanisms may be responsible for deregulation (e.g., point mutations, translocation, amplification). Increased copy number of specific members of the *myc* gene family (c,N,0-*myc*) have been found in human neuroblastoma, small cell cancer of the lung, breast cancer, and retinoblastoma [29, 43, 60]. It is possible that cancers with markedly elevated levels of c-*myc* expression, but no *myc* gene amplification (e.g., colon cancers, some small cell lung cancers) may have mutations in a regulatory region of the c-*myc* gene.

Gene Translocation

There are two major ways in which translocation may result in activation of a proto-oncogene. In the first, the translocation results in the moving of the proto-oncogene to another genetic locus and thus, under the influence of other regulatory elements. In Burkitt's lymphoma, the c-*myc* gene is moved to the vicinity of the promoters/enhancers of an immunoglobulin locus and in the process is deregulated (summarized in [10]).

The second potential consequence of a reciprocal translocation involving a proto-oncogene is the creation of a hybrid fused gene at a chromosome breakpoint. Thus, in chronic myelogenous leukemia, the c-*abl* gene on chromosome 9 is transferred from its normal position to the *bcr* gene on chromosome 22, resulting in a chimeric gene and a hybrid protein product [23]. The *abl-bcr* gene product has been found to have altered functional activity.

ras Oncogenes

The *ras* family of oncogenes are the most frequently identified genes capable of transforming NIH/3T3 cells in culture [4]. It is now recognized that there are at least three members of this gene family; Harvey-*ras* (Ha-*ras*), Kirsten-*ras* (Ki-*ras*) and N-*ras*. All three genes encode proteins of 189 amino acids with a molecular weight of 21 000 which are generally designated p21. In humans, Ha-*ras* has been mapped to the short arm of chromosome 11, Ki-*ras* to the short arm of chromosome 12, and N-*ras* to the short arm of chromosome 1 [40]. There is strong sequence similarity among these three family members, particularly at the amino terminal end of the protein. Genes distantly related to *ras* have been isolated in a variety of species and it is unclear if these genes perform the same cellular functions as the conserved *ras* family genes [31].

The importance of *ras* proto-oncogenes in normal cellular function is suggested by their highly conserved nucleotide sequence throughout evolution. There is less than 5% variability in amino acid sequence between p21 proteins in humans and rats, and probably less than 10% variation in the functional amino terminal portion of yeast and mammalian *ras* proteins. The *ras* genes appear to be expressed at low levels in most cells, although specific cell types (e.g., thyroid acinar cells, gastric parietal cells) express elevated levels of p21 normally [16]. Although *ras* p21 is expressed in high amounts in some non-neoplastic rapidly growing cells [20], p21 expression is not tightly linked to cell proliferation.

The precise biochemical role of p21 proteins remains unclear, but currently available information has provided some clues to their function. p21 is located on the inner surface of the plasma membrane [45], binds guanine nucleosides [42], and has intrinsic GTPase activity [19, 32, 33, 41]. In its location, biochemical properties (GTP binding, GTPase), and nucleotide sequence, p21 appears similar to G-proteins, a group of proteins which function as signal transducers [26]. G-proteins are "active" in their GTP-bound form and hydrolyze GTP to GDP with intrinsic GTPase activity, thus self-regulating their level of activity. It has been found that viral and tumor-associated mutations of *ras* p21 at specific sites (see later in this chapter) result in diminished GTPase activity (or diminished responsiveness to activating proteins), resulting in a p21 molecule which is always in the "active form." Therefore, it appears that *ras* p21 transduces specific ligand-cell receptor-generated signals to responsive intracellular pathways. In some cells (e.g., fibroblasts) the cell response to activated p21 is cell proliferation [12, 34], but other cell types may respond to activated p21 by cessation of cell division and undergo terminal differentiation [21]. The pathways p21 uses to transduce cell-type-specific signals are not clearly identified, but may involve phosphatidyl inositol turnover [13]. We have shown that activated p21 induces an obligatory rapid rise in intracellular pH in promoting the mitogenic response in fibroblasts [22].

Oncogenic forms of both Ha-*ras* and Ki-*ras* are found in the genomes of the acutely transforming strains of the Harvey and Kirsten mouse sarcoma viruses, respectively. N-*ras* has been found in some human cancers [5], but is not known to be carried by a transforming retrovirus. Mutated Ha-*ras* genes appear to derive their malignant potential from a change in the amino acid glycine in position 12 or glutamine in position 61. Substitutions at or around position 12 appear to alter the tertiary structure of p21 profoundly, and result in a molecule either with less GTPase activity or a p21 molecule which is unresponsive to cytoplasmic protein stimulators of its GTPase activity and, thus, unable to downregulate its own activity [37]. Substitutions at position 61 diminish GTPase activity also and increase the transforming ability of p21.

Animal Models

Several animal models exist which lend credence to the possible role of *ras* in mammary neoplasia. Zarbl [61] has reported that NMU (*N*-nitroso-*N*-methylurea) can directly induce mammary carcinomas during sexual development in rats by activating the Ha-*ras* locus. Since NMU is quite labile and induces tumors after a single injection, it is thought that mutagenesis occurs within hours, and that the transforming genetic event occurs at the same time.

The molecular specificity of *ras* activation in this system was demonstrated by the finding that nucleotide 35 in the 12th codon of c-Ha-*ras* underwent a G-A transition which activated the oncogene in 100% of tumors tested. In contrast, rat mammary tumors induced by dimethylbenzanthrene (DMBA) are associated with mutations in c-H-*ras* at codon 61 [4, 61]. These experiments show that the *ras* oncogene alterations may occur at an early step in carcinogenesis, and that the molecular lesion is determined by the carcinogenic agent, given the restrictions of the specific experimental system. Thus, in chemical carcinogen-induced breast cancer in rodents, the Ha-*ras* locus appears to be a susceptible target for mutation.

An activated *ras* oncogene linked to a hormone-responsive promoter has been introduced into transgenic mice [6]. Several strains were developed which express elevated levels of p21 constitutively in mammary and salivary glands. These animals developed enlarged hyperplastic salivary glands and adenocarcinomas of the breast. The latter tumors occurred in a stochastic fashion, suggesting that additional mutations were necessary to complement *ras* in order to cause tumor induction.

ras and Human Breast Cancer

ras Mutations

The most frequent method by which cellular *ras* genes attain transforming ability is by point mutation. *ras* mutations are most readily identified by transformation of murine NIH/3T3 cells. Such abnormal *ras* genes have been identified in 15% of a wide variety of primary tumors and cell lines derived from human carcinomas. However, when *ras* genes are assayed directly in tumors, either by mutation-specific hybridization assays or RNase mismatch assays, *ras* mutations were found in 45% of human colon cancers [6, 14]. However, *ras* mutation appears to be an infrequent event in human breast cancer [38]. In addition to the paucity of point mutations of *ras* found in breast cancer, *ras* genes are infrequently found to be rearranged or amplified in this cancer type.

ras Expression

Although there has been a lack of positive findings of structural alterations of *ras* genes in breast cancer, numerous studies have found enhanced expression of *ras* p21 in breast cancer. These studies are of importance since the normal *ras* proto-oncogene can transform NIH/3T3 cells if expressed in high amounts [7], and even transformation with the oncogenic *ras* genes is subject to a dosage effect [49].

The detection of *ras* expression at the single cell level has been made possible by the generation of murine monoclonal antibodies to p21. The most widely used of these are RAP-5 and Y13-259. The former was generated by a synthetic peptide identical to amino acids 10-17 of the *ras* oncogene from the human T24 bladder cancer cell line [24]. Although this oncogene contains a mutation at amino acid 12, RAP-5 has been shown to react with nonmutated cellular Ha-, Ki-, and N-*ras* proto-oncogene p21 [54]. Y13-259 was raised with v-Ha-*ras* p21 as the immunogen, and recognizes both Ha- and Ki-*ras* gene products as well as normal cellular *ras* [17].

These antibodies have now been used by several groups of investigators with somewhat conflicting results. Further work will be necessary to resolve these discrepancies, but some tentative conclusions are possible at the present time. Results of this work are summarized here.

Hand et al. [24] first examined RAP-5 immunohistochemical staining of formalin-fixed sections of lesions containing infiltrating duct carcinomas, fibroadenomas, fibrocystic disease, as well as normal breast tissue from the same patients. When 20% of total cells stained was considered a positive result, 19/30 carcinomas were shown to express p21. Although some overlap with benign lesions was noted, overall there was a clear distinction between benign and malignant lesions. Further work by this group has extended their original observations to include a wider spectrum of breast pathology [35]. In fibrocystic disease, p21 staining with RAP-5 was rare; hyperplastic lesions without atypia stained an average of 18% cells, while hyperplastic lesions with atypia averaged 34% cells positive. Carcinoma in situ and invasive ductal carcinomas had the highest reactivity, averaging 54% and 62%, respectively. Overall, 36/47 invasive cancers had staining in at least 50% of cells. Furthermore, there was good correlation between the immunohistochemical assay for p21 and its determination by liquid competition radioimmunoassay in a small number of patients. Expression of p21 was also similar in pattern, although less intense, when Y13-259 was used as the primary antibody. Lundy et al. [30] employed RAP-5 to stain breast cancer specimens; overall, 16/41 sections had more than 25% of cells staining at an antibody dilution which was consistently negative with normal cells. Further work by Fromowitz et al. [15] showed a correlation between staining in the primary breast tumor and that seen in tumor in regional lymph nodes. Staining of distant metastases was more variable; liver and bone metastases generally demonstrated less p21 than lung, skin, endocrine, and central nervous system metastases. A high level of p21 was noted in the invasive components of the primary tumor compared with the intraductal elements. Since the detection of mutated *ras* in human breast cancer is rare, it is presumed that RAP-5 is staining normal cellular *ras* p21 in these studies.

Increased levels of p21 have also been noted by Agnantis et al. [2] using Y13-259. Their results were similar to those of Hand et al. [24]. Increasing levels of p21 were detected in specimens of simple cystic disease, complex cysts, fibroadenomas, carcinoma in situ, and, finally, invasive carcinoma. This same group, however, has disputed the ability of RAP-5 to stain p21 specifically [39].

Other conflicting results were obtained by Ghosh et al. [18] using the RAP-5 antibody. These investigators also performed immunohistochemical staining of a variety of breast sections, and could find no dilution of antibody which consistently discriminated between benign and malignant lesions. They concluded that RAP-5 recognized a normal cellular product which is not expressed in increased amounts in hyperplastic or neoplastic conditions.

The reasons for the discrepancies among these studies are not clear. It is quite probable that technical factors are involved (e.g. fixation techniques) since several of the studies which gave positive results documented only minor disagreement in slide interpretation among multiple observers. It should also be noted that the results with RAP-5 have been corroborated by other evidence for enhanced *ras* expression (see later). Further work, however, will be necessary to clarify these findings with the RAP-5 antibody.

Enhanced *ras* expression in breast cancer was further substantiated by an analysis of *ras*-specific mRNA in surgically resected human breast cancer. By utilizing radio-labeled DNA probes for Ha-*ras*, Ki-*ras*, *and* N-*ras*, Theillet [52] found that 16/22 tumors had significant levels of Ha-*ras*-specific mRNA, comparable to that found in the T24 bladder cancer cell line and higher than that found in breast cancer cell lines. Very little expression of Ha-*ras* was found in the remaining six tumors, and no evidence for substantial expression of N-*ras* or Ki-*ras* was detected. Analysis of tumor DNA found no evidence of gene rearrangement, amplification, or point mutations. These data extended the original observations of Slamon et al. [47] and Agnantis et al. [1]. In the former study, increased levels of both Ha- and Ki-*ras*-specific mRNA, along with several other oncogenes, was noted in four patients with breast cancer. Agnantis et al. [1] analyzed 24 breast cancer specimens and found substantial increase in Ha-*ras*-specific mRNA transcripts compared with histologically normal tissue in the same patients. Although no correlation could be found with the TNM classification, patients with infiltrating duct cancer and those with lymph node metastases had the highest levels; patients with lymphocytic infiltration, higher grade tumors, and cancers of large size had the lowest values. Whittaker et al. [58] have also found increased steady state *ras*-specific RNA in breast carcinomas compared with normal and histologically benign breast tissue. In contrast to other studies, however, Ki- and N-*ras* RNA transcripts were detected, as opposed to Ha-*ras*. As in the study of Slamon et al., most tumors had evidence for increased transcription of several oncogenes.

Restriction Fragment Length Polymorphism at the Ha-ras locus

The human Ha-*ras* locus demonstrates a restriction fragment length polymorphism, as a result of a variable tandem reiteration (VTR) of a 28-base pair sequence 3′ to the Ha-*ras* locus. A number of common and rare alleles have been identified based on variable restriction fragment lengths. Kontiris et al. [27] first noted that cancer patients in general had a higher frequency of rare alleles of c-Ha-*ras* than do normal individuals. However, in a number of patient groups this finding has not been confirmed [53]. Lidereau et al. [28] subsequently examined DNA from breast cancer tissue and lymphocytes in 104 patients and compared the restriction fragment pattern with that of the DNA in lymphocytes of 56 normal individuals. They found that 51% of the normal subjects were heterozygous for the Ha-*ras* gene, a frequency similar to the patient population. However, there was a significant increase in the number of rare alleles (based on restriction fragment length size) among the breast cancer patients and a corresponding decrease in the common alleles. Overall, the four commonest alleles accounted for 91% of the restriction fragments in the normal population, but only 59% of the allele pool in breast cancer patients. The common 6.5 and an 8.0 kilobase fragment were significantly decreased in breast cancers and a rare 6.3 kilobase fragment significantly increased. There was no evidence for genetic rearrangements when lymphocyte DNA and tumor DNA were compared in a subset of 40 patients. This finding suggests a possible linkage of susceptibility to breast cancer development to a genetic locus within 20 million base pairs of c-Ha-*ras* on chromosome 11p. However, more extensive testing in other population samples is necessary.

A genetic locus which demonstrates a high frequency of restriction fragment length polymorphism (e.g., c-Ha-*ras*) is useful in demonstrating tumor-associated allele loss. Since both maternal and paternal alleles are readily demonstrated in constitutional DNA, comparison with tumor DNA may show loss of one parental allele. This phenomenon occurs in retinoblastoma, Wilms' tumor, and other embryonal cancers where the loss of the normal allele results in activation of a mutant recessive allele.

Allelic deletions at the c-Ha-*ras* locus have been reported in breast cancer by Yokota et al. [60], Cline et al. [9], as well as Lidereau et al. [28]. Yokota reported that deletions of one c-Ha-*ras* allele were seen in 15% of primary tumors and 29% of metastatic lesions (at a frequency similar to that reported by Lidereau et al.). In a subsequent study [9] designed to examine a variety of proto-oncogene abnormalities in breast cancer patients, allelic deletions of c-Ha-*ras* were noted in 15% of all breast cancers. However, since c-Ha-*ras* is rarely mutated in breast cancer, the deleted area may extend beyond the *ras* locus and activate other, as yet unidentified genetic loci (R. Callahan, 1987, unpublished work).

In summary, structural alterations of c-Ha-*ras* (point mutations, gene amplification, and chromosomal translocations) appear to be unusual events in breast cancer. This is in contrast to a number of experimental breast cancer systems. However, increased steady state *ras*-specific RNA and enhanced levels of the *ras* p21, as assessed by immunohistochemical staining, are quite common. In addition, in preliminary results the presence of rare c-Ha-*ras* alleles and deletions at this locus appear with increased frequency.

At the present time, the biological implications of these changes with respect to the initiation and progression of human breast cancer are far from clear. Carcinogenesis is a multistep process which likely takes place over several years in humans, a significant difference from the animal models. It is unlikely that activation of the *ras* proto-oncogene is solely responsible for carcinogenesis in any human or animal system. A number of clinical investigations have documented increased expression of several oncogenes within the same tumor. Further, the *ras* oncogene is incapable of transforming *primary* cells in culture without the complementary effect of a restricted group of other oncogenes. In transgenic mice experiments, activated *ras* alone will not induce cancer without additional genetic events occurring. Therefore, it is likely that *ras* activation is but one of many important changes in the biology of some human breast cancers. Our understanding of these issues is further complicated by our ignorance of the precise biochemical role of p21 in cell proliferation. It is possible, for example, that moderate elevations of *ras* p21 may be found in only some cells of an individual tumor, but that this expression may be critical for tumor progression. It should be noted that immunohistochemical staining for *ras* is generally quite heterogeneous at the single-cell level and that some investigators [15] have found the most intense p21 staining in the invasive components of the tumor. In this regard, mutated *ras* has been reported: (a) to increase the metastatic ability of some cancer cells [55]; (b) to enhance interaction with laminin in MCF-7 breast cells [3]; and (c) to affect collagen synthesis in a mouse mammary epithelial line [56]. The relevance of these findings to clinical oncology can only be clarified by a better understanding of the regulation of *ras* and the function of its protein product.

ras and Breast Cancer Prognosis

Although the biologic significance of *ras* proto-oncogene activation is unclear, there do appear to be increased levels of p21 and mRNA transcripts in breast cancer, and it has been postulated, therefore, that c-*ras* might serve as a prognostic indicator. Two areas of potential importance in this regard are identification of: (a) those patients with benign lesions who have a higher risk of developing subsequent neoplasia; and (b) those patients within the group of stage I and II cancers with the greatest risk of clinical recurrence.

There are only limited data regarding p21 as a marker of the malignant potential of preneoplastic lesions of the breast. Ohuchi et al. [35] reported a group of 18 patients with nonatypical ($N=8$) and atypical ($N=10$) hyperplasia of the breast, followed for 15 years. Four of ten patients with atypical hyperplasia and one of eight patients with nonatypical hyperplasia developed breast cancer. Immunohistochemical staining with RAP-5 distinguished those who subsequently developed cancer (40% cells positive) from those who did not (21% cells positive). Fromowitz et al. [15] noted both atypical hyperplasia and invasive carcinoma in the same specimens of two patients; staining with RAP-5 was present in both sections, but more intense in the invasive cancer. Lidereau et al. [28] suggested that women with rare alleles at the Ha-*ras* locus might be at greater risk for the development of breast cancer, but there are no data to confirm or refute this hypothesis. Unfortunately, the only data which exist at the present time are far too limited to draw any firm conclusions about this problem.

Several studies have examined the prognostic significance of abnormalities of *ras* oncogenes in patients with documented cancer. Lundy et al. [30] compared immunohistochemical staining of breast cancer specimens with RAP-5 in node-negative patients with a group of breast cancer patients with four or more positive nodes. Both the intensity of staining and the percentage of positive cells were significantly greater in the node-positive group. Although long-term follow-up data were not available on this patient group, prior experience would suggest that the node-positive group would have a poorer clinical outcome. A similar correlation of p21 levels with prognosis was reported by Clair et al. [8], using a different method of p21 quantitation.

Clinicopathologic correlates with the loss of one allele at the Ha-*ras* locus have been presented by Theillet [53]. In a small group of patients, this finding was statistically associated with higher grade tumors, lack of estrogen and progesterone receptors, but not with axillary node metastases. Follow-up for 1-5 years on these patients has shown an increased frequency of distant metastases, but similar rates of local recurrence compared with a control group of patients with a normal heterozygous phenotype. Cline et al. [9] have also presented clinical data in 54 primary breast cancer patients with a variety of proto-oncogene abnormalities. Allelic deletions of Ha-*ras* occurred in 15% of patients; this was strongly correlated with high grade tumors and clinical progression of cancer within 2 years, but not with axillary node metastases. Much larger studies and longer follow-up are needed to confirm these preliminary observations.

Additional Oncogene Abnormalities in Breast Cancer

As noted already, it is likely that *ras* proto-oncogene activation is only one of many changes occurring in some human breast cancers. In this regard it should be emphasized that several other proto-oncogene abnormalities have been found in patients with breast cancer. The study by Cline et al. [9] demonstrated proto-oncogene abnormalities in 58% of 53 patients with primary breast cancer. Three patients had more than one abnormality. In addition to allelic deletions of c-Ha-*ras*, the most frequent findings were amplifications of c-*myc* and c-*erb*-B2, and allelic deletions of c-*myb*. Cancer progression or recurrence was strongly correlated with the presence of multiple proto-oncogene abnormalities. Slamon et al. [48] have also found amplifications of c-*erb*-2 (*neu*/HER-2) in 189 patients with breast cancer. This oncogene was amplified 2- to 20-fold in 30% of tumors, and its expression was significantly associated with overall survival and time to relapse. The relationship of an increased expression of *ras* to alterations of structure and expression of other oncogenes is unknown and can only be determined by further studies which look for multiple abnormalities in the same tumor specimens.

Conclusions

Recent developments in the field of oncogene research have provided important clues to the pathogenesis and progression of cancer, including human breast cancer. As basic research continues, it is likely that our knowledge of the roles of the various oncogenes in the evolution and progression of malignant cell populations will increase and perhaps provide the basis for new therapeutic strategies.

The use of oncogene activation and expression as biological markers of aggressive breast cancer is preliminary, but promising. Additional investigations of larger groups of patients with longer follow-up will be necessary to confirm early expectations.

Acknowledgment. The work reported in this chapter was supported by Grant CA 3940802 (MVV) from the National Institutes of Health.

References

1. Agnantis NJ, Parissi P, Anagnostakis D, Spandidos DA (1986) Comparative study of Harvey-*ras* oncogene expression with conventional clinicopathologic parameters of breast cancer. Oncology 43: 36-39
2. Agnantis NJ, Petraki C, Markoulatos P, Spandidos DH (1986) Immunohistochemical study of the *ras* oncogene expression in human breast lesions. Anticancer Res 6: 1157-1160
3. Albini A, Graf J, Kitten GJ, Kleinman HK, Martin GR, Veillette A, Lippman ME (1986) 17β-estradiol regulates and v-Ha-*ras* transfection constitutively enhances MCF-7 breast cancer cell interactions with basement membrane. Proc Natl Acad Sci USA 83: 8182-8186

4. Barbacid M (1986) Oncogenes and human cancer. cause or consequence? Carcinogenesis 7: 1037-1062
5. Barbacid M (1986) Human oncogenes. In: Devita V, Hellman S, Rosenberg S (eds) Important advances in oncology 1986. Lippincott, Philadelphia, pp 3-22
6. Bos JL, Fearon ER, Hamilton SR, Verlaan-de Vries M, van Boom JH, van der Eb AJ, Vogelstein B (1987) Prevalence of *ras* gene mutations in human colorectal cancers. Nature 327: 293-297
7. Chang EH, Furth ME, Scolnick EM, Lowy DR (1983) Tumorigenic transformation of mammalian cells induced by a normal human gene homologous to Harvey murine sarcoma virus. Nature 297: 479-483
8. Clair T, Miller W, Cho-Chung Y (1987) Prognostic significance of the expression of a *ras* protein with a molecular weight of 21000 in human breast cancer. Cancer Res 47: 5290-5295
9. Cline M, Battifora H, Yokota J (1987) Proto-oncogene abnormalities in human breast cancer: correlations with anatomic features and clinical course of disease. J Clin Oncol 5: 999-1006
10. Croce C (1987) Role of chromosome translocations in human neoplasia. Cell 49: 155-156
11. Downward J, Yarden Y, Mayes E, Scroce C, Totty W, Stockwell P, Ullrich A, Schlessinger J, Wallenfield M (1984) Close similarity of the epidermal growth factor receptor and v-*erb*-B oncogene protein sequences. Nature 307: 521-527
12. Feramisco JR, Gross M, Kamota T, Rosenberg M, Sweet RW (1984) Microinjection of the oncogene form of the human H-*ras* (T24) protein results in rapid proliferation of quiescent cells. Cell 38: 109-117
13. Fleischman L, Chahwala S, Cantley L (1986) *ras* transformed cells: altered levels of phosphatidyl-inositol 4-5 biphosphate and catabolites. Science 231: 407-410
14. Forrester K, Almoguera C, Han K, Grizzle WE, Perucho M (1987) Detection of high incidence of K-*ras* oncogenes during human colon tumorigenesis. Nature 327: 298-303
15. Fromowitz F, Viola M, Chao S, et al (1987) *ras* p21 expression in the progression of breast cancer. Hum Pathol 18: 1268-1276
16. Furth M, Aldrich T, Cordon-Cardo C (1987) Expression of *ras* proto-oncogene proteins in normal human tissue. Oncogene 1: 47-58
17. Furth ME, David LT, Fleurdelys B, Scolnick EM (1982) Monoclonal antibodies to the p21 products of the transforming gene of Harvey murine sarcoma virus and of the cellular *ras* gene family. J Virol 43: 294-304
18. Ghosh A, Moore M, Harris M (1986) Immunohistochemical detection of *ras* oncogene p21 product in benign and malignant mammary tissue in man. J Clin Pathol 39: 428-434
19. Gibbs JR, Sigal IS, Poe M, Scolnick EM (1984) Intrinsic GTPase activity distinguishes normal and oncogenic *ras* p21 molecules. Proc Natl Acad Sci USA 81: 5704-5708
20. Goyette M, Petropoulos C, Shank P, Fausto N (1983) Expression of a cellular oncogene during liver regeneration. Science 219: 510-512
21. Hagag N, Haleguoa S, Viola M (1986) Inhibition of growth factor induced differentiation of PC12 cells by microinjection of antibody to *ras* p21. Nature 319: 680-682
22. Hagag N, Lacal JC, Graber M, Aaronson S, Viola M (1987) Microinjection of *ras* p21 induces a rapid rise in intracellular pH. Mol Cell Biol 7: 1984-1988
23. Heistercamp N, Stephenson JR, Croffen J, Hausen PF, deKlein A, Bartram CR, Grosocid G (1983) Localization of the c-*abl* oncogene adjacent to a translocation breakpoint in chronic myelogenous leukemia. Nature 306: 239-242
24. Hand PH, Thor A, Wunderlich D, Muraro R, Caruso A, Schlom J (1984) Monoclonal antibodies of predefined specificity detect activated *ras* gene expression in human mammary and colon carcinomas. Proc Natl Acad Sci USA. 81: 5227-5231

25. Hunter T (1987) A tail of two *src*'s: mutatis mutandis. Cell. 49: 1-4
26. Hurley J, Simon M, Teplow D (1984) Homologies between signals transducing G proteins and *ras* gene products. Science 226: 860-862
27. Krontiris TG, DiMartino NA, Colb M, Parkinson DR (1985) Unique allelic restriction fragment of the human Ha-*ras* locus in leukocyte and tumor DNAs of cancer patients. Nature 313: 369-374
28. Lidereau R, Escot C, Theillet C, Champene MH, Brunet M, Gest J, Callahan R (1986) High frequency of rare alleles of the human c-Ha-*ras*-1 proto-oncogene in breast cancer patients. JNCI 77: 697-701
29. Little CD, Nau MM, Carney DM, Gazdar AF, Minna JD (1983) Amplification and expression of the c-*myc* oncogene in human cancer cell lines. Nature 306: 194-196
30. Lundy J, Grimson R, Mishriki Y (1986) Elevated *ras* oncogene expression correlates with lymph node metastases in breast cancer patients. J Clin Oncol 4: 1321-1325
31. Madaule P, Axel R (1985) A novel *ras*-related gene family. Cell 41: 31-40
32. Manne V, Bekesi E, Kung H (1985) Ha-*ras* proteins exhibit GTPase activity: point mutations that activate Ha-*ras* gene product result in decreased GTPase activity. Proc Natl Acad Sci USA 82: 376-380
33. McGrath J, Capon D, Goeddel D, Levins AD (1984) Comparative biochemical properties of normal and activated human *ras* p21 protein. Nature 310: 644-649
34. Mulcahy L, Smith M, Stacy D (1985) Requirement for *ras* proto-oncogene function during serum stimulated growth of NIH 3T3 cells. Nature 313: 241-248
35. Ohuchi N, Thor A, Page DL, Hand PH, Halter SA, Schlom J (1986) Expression of the 21 000 molecular weight *ras* protein in a spectrum of benign and malignant human mammary tissues. Cancer Res 46: 2511-2519
36. Pellicci PG, Knowles D, MacGrath I, Della-Favera R (1986) Chromosomal breakpoints and structural alterations of the c-*myc* locus differ in endemic and sporadic forms of Burkitt's lymphoma. Proc Natl Acad Sci USA 83: 2984-2988
37. Pincus MR, van Renswoude J, Harford JB, Chang EH, Carty RP, Klausner RD (1983) Prediction of the three-dimensional structure of the transforming region of the EJ/T24 human bladder oncogene product and its normal cellular homologue. Proc Natl Acad Sci USA 80: 5253-5257
38. Pulciani S, Santos E, Lanver A, Long LK, Aaronson SA, Barbacid M (1982) Oncogenes in solid human tumors. Nature 300: 539-542
39. Robinson A, Williams ARW, Piris J, Spandidos DA (1986) Evaluation of a monoclonal antibody to *ras* peptide, RAP-5, claimed to bind preferentially to cells of infiltrating carcinomas. Br J Cancer 54: 877-883
40. Ryan J, Barker PE, Shimizu K, Wigler M, Ruddle FH (1983) Chromosomal assignment of a family of human oncogenes. Proc Natl Acid Sci USA 80: 4460-4464
41. Sap J, Munoz A, Damm K, Goldberg Y, Ghysdael J, Leutz A, Beug H, Vennstrom B (1986) The c-*erb*-A protein is a high affinity receptor for thyroid hormone. Nature 324: 635-640
42. Scolnick EM, Papageorge AG, Shih TY (1979) Guanine nucleotide-binding activity as an assay for the *src* protein of rat-derived murine sarcoma viruses. Proc Natl Acad Sci USA 76: 5355-5359
43. Seeger RC, Brodeur GM, Sather H, Dalton A, Siegel SE, Wong KY, Hammond D (1985) Association of multiple copies of the N-*myc* oncogene with rapid progression of neuroblastoma. N Eng J Med 313: 1111-1116
44. Sherr C, Rettenmier C, Sacca R, Roussel M, Look A, Stanley E (1985) The c-*fms* proto-oncogene product is related to the receptor for mononuclear phagocyte growth factor (CSF-1). Cell 41: 665-676

45. Shih TY, Weeks MO, Gruss P, Dhar R, Oroszlan S, Scolnick EM (1982). Identification of a precursor in the biosynthesis of the p21 transforming protein of Harvey murine sarcoma virus. J Virol 42: 253-261
46. Sinn E, Muller W, Pattengale P, Tepler I, Wallace R, Leder P (1987) Co-expression of MMTV/v-Ha-*ras* and MMTV/c-*myc* genes in transgenic mice: synergistic action of oncogenes in vivo. Cell 49: 465-475
47. Slamon DJ, de Kernion JB, Verma I, Cline MJ (1984) Expression of cellular oncogenes in human malignancies. Science 224: 256-262
48. Slamon DJ, Clark GM, Wong SG, Levin WJ, Ullrich A, McGuire WL (1987) Human breast cancer: correlation of relapse and survival with amplification of the HER-2/*neu* oncogene. Science 234: 177-182
49. Spandidos D, Wilkie N (1984) Malignant transformation of early passage rodent cells by a single mutated human oncogene. Nature 310: 469-475
50. Studzinski G, Brelvi Z, Feldman S, Watt R (1986) Participation of the c-*myc* protein in DNA synthesis of human cells. Science 234: 467-470
51. Sweet RW, Yokoyama S, Kamata T, Feramisco JR, Rosenberg M, Gross M (1984) The product of *ras* is a GTPase and the T24 oncogenic mutant is deficient in this activity. Nature 311: 273-275
52. Theillet C, Lidereau R, Escot C, Hutzell P, Brunet M, Gest J, Callahan R (1986) Loss of a c-H-*ras*-1 allele and aggressive human primary breast carcinomas. Cancer Res 46: 4776-4781
53. Thein SL, Oscier DG, Flint J, Wainscoat JS (1986) H-*ras* hypervariable alleles in myelodysplasia. Nature 321: 84-85
54. Thor A, Ohuchi N, Hand PH, Callahan R, Weeks MD, Theillet C (1986) *ras* gene alterations and enhanced levels of *ras* p21 expression in a spectrum of benign and malignant human mammary tissues. Lab Invest 55: 603-615
55. Vousden KH, Eccles SA, Purvies H, Marshall CJ (1986) Enhanced spontaneous metastasis of mouse carcinoma cells transfected with an activated c-Ha-*ras*-1 gene. Int J Cancer 37: 425-433
56. Warburton M, Ferns S, Hynes N (1986) Collagen processing in *ras*-transformed mouse mammary epithelial cells. Biochem Biophys Res Commun 137: 161-166
57. Watterfield MD, Scrace GT, Whittle N, Stroobant P, Johnsson A, Wasteson A, Westermark B, Heldin CH, Huang JS, Deuel TF (1984) Platelet derived growth factor is structurally related to the putative transforming protein $p28^{sis}$ of simian sarcoma virus. Nature 304: 35-39
58. Whittaker J, Walker R, Varley J (1986) Differential expression of cellular oncogenes in benign and malignant human breast tissue. Int J Cancer 38: 651-655
59. Yarden Y, Kuang WJ, Yang-Feng T, Coussens L, Munemitsu S, Dull TJ, Chen E, Schlessinger J, Francke U, Ullrich A (1987) Human proto-oncogene c-*kit*: a new surface receptor tyrosine kinase for an unidentified ligand. EMBO J 6: 3341-3351
60. Yokota J, Tsunetsugu-Yokota Y, Battifora H, LeFevre C, Cline MJ (1986) Alterations of *myc*, *myb*, and *ras*-Ha proto-oncogenes in cancers are frequent and show clinical correlation. Science 231: 261-265
61. Zarbl H, Sukumar S, Arthur AV, Martin-Zanca D, Barbacid M (1985) Direct mutagenesis of Ha-*ras*-1 oncogenes by *N*-nitroso-*N*-methylurea during initiation of mammary carcinogenesis in rats. Nature 315: 382-385

Flow Cytometry

Measurement of DNA Content of Archival Material as a Guide to Prognosis

D.W. Hedley

Ludwig Institute for Cancer Research (Sydney Branch), University of Sydney, Blackburn Building, N.S.W. 2006, Australia

Introduction

Flow cytometry is capable of measuring total DNA content of tens of thousands of cancer cells in minutes, with high precision. From such analyses two distinct and potentially important pieces of information are obtained; tumour DNA index (ploidy) and the percentage of cells in S-phase (% S-phase). There is currently optimism that this information will help in the identification of high risk breast cancer patients, and DNA flow cytometry is indeed now being offered on a routine clinical basis in the United States. Unfortunately, most of the published studies used fresh frozen material submitted for steroid hormone receptor analysis, and clinical follow-up is at best incomplete. The use of paraffin-embedded archival material allows the retrospective analysis of DNA content from defined cohorts of patients with known clinical outcome. This chapter outlines the techniques of DNA flow cytometry, with emphasis on the use of paraffin-embedded material, and reviews the results from three large, recently published series. Although DNA index appears to be a relatively weak prognostic indicator, preliminary results show that % S-phase, which is strongly linked to both nuclear grade and labelling index, could prove a clinically valuable measure of inherent biological aggression.

Background

Aneuploidy

An association between gross chromosomal imbalance (aneuploidy) and poor prognosis of a range of tumour types has been recognised for many years [48, 49]. Despite recent technical advances however, detailed chromosome analysis of human solid tumours remains difficult. Because of this, cytometric methods have been developed which allow total cellular DNA content to be measured. This correlates with modal chromosome content, although obviously it gives no information about which specific chromosomes are abnormal [8, 56]. Early studies using static, microscope-based cytometry confirmed that aneuploidy is indeed frequently seen in solid tumours, and in some instances correlated with prognosis [1, 2, 23]. It should be noted that because static cytometry is time-consuming, many

Ragaz/Ariel (Eds.), High-Risk Breast Cancer

of the early papers deal with small numbers of cases, and detailed clinicopathologic staging techniques were often not employed, thus ignoring the possibility that the prognostic significance of aneuploidy might be linked to a correlation with other, more powerful prognostic features.

% S-Phase

Independently of cytometric measurement of DNA content, the availability of tritium-labelled thymidine in the late 1950s allowed the estimation of proliferative activity by autoradiography of tumour cells briefly exposed to labelled DNA precursor. Thymidine labelling index (TLI) in breast cancer has been investigated by a number of groups, and shown to be a major prognostic variable in both early and recurrent disease [44, 45, 51, 58]. More recently, preliminary data have suggested that high labelling index identifies a subgroup of premenopausal, oestrogen receptor (ER)-negative patients with an unusually poor prognosis despite having node-negative disease. Adjuvant chemotherapy may be of particular benefit in this subgroup [11]. Despite the fact that TLI is a major prognostic indicator in breast cancer, its measurement is not in regular clinical use, probably because the technical problems of autoradiography are outside the scope of routine pathology laboratories.

Flow Cytometry

Although flow cytometry came into widespread use as a research tool during the 1970s, the systematic investigation of neoplastic diseases goes back only a few years [6, 8, 37, 56]. Flow cytometric measurement of cellular DNA content has the advantages over static cytometry in being fast (results in less than 1 h of tumour excision) and of allowing tens of thousands rather than hundreds of cells to be examined. Not only does this improve the resolution of near diploid or small aneuploid populations, but it also allows an estimate of % S-phase to be measured in most cases, by integration of DNA histograms. It has been shown that % S-phase correlates with TLI measured in the same primary breast cancer [40, 41]. Thus, flow cytometric measurement of cellular DNA content gives potentially important information about proliferative activity as well as tumour ploidy.

Flow Cytometric Technique

Sample Preparation

An obligatory first step is the preparation of a suspension of single cells or nuclei. Various techniques exist, the choice being dictated by the nature of the sample and the cellular properties to be studied (e.g. single-parameter DNA analysis or correlated DNA versus light scatter or surface marker). In the study of breast cancer, fresh frozen tissue submitted for steroid hormone receptor analysis is a popular source of material, and the rapid staining technique described by Taylor [52], which involves detergent lysis in the presence of DNA fluorochrome, is particularly well suited. For % S-phase estimates it has been reported that disaggregation of fresh, nonfrozen, tissue by collagenase yields results with the closest correlation with TLI [40].

A range of DNA fluorochromes exists [53]. At suitable concentrations all bind to DNA stoichiometrically, i.e. for a given intensity of illumination, fluorescence is directly proportional to DNA content. For routine clinical application the intercalating agents propidium iodide and ethidium bromide are suitable, since they are excited at readily available wavelengths and produce intense nuclear fluorescence.

Machines and Computers

Flow cytometers incorporate a fluidics system, with which the stained cell suspension is made to stream in single file through an optical system comprising a light source (laser or arc lamp), suitable filters and one or more photomultiplier tubes. Analogue pulses produced as cells flow through the optical system are digitised, assigned a numerical value and stored by an electronics system [50]. Flow systems are routinely capable of examining several hundreds of cells per second, and frequency distribution histograms of cellular DNA content are typically based on tens of thousands of cells. Following acquisition and storage of data, the final step is analysis. With single-parameter DNA flow cytometry this yields two pieces of information, namely DNA index (ploidy) and % S-phase. DNA index is the ratio of tumour G_1 DNA content to normal diploid G_1. Nearly all clinical cancer samples contain normal host cells, which can be identified by reference to an internal biological standard such as chicken red blood cells. For homogeneous populations such as cell lines grown in tissue culture, estimation of % S-phase should theoretically be simply a matter of counting cells with a DNA content lying between the G_1 and G_2/mitosis peaks. In practice there is uncertainty about assigning a cell to these peaks, because of staining and instrumental factors rather than true variance in G_1 DNA content. Some G_1 or G_2/mitosis cells will therefore overlie S-phase cells and vice versa. Estimates of % S-phase are more difficult with tumour tissue, mainly because of variable admixture of normal host cells, and partly because of these problems they have received less attention than DNA index. In published series examining % S-phase, roughly two-thirds of samples overall have been considered to give a valid estimate [7, 34, 54, 55, 59].

Flow Cytometric Measurement of DNA Content of Human Cancers

Prognostic Significance of Cellular DNA Content: An Overview

Tumour types where abnormal DNA index is clearly associated with a poor prognosis include carcinomas of the ovary, bladder, lung (non-small cell), kidney and thyroid [24, 33, 46, 57, 59]. In some other cases DNA content is probably not related to outcome. Examples include small cell lung cancer, colon and metastatic adenocarcinoma of unknown primary site [12, 22, 30]. Finally, in childhood acute leukaemia and neuroblastoma DNA aneuploidy is a favourable prognostic feature [25, 38, 39].

In at least some instances DNA index is correlated with other important features such as stage, histological grade or patient's age, and this could account in part for the prognostic significance of DNA index. Whether or not tumour ploidy relates to prognosis probably depends to some extent on the selection criteria used. For example, although DNA index is reported not to have prognostic significance in gastric cancer, measurement of DNA content of very early cancers by single-cell microdensitometry shows a large proportion to be diploid. Since these early stages have a favourable prognosis, their inclusion with advanced cases would give the overall impression that ploidy was after all prognostically important. Allowance for correlations with prognostic features can be made by multivariate analysis, along the lines now standard when assessing the effects of treatment on patient outcome in randomised clinical trials.

Prognostic Significance of DNA Content in Breast Cancer

Because fresh frozen tissue is suitable for DNA flow cytometry there have been a number of large studies of breast cancer, utilising material sent to the laboratory for steroid hormone receptor analysis [17, 19, 20, 32, 35, 36, 54]. Most of these studies have concentrated on the relationship between DNA index and recognised prognostic features such as stage, grade and receptor status. Generally speaking, the correlations with stage and receptor status are weak, but probably real, with a trend for aneuploid tumours to be of higher stage and receptor negative.

Although it is probable that more breast cancers have been examined by DNA flow cytometry than any other tumour type, the prognostic significance of aneuploidy remains uncertain. This is because most series include all disease stages, with patients treated in various ways and with follow-up relatively short for a disease which characteristically relapses late. Because of this problem of follow-up we looked at the possibility of using formalin-fixed, paraffin-embedded tissue as a source of material for DNA flow cytometry [27, 29].

Method for Measuring DNA Content in Paraffin-Embedded Tissue

The first step is to select a block containing an adequate proportion of tumour cells. If DNA index is all that is required, a few percent tumour cells would probably be sufficient to give an identifiable aneuploid G_1 peak. Measurement of % S-phase would however be more reliable if the proportion of nonmalignant cells were kept to a minimum. With a conventional tissue section as a plan it is possible to trim away areas of nonmalignant tissue in a parallel thick section intended for flow cytometry.

The actual method has been given in detail, and in brief involves the cutting of thick microtome sections (to minimise debris from partially sectioned nuclei), followed by dewaxing and rehydration [27, 29]. Nuclei can then be extracted by incubation with acidic pepsin, washed and stained for flow cytometry. In our laboratory we use an ICP22 flow cytometer for single-parameter DNA work. This gives excellent DNA histograms with the added advantage of using mercury arc lamp illumination, so allowing the ultraviolet-excited fluorochrome DAPI to be used. In our hands DAPI gives better resolution than the intercalating dyes, although other laboratories use propidium iodide, which can be excited by a readily available emission line from an argon ion laser.

Representative DNA histograms are shown in Fig. 1. The simplest are made up of diploid tumours. These show a single major peak with a DNA content corresponding to G_0/G_1 of the cell cycle. Cells in G_2 or mitosis form a second peak with twice this DNA content, while cells in the process of replicating their DNA appear as an S-phase plateau between the two peaks. The majority of human solid tumours are aneuploid, usually containing a second G_1 peak of greater than diploid

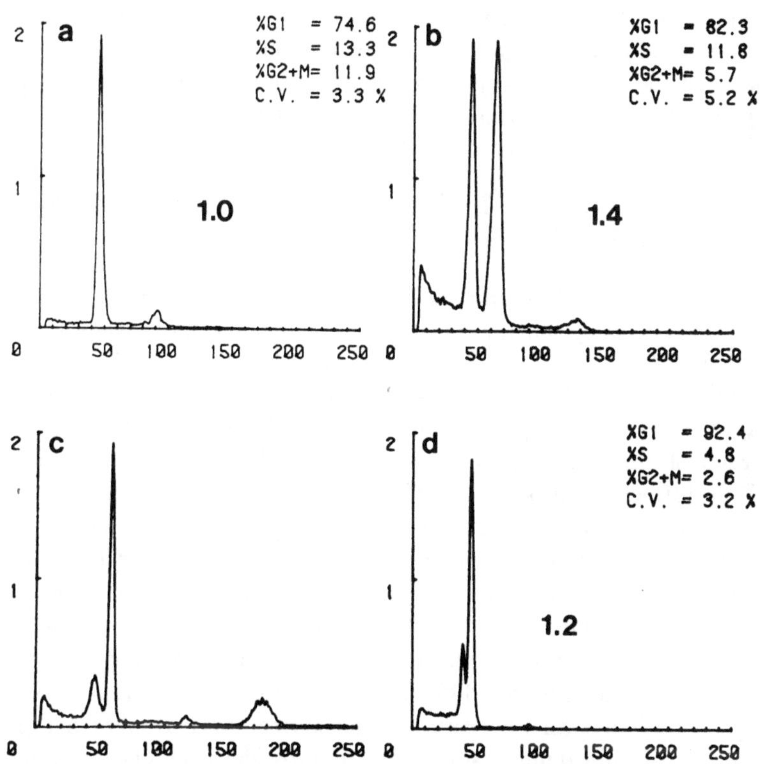

Fig. 1a-d. DNA histograms obtained from paraffin-embedded material. Numbers in bold type are DNA indices; histogram **a** (DNA index = 1.0) is diploid, **b-d** show DNA aneuploidy. Cell cycle phase distribution and coefficient of variance (C.V.) of diploid G_1 peak are given for three histograms (**a**, **b**, **d**). Histogram **c** is multiple aneuploid, and cell cycle analysis could not therefore be performed. *Horizontal axis* DNA content; *vertical axis* cell count × 10^{-3}

DNA content, while a significant proportion (roughly 10%) of breast cancers contain more than one aneuploid population. Estimates of % S-phase can be made with computer programs. Most of these use algorithms intended for homogeneous populations, and not all are suitable for tumour biopsies. Multiple aneuploid tumours are unsuitable for S-phase estimates, and paraffin-embedded tissue is probably not as good as fresh material because it is less easy to trim away nonmalignant tissue. Despite these problems % S-phase should be taken seriously because it is related to the major prognostic feature, TLI.

Results in Paraffin-Embedded Tissue

DNA Index

To date three large series have been published describing prognostic significance of DNA index measured in paraffin-embedded tissue. Detailed statistical analysis, including the use of Cox proportional hazard models, was performed in all cases. Details of relations between DNA index and other prognostic features are summarised in Table 1, which also gives an outline of the study population and the dates of the samples. Although all three studies are of operable primary breast cancer, they have important differences in detail.

Leiden, Netherlands. This is the largest study [16], a total of 685 breast cancers being examined. Of these 233 were analysed in fresh tissue and the remainder in paraffin blocks. A total of 120 were excluded from detailed analysis, the main reasons being the development of a second primary cancer or insufficient material for DNA flow cytometry. Of the remaining 565, there were 118 UICC stage I patients, 291 stage II, 118 stage III and 12 stage IV. The patients were also subdivided by pathological staging of the axilla as shown in Table 1. There was a higher incidence of diploid tumours in paraffin-embedded tissue (34%) compared with fresh tissue (22%), probably because of the lower resolution usually obtained for the former. Postoperatively 355 received radiotherapy, but adjuvant chemotherapy was only used in 58 premenopausal node-positive patients.

There was a significant trend for small (< 2 cm diameter) tumours to be diploid, while extensive axillary lymph node involvement (i.e. ten or more nodes involved) was associated with a very high incidence of aneuploidy. Overall there were no significant associations between DNA index and TNM stage or ER status. Ploidy was not associated with a difference in locoregional recurrence rates. As shown in Fig. 2, both overall and distant relapse-free survival were better with diploid tumours. Within defined subgroups a statistically significant trend in favour of diploid tumours was observed for node-positive postmenopausal, four or more positive nodes and for stage III disease. For premenopausal node-positive patients and for patients with disease recurrence, DNA index was not prognostically significant. Multivariate analysis with a Cox proportional hazard model showed that DNA index was an independent prognostic variable for overall survival,

Table 1. DNA content in operable breast cancer. Numbers refer to % diploid within groups

Study	Number of cases	Dates of samples	% Diploid	% Multiple aneuploid	Nodal status (%)	Menopausal status (%)	ER status (%)	Grade	Size (cm)	(%)
Leiden, Netherlands [16]	565	1975-1984	29[a]	10	0 (28)	N.S.[b]	+ve (30)	N.S.	<2	(33)
Node −ve	263				1-3 (25)		−ve (23)		2-5	(24)
Node +ve	302				4-9 (36)				>5	(31)
					>10 (7)					
Nottingham, England [18]	354	1974-1979	40	N.S.	−ve (45)	Pre (52)[b]	+ve (41)	I (77)	<2	(49)
Node −ve	184				+ve (34)	Post (33)	−ve (34)	II (45)	2-5	(34)
Node +ve	166							III (22)	>5	(31)
Sydney, Australia [28, 31]	473[c]	1979-1981	35	11	1-3 (31)	Pre (33)	+ve (33)	I (41)	<2	(29)
(all node +ve)					4-9 (29)	Post (21)	−ve (23)	II (29)	2-5	(29)
					>10 (15)			III (17)	>5	(18)

[a] 34% and 22% for paraffin-embedded or fresh tissue respectively.
[b] Prognostic significance of DNA ploidy greater in postmenopausal patients.
[c] 45 Diploid samples with coefficient of variance >5% excluded from some analyses.

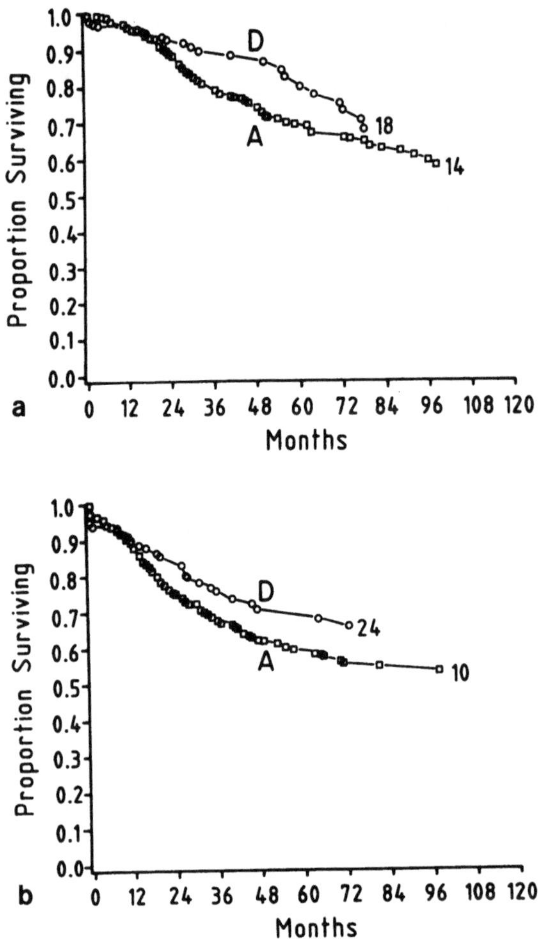

Fig. 2 a, b. Leiden series. **a** Overall; **b** distant disease-free survival. *D* diploid; *A* aneuploid. Time to local recurrence was not influenced by DNA ploidy (not shown). Reproduced by permission, Alan R. Liss Inc

although of only borderline significance for distant relapse-free survival. This impact appeared to be confined to postmenopausal patients.

Nottingham, England. This study [18] has the longest median follow-up, the patients comprising a consecutive series under the care of a single surgeon. They represent a particularly well-studied group where a detailed investigation of various clinicopathological features has been previously used to derive the Nottingham Prognostic Index. The tumours were subsequently examined to see whether DNA index was an additional prognostic feature. Lymph node status was available in 350 patients, and 166 had at least one positive node. There were 123 premenopausal and 225 postmenopausal patients. No patients received systemic adjuvant treatment.

There was a strong correlation between DNA index and histological grade (modified Bloom and Richardson) and also with menopausal status. The presence of a diploid DNA index correlated with small size ($P<0.02$) and there were nonsignificant trends for lymph node-negative or ER-positive tumours to be diploid. Overall there was a strong correlation between DNA index and grouping by the Nottingham Prognostic Index (which takes into account size, histological grade and lymph node status). Overall and disease-free survival curves are shown in Fig. 3. When overall survival was measured at 3 years, or when the aneuploid group was limited to those with DNA index = 1.2-1.9, there was a statistically significant survival advantage for patients with tumours of DNA index = 1.0. Similarly, for small (< 2.0 cm diameter) tumours and for postmenopausal patients, diploidy was a favourable predictor of survival. It should be noted, however, that even within these selected subgroups the impact of DNA index on survival only just reached conventional statistical significance.

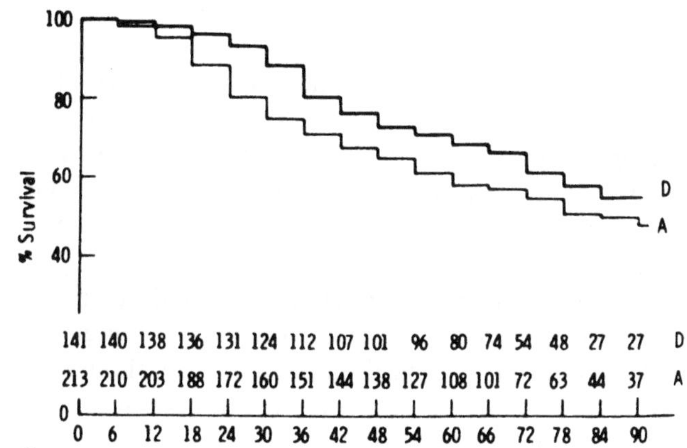

a

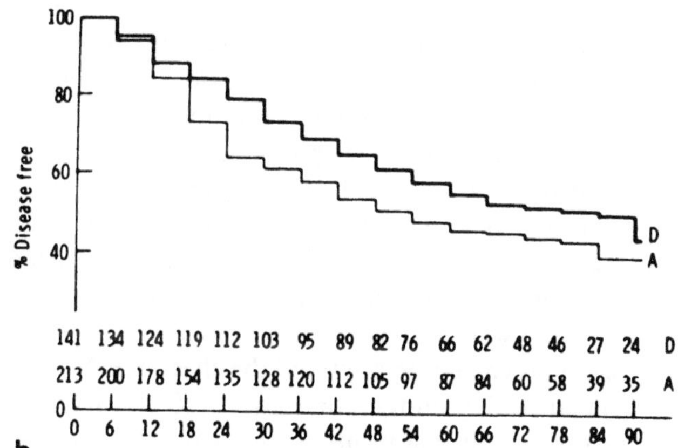

b

Fig. 3a, b. Nottingham series. **a** Overall survival; **b** disease-free survival. *D* diploid; *A* aneuploid. Reproduced by permission, Butterworth Ltd

Sydney, Australia. The unique features of this particular study [28, 31] are that all patients had positive axillary lymph nodes and all were randomised onto one of a series of interrelated trials of adjuvant treatment (Ludwig Breast Cancer Study Group Trials I-IV). Of the 490 blocks examined only 106 came from Sydney, the remainder being from Ljubljana, Yugoslavia (244 blocks), Wellington, New Zealand [54], Cape Town, South Africa [54] and Göteborg, Sweden [32]. The ability to amass samples from five different countries emphasises the utility of using paraffin-embedded tissue. Of the 490 blocks received, DNA histograms were obtained for all but 5. Subsequently, 12 patients were found to be ineligible for the trial, leaving 473 for detailed analysis. Of these, 165 were diploid, 51 multiple aneuploid and the remainder single aneuploid. As was noted with the Leiden series, the incidence of diploid tumours (35%) was noticeably higher than the 21% reported by this group in an earlier series with fresh tissue [54]. Of the diploid samples, 45 produced G_1 peaks with a coefficient of variance >5%, and might therefore have been composites of diploid plus a near diploid tumour cell population. Although in some instances these samples were treated as a separate group, the distinction was probably too strict; nearly all had a coefficient of variance <8%, their clinical correlates and outcome were similar to the better quality diploid histograms. It is in a sense unrealistic to set a cutoff, given that even good quality "diploid" histograms could harbour chromosomal defects such as translocations, deletions or double minutes, known to be associated with profound alterations of cell function in some instances.

The relationship between DNA index and other variables is shown in Table 1. There was a highly significant correlation between tumour ploidy and tumour grade (Bloom and Richardson), and weaker though still significant correlations with oestrogen and progesterone receptor status and with the number of positive axillary lymph nodes. In particular, heavy (i.e. ten or more) lymph node involvement was strongly correlated with an abnormal DNA index, as was found in the Leiden series. There was a highly significant tendency for aneuploidy to predominate in the postmenopausal patients, similar to that found in Nottingham.

When disease-free and overall survival were examined, patients with diploid tumours fared better than those with aneuploid tumours (Fig. 4). Subdividing the aneuploid group by actual DNA index not reveal any significant differences, and in particular, survival for patients with multiple aneuploid tumours was no worse than that of the rest of the aneuploid group. Multivariate analysis with a Cox proportional hazard model shows that tumour ploidy does not have independent prognostic significance – nodal status and menopausal status being more important prognostic factors. It should be noted that all premenopausal patients received adjuvant chemotherapy, and this may have influenced the results. The postmenopausal patients were examined by randomised treatment (observation, tamoxifen or tamoxifen plus chemotherapy), and the effect of DNA index on survival was found to be similar in all groups. In other words, DNA index did not identify a subgroup for whom adjuvant treatment was particularly beneficial.

Conclusions. Together the three series comprise 1392 patients with a median follow-up in excess of 5 years, and although the survival curves cannot be directly

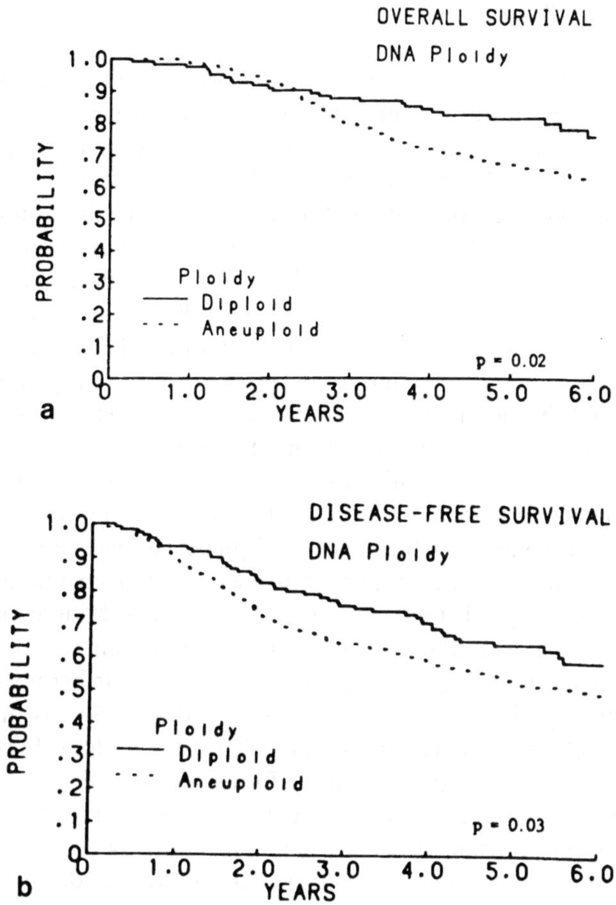

Fig. 4a, b. Sydney series. **a** Overall survival; **b** disease-free survival

compared because of differences in selection criteria and treatment, it is interesting to note some striking similarities. All three show weak trends for diploid tumours to be small, ER-positive and to have a lesser degree of axillary lymph node involvement. There were stronger trends for aneuploid tumours to be associated with involvement of ten or more axillary lymph nodes, to occur in postmenopausal patients and to be of higher histological grade. Disease-free and overall survival was somewhat better for diploid tumours in all series and there were no instances of a subgroup where aneuploidy was a favourable prognostic feature. It should be noted however that multivariate analysis indicated that DNA index was not a major prognostic feature, and that no study was able to identify a subgroup where DNA index had a particularly powerful impact on survival. Both the Leiden and the Nottingham studies showed that DNA index had a greater effect on survival in postmenopausal patients. However, the results from the Sydney study do not suggest that adjuvant endocrine or chemoendocrine therapy is of particular value in node-positive postmenopausal patients with aneuploid tumours.

% S-Phase

In contrast to tumour ploidy, surprisingly little has been published about flow cytometrically determined % S-phase and prognosis in the solid tumours, although it is now recognised that high % S-phase is a bad prognostic feature in non-Hodgkin's lymphomas [9, 13, 42]. A correlation between high % S-phase and receptor negativity or high tumour grade has been noticed in some studies with fresh frozen breast cancers, as has a strong relationship between diploid DNA content and low % S-phase [34, 36, 41, 47], although how far this simply reflects the dilutional effect of nonmalignant cells remains to be established. Intuitively one would expect % S-phase to correlate with TLI, and this has now been demonstrated [40, 41]. This is an important result, because % S-phase estimates are much faster (and cheaper) than TLI. Because labelling index is a powerful prognostic determinant in both early and advanced breast cancer one would expect the same for % S-phase, and this was investigated in the Sydney study, with the DNA histograms originally generated for determining tumour ploidy.

The major problem with % S-phase estimates for clinical samples is admixture of nonmalignant cells, which is only partly overcome by selecting paraffin blocks containing substantial amounts of tumour. Additional problems are variability of % S-phase at different sites within a tumour and the presence of excessive cellular debris or multiple aneuploid populations. Furthermore, Mauro et al. [43] have published preliminary data suggesting that % S-phase might after all overestimate labelling index, perhaps because of arrest in S-phase. In contrast to DNA index, it is difficult to give precise criteria for accepting a % S-phase estimate as valid. In the Sydney series 285 of 473 histograms were judged to give a reliable % S-phase [31], a proportion similar to that reported by others [7, 34, 55, 59]. Unlike DNA index, a high % S-phase was not associated with nodal or receptor status, but there was a strong correlation with tumour grade, as has previously been observed for TLI (44). The prognosis for high % S-phase tumours was significantly worse than for low % S-phase (Fig. 5), multivariate analysis showing that this was largely explained by its correlation with tumour grade. It is of interest, however, that within the tumours with % S-phase > 10, the grade did not give additional prognostic information. These results suggest that further refinements in % S-phase measurements might be of considerable clinical utility. A recent series of 93 patients from Tampere, Finland [34] produced results remarkably similar to the Sydney series, and likewise concluded that % S-phase was a more powerful prognostic indicator than DNA index.

Role of Image Analysis

The earliest studies of cellular DNA content in breast cancer used single-cell microdensitometry of Feulgen-stained slide preparations. In contrast to flow cytometry, individual cells are selected for measurement by a microscope-based system. This has the advantage of confining measurements to the malignant cell population, the normal diploid standard being derived from adjacent normal duct

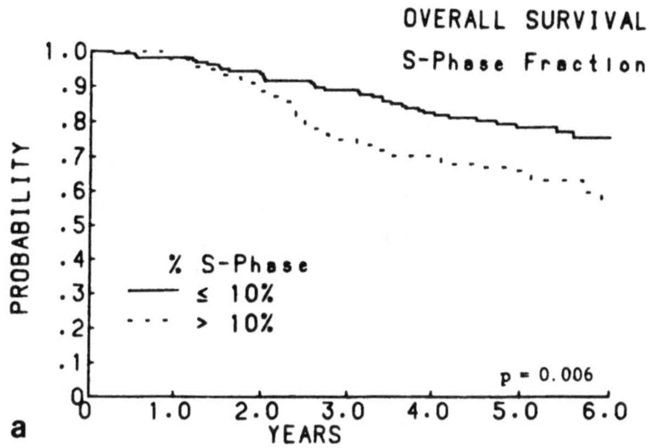

a

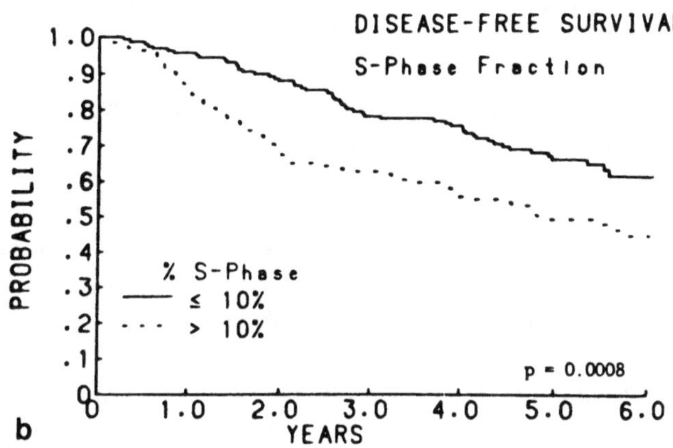

b

Fig. 5 a, b. Sydney series. Effect of % S-phase on prognosis. **a** Overall survival; **b** disease-free survival. Note that fewer samples could be assessed for % S-phase than for DNA index

epithelial cells. Because the technique is somewhat time-consuming, DNA histograms produced in this way typically contain at most a few hundred cells, and the resolution is therefore less than that seen with flow cytometry.

Atkin's 1972 study [1] showed that patients with near diploid tumours had a significantly better 8-year survival when compared with those with triploid-tetraploid tumours. A greater proportion of triploid-tetraploid tumours showed involvement of axillary nodes or were of "poor" histological differentiation, a finding reminiscent of the more recent flow cytometry studies.

Comparison of flow cytometry and image analysis of the same specimen shows good overall agreement, although flow cytometry proved better at resolving near diploid aneuploid populations, whereas image analysis detected small numbers of cells with gross aneuploidy not identified by flow cytometry [14, 15]. Aneuploid DNA histograms obtained by image analysis also contain fewer accessory diploid cells than those obtained with flow cytometry, because of the rejection of nonmalignant cells.

The value of image analysis-derived DNA cytometry as a guide to prognosis in breast cancer has been re-evaluated in detail by Auer and co-workers in Stockholm [3, 5]. The material used comprises archival fine needle aspiration biopsy samples, which has the advantages of providing well-dispersed single cells with a relatively small admixture of nonmalignant cells. Histograms of DNA content are subdivided into four classes. Type I are characterised by a diploid modal DNA content; type II either tetraploid or tetraploid plus diploid, but with a low % S-phase; type III a diploid peak with a second peak lying between diploid and tetraploid; type IV a very pronounced and irregular aneuploidy, with DNA amounts per cell ranging from levels near 2 c up to values beyond 6 or even 8 c [3]. Although a high proportion of small primary tumours detected by mammographic screening were diploid [21], more advanced tumours showed remarkable stability of DNA content, repeat samples of recurrences taken up to 12 years after original biopsy showing in nearly all cases an identical type of DNA histogram, i.e. when clinically apparent, diploid tumours did not evolve into aneuploid tumours [4]. In contrast to the flow cytometric studies of archival material, DNA content determined by single-cell microdensitometry of the fine needle aspirates was found to be of major prognostic significance in breast cancer patients selected for either death from cancer within 2 years or survival beyond 15 years [5]. Of the 36 patients surviving beyond 15 years, 78% showed either type I or type II tumours, whereas 91% of 42 short-term survivors had either type III or type IV tumours. A recent study from Perth, Australia, which subdivided tumours simply into diploid or aneuploid, shows a similar strongly favourable outcome for patients with diploid tumours [26].

The apparent contradiction, that DNA content measured by static cytometry is of major prognostic significance while flow cytometric measurement does not, needs explaining. Image analysis, although slower than flow cytometry, has the advantage of examining cancer cells only, without admixture from normal host cells. It is possible that some "highly aneuploid" samples might in fact be high % S-phase hyperdiploid tumours, and that proliferation rather than chromosome content is the main reason for their bad prognosis. In any event, image analysis might receive greater attention in the near future. With recent technical refinements equipment is cheaper and easier to maintain than flow systems, and may well be acquired by routine pathology laboratories for quantitating oestrogen receptor status measured immunocytochemicaly. It should also be possible simultaneously to produce rapid and reliable labelling index data by brief exposure of fresh tumour tissue to the thymidine analogue bromodeoxyuridine (BrUdR) followed by immunocytochemical staining with monoclonal antibodies to BrUdR.

Conclusions: Prognostic Significance of Cellular DNA Content in Early Breast Cancer

We have seen how, despite early optimism, flow cytometrically determined tumour ploidy has not proved a useful guide to prognosis. It is interesting to speculate why this is the case. All cancers must start from diploid cells, and indeed very early breast cancers detected by mammographic screening are reportedly mainly diploid [21]. Despite the presence of gross chromosomal imbalance or multiple stem lines, aneuploid tumours do not behave in a particularly aggressive fashion when allowance is made for their association with more advanced stages, and this suggests that aneuploidy is something which happens to tumours as they evolve, rather than being a driving force in neoplastic progression. Recent evidence from recombinant DNA technology suggests that biological aggression might be related to abnormal functions of a limited number of genes [10], and major alterations in the genetic constitution of cancer cell lines might therefore be found in tumours with an apparently diploid DNA content.

In contrast to DNA index, % S-phase shows considerable promise as a useful clinical marker for bad prognosis breast cancer. It would be of interest to examine its impact on survival in node-negative patients, particularly since the Milan group report that high TLI, ER-negative premenopausal patients have a particularly bad prognosis unless treated with adjuvant chemotherapy [11]. However, before flow cytometric measurement of % S-phase can be used generally, further technical refinements as needed to allow analysis of multiploid tumours and more importantly to gate out nonmalignant cells. To do so will probably require the development of multiparametric staining, with a second parameter specific for malignant cells. Considerable progress is being made in this field, for example with monoclonal antibodies to oncogene products [60], and the clinical investigation of flow and image cytometry should be pursued with vigour.

Acknowledgments. I wish to thank Dr C.J. Cornelisse and Mr. C.S. Dowle for their permission to reproduce their data and Miss J. Hood for preparing this manuscript.

References

1. Atkin NB (1972) Modal deoxyribonucleic acid value and survival in carcinoma of the breast. Br Med J 1: 271-272
2. Atkin NB, Kay R (1979) Prognostic significance of modal DNA value and other factors in malignant tumours, based on 1465 cases. Br J Cancer 40: 210-221
3. Auer GU, Caspersson TO, Wallgren AS (1980) DNA content and survival in mammary carcinoma. Anal Quant Cytol 2: 161-165
4. Auer GU, Eriksson E, Azavedo E, Caspersson T, Wallgren A (1984a) Prognostic significance of nuclear DNA content in mammary adenocarcinomas in humans. Cancer Res 44: 394-396
5. Auer GU, Fallenius AG, Erhardt KY, Sundel in BSB (1984b) Progression of mammary adenocarcinomas as reflected by nuclear DNA content. Cytometry 5: 420-425
6. Barlogie B, Gohde W, Johnston DA, Smallwood L, Schumann J, Drewinko B, Freireich EJ (1978) Determination of ploidy and proliferative characteristics of human solid tumours by pulse cytophotometry. Cancer Res 38: 3333-3339
7. Barlogie B, Johnston DA, Smallwood L, Raber MN, Maddox AM, Latreille J, Swartzendruber DE, Drewinko B (1982) Prognostic implications of ploidy and proliferative activity in human solid tumours. Cancer Genet Cytogenet 6: 17-28
8. Barlogie B, Raber MN, Schumann J, Johnson TS, Drewinko B, Swartzendruber DE,

Gohde W, Andreef M, Freireich EJ (1983) Flow cytometry in cancer clinical research. Cancer Res 43: 3982-3997
9. Bauer KD, Merkel DE, Winter JN, Marder RJ, Hauck WW, Wallemark CB, Williams TS, Variakojis D (1986) Prognostic implications of ploidy and proliferative activity in diffuse large cell lymphomas. Cancer Res 46: 3173-3178
10. Bishop JM (1987) The molecular genetics of cancer. Science 235: 305-311
11. Bonadonna G, Valagussa P, Tancini G, Rossi A, Brambilla C, Zambetti M, Bignami P, diFronzo G, Silvestrini R (1986) Current status of Milan adjuvant chemotherapy trials for node-positive and node-negative breast cancer. Natl Cancer Inst Monogr 1: 45-49
12 Bunn PA, Carney DN, Gazdar AF, Whang-Peng J, Matthews MJ (1983) Diagnostic and biological implications of flow cytometric DNA content analysis in lung cancer. Cancer Res 43: 5026-5032
13. Christensson B, Tribukait B, Linder I-L, Ullman B, Biberfeld P (1986) Cell proliferation and DNA content in non-Hodgkin's lymphoma. Flow cytometry in relation to lymphoma classification. Cancer 58: 1295-1304
14. Cornelisse CJ, deKoning HR, Moolenaar AJ, van de Velde CJ, Ploem JS (1984) Image and flow cytometric analysis of DNA content in breast cancer. Relation to estrogen receptor content and lymph node involvement. Anal Quant Cytol Histol 6: 9-18
15. Cornelisse CJ, van Driel-Kulker AM (1985) DNA image cytometry on machine-selected breast cancer cells and a comparison between flow cytometry and scanning cytophotometry. Cytometry 6: 471-477
16. Cornelisse CJ, van de Velde CJH, Caspers RJC, Moolenaar AJ, Hermass J (1987) DNA ploidy and survival in breast cancer patients. Cytometry 8: 225-234
17. Coulson PB, Thornthwaite JT, Wolley TW, Sugarbaker EV, Seckinger D (1984) Prognostic indicators including DNA histogram type, receptor content, and staging related to human breast cancer patient survival. Cancer Res. 44: 4187-4196
18. Dowle CS, Owainati A, Riobirns A, Burns K, Ellis IO, Elston CW, Blamey RW (1987) Prognostic significance of the DNA content of human breast cancer. Br J Surg 74: 133-136
19. Dressler LG, Owens M, Seamer L, McGuire WL (1986) Identifying breast cancer patients for adjuvant therapy by DNA flow cytometry and steroid receptors: a 1000 patient study. Proc Am Soc Clin Oncol 5: 61
20. Ewers SB, Langstrom E, Baldetorp B, Killander D (1984) Flow cytometric DNA analysis in primary breast carcinoma and clinicopathological correlations. Cytometry 5: 408-419
21. Fallenius AG, Skoog LK, Svane GE, Auer (1984) Cytophotometrical and biochemical characterization of nonpalpable, mammographically detected mammary adenocarcinomas. Cytometry 5: 426-429
22. Finan PJ, Quirke P, Dixon MF, Dyson JED, Giles GR, Bird CC (1986) Is DNA aneuploidy a good prognostic indicator in patients with advanced colorectal cancer? Br J Cancer 54: 327-330
23. Friedlander ML, Hedley DW, Taylor IW (1984) Clinical and biological significance of aneuploidy in human tumours, a review. J Clin Pathol 37: 961-974
24. Friedlander ML, Hedley DW, Taylor IW, Russell P, Coates AS, Tattersall M (1984) Influence of cellular DNA content on survival in advanced ovarian cancer. Cancer Res 44: 397-400
25. Gansler T, Chatten J, Varello M, Bunin GR, Atkinson B (1986) Flow cytometric DNA analysis of neuroblastoma. Correlation with histology and clinical outcome. Cancer 58: 2453-2458
26. Harvey J, deKlerk N, Berryman I, Sterrett G, Byrne M, Papadimitriou J (1987) Nuclear DNA content and prognosis in human breast cancer. Breast Cancer Res Treat (In press)

27. Hedley DW, Friedlander ML, Taylor IW, Rugg CA, Musgrove EA (1983) Method for analysis of cellular DNA content of paraffin-embedded pathological material using flow cytometry. J Histochem Cytochem 31: 1333-1335
28. Hedley DW, Rugg CA, Ng ABP, Taylor IW (1984) Influence of cellular DNA content on disease-free survival of stage II breast cancer patients. Cancer Res 44: 5395-5398
29. Hedley DW, Friedlander ML, Taylor IW (1985) Application of DNA flow cytometry to paraffin-embedded archival material for the study of aneuploidy and its clinical significance. Cytometry 6: 327-333
30. Hedley DW, Leary JA, Kirsten F (1985) Metastatic adenocarcinoma of unknown primary site: abnormalities of cellular DNA content and survival. Eur J Cancer Clin Oncol 21: 185-189
31. Hedley DW, Rugg Ca, Gelber RD (1987) Association of DNA index and S-phase fraction with prognosis of nodes positive early breast cancer. Cancer Res 47: (In press)
32. Jakobsen A, Poulsen S, Madsen EL, Petersen SE, Hansen HS (1984) Ploidy level of human breast carcinoma. Relation to histopathologic features and hormone receptor content. Acta Radiol [Oncol] 23 (2-3): 103-107
33. Joensua H, Klemi P, Eerola E, Tuominen J (1986) Influence of cellular DNA content on survival in differentiated thyroid cancer. Cancer 58: 2462-2467
34. Kallioniemi O-P, Hietanen T, Mattila J, Lehtinen M, Lauslahti K, Koivula T (1987) Aneuploid DNA content and high S-phase fraction of tumour cells are related to poor prognosis in patients with primary breast cancer. Eur J Cancer Clin Oncol 23: 277-282
35. Kute TE, Muss HB, Anderson D, Crumb K, Miller B, Burns D, Drube LA (1981) Relationship of steroid receptor, cell kinetics and clinical status in patients with breast cancer. Cancer Res 41: 3524-3529
36. Kute TE, Muss HB, Hopkins M, Marshall R, Case D, Kammire L (1985) Relationship of flow cytometry results to clinical and steroid receptor status in human breast cancer. Breast Cancer Res Treat 6: 113-121
37. Laerum OD, Farsund T (1981) Clinical application of flow cytometry: a review. Cytometry 2: 1-13
38. Look AT, Hayes A, Nitschke R, McWilliams NB, Green AA (1984) Cellular DNA content as a prediction of response to chemotherapy in infants with unresectable neuroblastoma. N Engl J Med 311: 231-235
39. Look AT, Robertson RK, Williams DL (1985) Prognostic importance of blast cell DNA content in childhood acute lymphoblastic leukaemia. Blood 65: 1079-1086
40. McDivitt RW, Stone KR, Meyer JS (1984) A method for dissociation of viable human breast cancer cells that produces flow cytometric kinetic information similar to that obtained by thymidine labelling. Cancer Res 44: 2628-2633
41. McDivitt RW, Stone UR, Craig RB, Palmer OS, Meyer JS, Bauer WC (1986) A proposed classification of breast cancer based on kinetic information. Derived from a comparison of risk factors in 168 primary operable breast cancers. Cancer 57: 269-276
42. Macartney JC, Camplejohn RS, Alder J, Stone MG, Powell G (1986) Prognostic importance of DNA flow cytometry in non-Hodgkin's lymphomas. J Clin Pathol 39: 542-546
43. Mauro F, Teodori L, Schumann J, Gohde W (1986) Flow cytometry as a tool for the prognostic assessment of human neoplasia. Int J Radiat Oncol Biol Phys 12: 625-636
44. Meyer JS, Lee JY (1980) Relationship of S-phase fraction of breast carcinoma in relapse to duration of remission, estrogen receptor content, therapeutic responsiveness, and duration of survival. Cancer Res. 40: 1890-1896
45. Meyer JS, Friedman E, McCrate M, Bauer WG (1983) Prediction of early course of breast carcinoma by thymidine labeling. Cancer 51: 1879-1886

46. Otto U, Baisch H, Huland H, Kloppel G (1984) Tumour cell deoxyribonucleic acid content and prognosis in human renal cell carcinoma. J Urol 132: 237-239
47. Raber MN, Barlogie B, Latreille J, Bedrossian C, Fritsche H, Blumenschein G (1982) Ploidy, proliferative activity and estrogen receptor content in human breast cancer. Cytometry 3: 36-41
48. Sandberg AA (1980) The chromosomes in human cancer and leukaemia. Elsevier/North Holland, New York
49. Sandberg AA, Turc-Carel C (1987) The cytogenetics of solid tumors. Relation to diagnosis, classification and pathology. Cancer 59: 387-395
50. Shapiro H (1985) Practical flow cytometry. Liss New York
51. Silvestrini R, Daidone MG, Gasparini G (1985) Cell kinetics as a prognostic marker in node-negative breast cancer. Cancer 56: 1982-1987
52. Taylor IW (1980) A rapid single step staining technique for DNA analysis by flow microfluorimetry. J Histochem Cytochem 28: 1021-1024
53. Taylor IW, Milthorpe BK (1980) An evaluation of DNA fluorochromes, staining techniques and analysis for flow cytometry. J Histochem Cytochem 28: 1224-1232
54. Taylor IW, Musgrove EA, Friedlander ML, Foo MS, Hedley DW (1983) The influence of age on the DNA ploidy levels of breast tumours. Eur J Cancer Clin Oncol 19: 623-628
55. Tribukait B, Hammarberg C, Rubio C (1983) Ploidy and proliferation patterns in colorectal adenocarcinomas related to Duke's classification and to histopathological differentiation. A flow cytometric DNA study. Acta Pathol Microbiol Immunol Scand [A] 91: 89-95
56. Tribukait B (1984a) Clinical DNA flow cytometry. Med Oncol Tumor Pharmacother 1: 211-218
57. Tribukait B (1984b) Flow cytometry in surgical pathology and cytology of tumors of the genito-urinary tract. In: Koss LG, Coleman DV (eds) Advances in clinical cytology, vol 2. Masson, New York, pp 163-189
58. Tubiana M, Pejovic MH, Chavaudra N, Contesso G, Malaise E (1984) The long-term prognostic significance of thymidine labelling index in breast cancer. Int J Cancer 33: 441-445
59. Volm M, Drings P, Mattern J, Sonka J, Vogt-Moykopf I, Wayss K (1985) Prognostic significance of DNA patterns and resistance-predictive tests in non-small cell lung carcinoma. Cancer 56: 1396-1403
60. Watson JV (1986) Oncogenes, cancer and analytical cytology. Cytometry 7: 400-410

Flow Cytometry in the Management of Breast Cancer

H.B. Muss and T.E. Kute

Cancer Center of Wake Forest University, Winston-Salem, NC 27103, USA

Introduction

There is a pressing need for the further definition of prognostic factors capable of defining the clinical course of patients with primary breast cancer. Current data suggest that approximately 50% of women will present with node-negative (N−) disease, 35% with node-positive (N+) disease, and 15% with metastases [37]. Of these patients, 25% with N− and 60% with N+ will develop locally recurrent or metastatic disease over a 10-year follow-up period. Adjuvant chemotherapy and/or endocrine therapy following primary treatment provides potentially curative treatment for an additional 10%-25% of patients with N+ disease, and current trials suggest benefit in N− patients [35]. For patients with primary operable breast cancer, a continuing clinical dilemma related to the use of adjuvant therapy is the need to treat all patients of a given stage in order to provide effective treatment for only a small proportion of the population. Although tumor size, histologic grade, and steroid receptor status provide information suggesting recurrence risk for large groups of patients, there remains no satisfactory tool for accurate prediction of recurrence in the individual.

The utilization of thymidine labeling (H^3) studies to define tumor kinetic parameters was a major step forward in tumor biology [29, 38, 39]. This procedure however, requires fresh tissue, radioactive materials, and is time-consuming, making wide usage unlikely. Nevertheless, [H^3] thymidine-derived kinetic parameters clearly are related to breast cancer recurrence and excellent reviews are presented in this monograph. More recently, flow cytometry (FC) techniques have been used to characterize malignant tumors [5, 16]. Flow cytometry is a rapid, highly automated procedure which allows calculation of tumor ploidy as well as cell cycle parameters. Recent studies have demonstrated that paraffin-embedded specimens as well as frozen or fresh tissues can all be used for FC analysis [17, 18]. In this chapter we will present the results of our FC studies on both fresh frozen and paraffin-embedded tissues, will compare our results with those of others, and will attempt to define the current role for this methodology in patient management.

Ragaz/Ariel (Eds.), High-Risk Breast Cancer

Materials and Methods

Flow Cytometry Analysis

Breast cancer tissue that remained after removal of a sample used for steroid receptor assay was frozen (−70°C), stored, and later used for cell kinetic and DNA analysis. The procedure used was a modification of that described by Thornthwaite et al. [42]. Frozen tissues were thawed and cut into small pieces in a nuclear isolation medium containing standard Dulbecco's phosphate-buffered saline with 50 μg/ml propidium iodide (specific DNA fluorescent stain), 0.6% NP-40, and 37 μg/ml RNAase. The suspension was passed through a nylon mesh to remove unfractionated tissues and other large debris, diluted to approximately 10^6 nuclei per milliliter nuclear isolation medium, and analyzed in a TPS-1 or TPS-2 flow cytometer (Coulter Electronics). The nuclei were excited by a 488-nm beam from a Spectra Physics argon ion laser, and the red fluorescent emission was measured with a 510-nm barrier filter and a 520-nm absorbance filter. The resulting DNA histogram was generated by counting at least 50000 nuclei.

For paraffin-embedded fixed tissues the procedure used was that of Hedley et al. [17] as modified in our laboratory. Fixed tissues were cut into 30- to 50-μm sections and deparaffinized with two changes of 3-4 ml xylene for 10 min at room temperature. The samples were vortexed well during incubation and 3-4 ml of 100% ethanol were added for 10 min. After the tissue had sedimented to the bottom of the tube, the supernate was discarded and the same procedure repeated with 95%, 70%, and 50% ethanol. The last ethanol dilution was removed and the cells washed with 5 ml water; water was then removed and 1 ml 0.5% pepsin in 0.9% NaCl pH 1.8 added. The sample was then incubated at 37°C for 30 min in a rapid-shaking water incubator. Afterwards, 3-4 ml Dulbecco's phosphate-buffered saline (PBS-A) was added to increase the pH (and inhibit pepsin) and the debris was allowed to settle for 1 min. The supernate containing the cell suspension was then removed and centrifuged at 200 *g* for 10 min at 4°C. The supernate was again removed and a second 3-4 ml PBS-A was added and this step repeated. To the final pellet of cells, 1-2 ml nuclear isolation medium was added and the mixture analyzed on the Coulter TPS-2 fluorescent activated cell sorter.

For both frozen and paraffin-embedded tissue, ploidy and cell kinetic status were determined by mixing propidium iodide with prepared nuclei. A comparison of the tumor histogram with the histogram containing normal diploid nuclei (normal white blood cell nuclei for frozen tissue analysis and nuclei from deparaffinized normal human liver tissue for paraffin-embedded samples) allowed for the detection of aneuploidy (Fig. 1).

If an aneuploid peak was observed, the ratio of the $G_{1/0}$ tumor DNA channel peak to the $G_{1/0}$ diploid channel peak was defined as the DNA index. A DNA index of 1.00 ± 0.04 was defined as a diploid tumor.

The cell kinetic activity for frozen tissues was determined from the DNA histogram data by the Fried program [14, 15] which fits the data to a gaussian distribution. The S-phase activity was the percentage of S-phase nuclei in the DNA histogram, while the proliferative index (PI) was the percentage of $S+G_2$ nuclei in

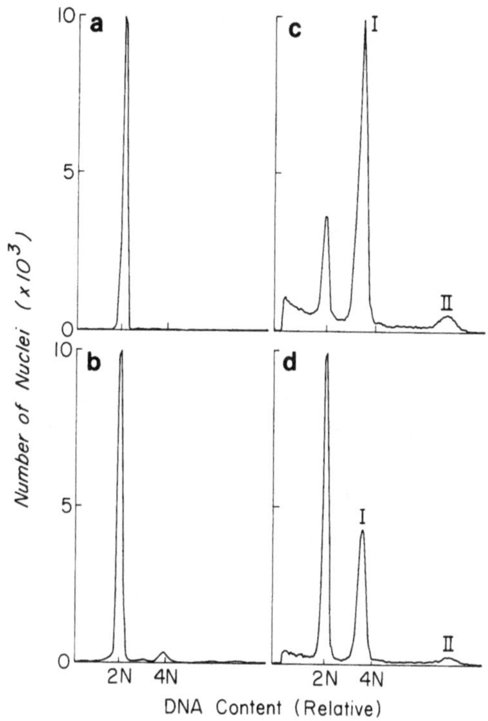

Fig. 1a-d. DNA histograms. **a** Benign breast tissue. **b** Diploid breast cancer; *2 N*, diploid DNA content; *4 N*, normal tetraploid DNA (G_2, M). **c** Aneuploid breast cancer; *I*, $G_{1/0}$ peak for aneuploid tumor; *II*, G_2/M peak for aneuploid tumor. **d** Aneuploid breast cancer in **c** after addition of normal human diploid WBC. Note increase in diploid peak and decrease in aneuploid $G_{1/0}$ and G_2/M peaks due to dilution by normal cells

the DNA histogram. For paraffin-embedded sections the method of Baisch et al. was used which calculates histogram areas by a rectangular fit program [4].

Steroid Receptor Assay

Tumor samples submitted for steroid receptor analysis were received under dry ice from local and surrounding areas and were processed by the steroid receptor laboratory at the Bowman Gray School of Medicine. The steroid receptor assays were performed by either the sucrose density gradient or the dextran-coated charcoal procedure as described previously [23]. Receptor activity $\geq$10 fmol per milligram protein was defined as a steroid receptor-positive value for both estrogen and progesterone receptor (ER and PR). Quality control of the assay procedure was maintained by analyzing reference standards in conjunction with the tumor assay.

Histologic Review

When possible representative sections of tissues received by the steroid receptor laboratory were reviewed histologically to determine percentage tumor (tumor cells divided by the sum of tumor cells plus stromal cells) by standard staining procedures [3]. In addition, a random sample from each group was selected and compared with the original histologic material used for diagnosis. Tumor grading criteria were those established by the National Surgical Adjuvant Breast Project; grade 1 tumors were well differentiated and grade 3 tumors were poorly differentiated [12].

Clinical Evaluation

For studies done on frozen tissues, clinical information was obtained from review of the patient's chart or from questionnaires sent to referring physicians. When possible all original pathology reports were reviewed, and information related to histologic type and grade, tumor size, and nodal status were recorded. Follow-up data for patients with stage I and stage II disease were obtained by submitting questionnaires at intervals of 6 months or less to referring physicians.

For analysis of archival, paraffin-embedded material from patients with N− breast cancer, a list of appropriate patients who had at least a 3-year follow-up was obtained from the North Carolina Baptist Hospital tumor registry. An equal amount of disease-free and relapsed patients were randomly selected for review and the clinical data obtained from chart follow-up and tumor registry data.

Results

DNA Distribution, % S-Phase, and Proliferative Index

FC studies were done on 226 patients with fresh frozen tissues [37]. Of the 226 samples, 10 were removed from analysis as histologic evaluation of submitted tissue failed to reveal malignancy. Of note, one of these patients had aneuploidy and a DNA index of 0.86. In review, this proved to be a cystosarcoma phylloides lesion. Of the remaining 216 patients, 27 had tumor tissue which contained between 1% and 10% malignant cells. All patients had ER assays, 92% had PR assays, all had analysis of ploidy status, and 177 had analysis for S-phase and PI. A total of 39 DNA histograms were not suitable for cell kinetic determination owing either to inadequate separation of diploid and aneuploid peaks or to the interface between G_1 and S or S and G_2. We prefer to use PI, the sum of S- and G_2-phases divided by the entire area under the histogram, as a measure of cell kinetic activity. PI only requires distinguishing the G_1/S interphase and not the S/G_2 interface; the measurement of S-phase activity requires two discrimination points (i.e., the G_1/S interface and S/G_2 interface). PI therefore, might be less prone to errors. In addition, correlation between S and PI values for our data was 0.91 ($P<0.05$). Scattergrams of the comparisons of % S-phase versus PI, % G_2-phase versus PI and % S-phase versus % G_2-phase are presented in Fig. 2. Since the major component of PI consists of cells in S-phase, the highly significant correlations between S and PI, and G_2 and PI are not unexpected. There is no correlation between the percentage of cells in G_2 and the percentage of cells in S. Both % S-phase and PI values are

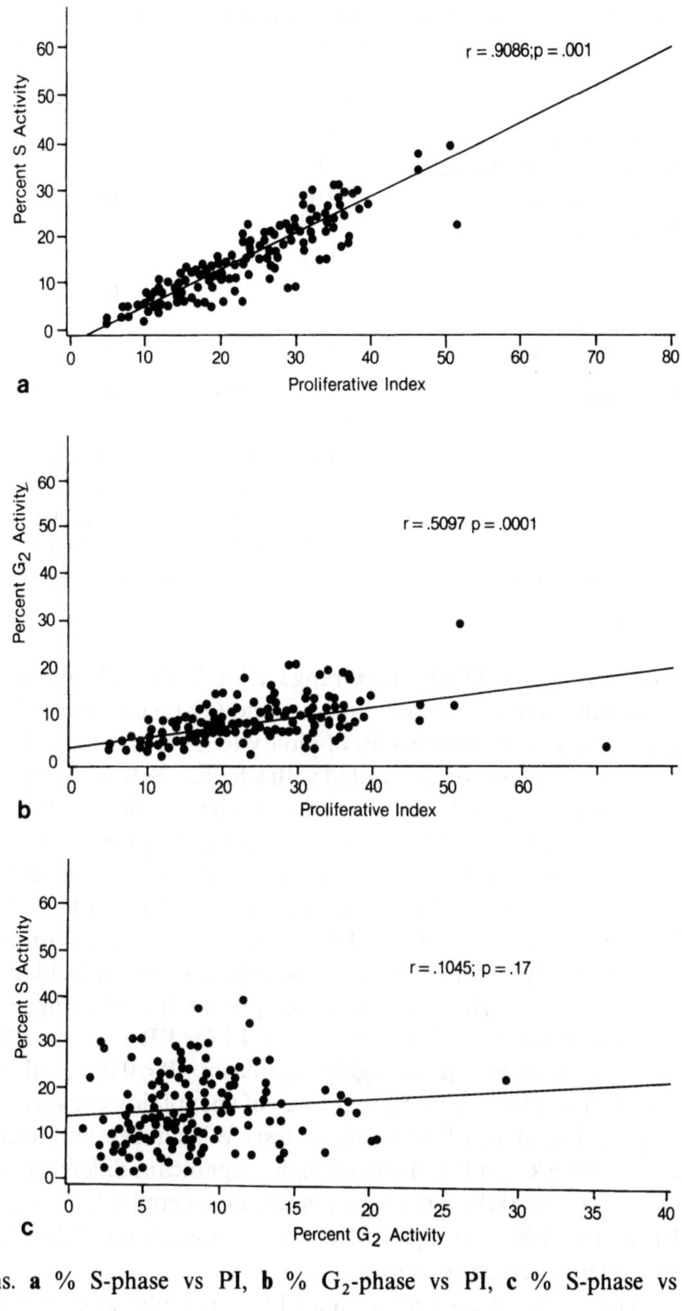

Fig. 2a-c. Scattergrams. **a** % S-phase vs PI, **b** % G_2-phase vs PI, **c** % S-phase vs % G_2-phase

presented in this chapter to facilitate comparison of our data with those of other investigators.

The results of ploidy and cell cycle analysis for frozen tissues are summarized in Table 1. In all, 54% of patients had aneuploid cell lines whose predominant clonal

Table 1. Frozen tissue-ploidy and cell kinetic analysis

	n	(%)
Total patients studied	226	—
No tumor tissue in specimen	10	—
Total evaluable	216	(100)
Ploidy status		
Diploid	100	(46)
Aneuploid	116	(54)
Cell kinetic data		
Number evaluable	178	(100)
Cell cycle phase	Mean ±SD (%)	Range (%)
$G_{1/0}$	76.8±10.0	28.5-95.1
S	15.4± 8.6	1.6-69
G_2	7.7± 4.2	1.0-29.1
$S+G_2$	23.1±10.0	4.9-71.5

form was in the DNA index range 1.5-1.9. For 177 patients with interpretable histograms, the $G_{1/0}$-phase, S-phase, and G_2-phase were 76.8%, 15.4%, and 7.7%, respectively. The relationship of ploidy to % S-phase or PI is presented in Fig. 3. Aneuploid tumors are associated with a higher % S-phase or PI ($P<0.05$), but there is a wide overlap in the distribution of S-phase activity within each ploidy category.

A comparison of PI, ploidy, and steroid receptor status is presented in Table 2 which shows that 53% of patients had ER-positive and 46% PR-positive malignancies. Moreover, 30% of the patients were ER+/PR+, 16% ER+/PR−, 9% ER−/PR+, and 30% ER−/PR−, percentages comparable to the distribution of steroid receptors from other published studies. Tumor lacking steroid receptors had a significantly higher PI and higher probability of being aneuploid than tumor containing receptors. The difference in PI for ER+ versus ER− and PR+ versus PR− receptor groups is highly significant ($P<0.001$ and $P<0.05$, respectively, *t*-test). The difference in the frequency of aneuploidy between the receptor groups is only significant for ER ($P=0.02$, χ^2-test). When receptor data are analyzed in paired groups for ER and PR, there is a highly significant difference in PI between the four groups ($P<0.0001$), but not in percentage aneuploidy ($P=0.12$). However, within ER+ and ER− groups, there are no significant differences in PI related to progesterone receptor status.

The relationship of ploidy and PI to age, tumor size, histologic grade, and stage is presented in Table 3. Unfortunately, complete information was not available for many patients. There was a statistically significant difference in PI ($P=0.03$), but not ploidy status ($P=0.73$), when patients were stratified into age groups above or below 50 years. Tumors greater than 2 cm tended to have a higher PI and were more frequently aneuploid, but the numbers of patients are too small to draw firm conclusions. For tumor grade, however, analysis revealed that poorly differentiated

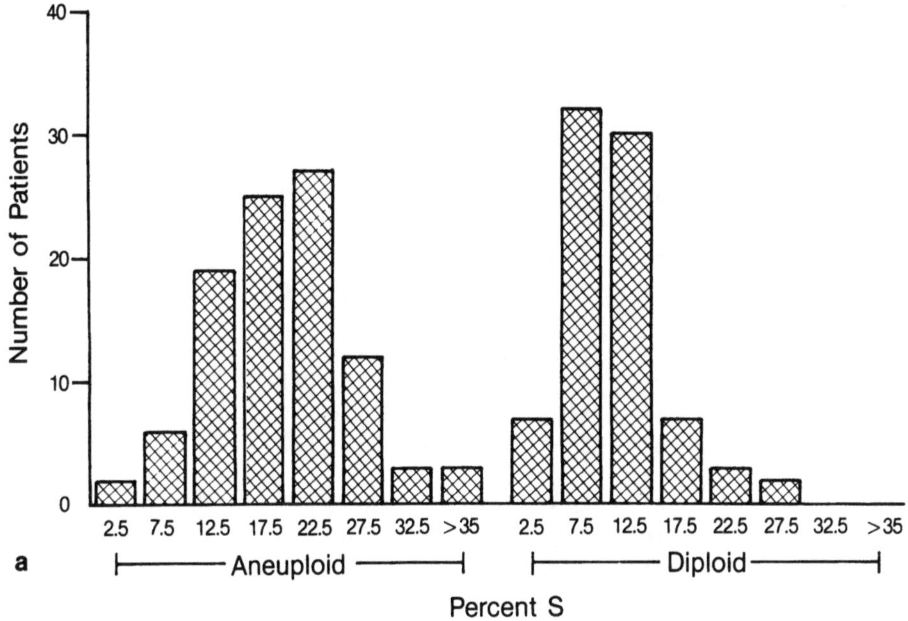

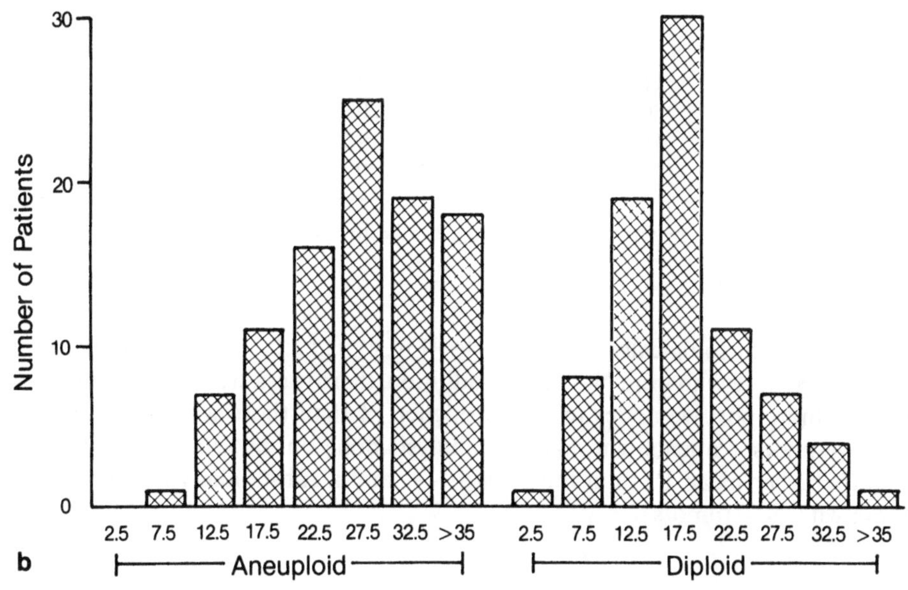

-**Fig. 3a, b.** Histograms. **a** Ploidy vs % S-phase, **b** ploidy vs PI

tumors had a significantly higher **PI** ($P = 0.01$), but similar ploidy status to tumors which were well differentiated. Finally, a comparison of flow characteristics for N+, N−, and metastatic lesions was conducted. The distribution of the DNA index for these three groups are presented in Fig. 4 and reveal similar ploidy status.

Table 2. Receptor status vs flow cytometry data

	S-phase		Proliferative index		Ploidy status	
	n	Mean ± SD	n	Mean ± SD	n	% Aneuploid
Receptor status						
ER+	93	12.9 ± 6.8	93	19.8 ± 7.7	114	46
ER−	85	18.1 ± 9.0	85	26.8 ± 10.9	102	63
PR+	76	13.5 ± 6.4	76	20.3 ± 7.5	92	46
PR−	88	17.3 ± 9.9	88	25.0 ± 11.0	107	62
ER/PR status						
ER+/PR+	62	12.4 ± 6.2	62	19.0 ± 7.1	74	43
ER+/PR−	25	14.5 ± 8.4	25	20.6 ± 9.1	32	50
ER−/PR+	14	18.0 ± 5.3	14	26.3 ± 6.6	18	56
ER−/PR−	63	18.5 ± 10.?	63	26.7 ± 11.2	75	67
ER (fmol/mg protein)[a]						
0-3	67	18.3 ± 10.0	67	26.8 ± 11.5	80	65
3-10	18	17.4 ± 7.7	18	27.0 ± 8.5	22	55
10-50	51	13.1 ± 6.6	51	20.0 ± 7.3	64	48
50-100	19	12.2 ± 5.7	19	18.7 ± 7.2	24	38
>100	23	13.1 ± 8.3	23	20.1 ± 8.9	26	46
PR (fmol/mg protein)						
0-3	91	17.0 ± 10.0	91	25.2 ± 11.4	112	61
3-10	11	16.0 ± 6.9	11	25.4 ± 8.0	12	50
10-50	30	13.6 ± 5.9	30	20.9 ± 7.4	35	51
50-100	19	13.0 ± 5.1	19	19.3 ± 6.7	26	38
>100	27	13.6 ± 7.8	27	20.5 ± 8.3	31	45

[a] 0-3 fmol/mg protein, negative; 3-10 fmol/mg, borderline; >10 fmol/mg, positive.

Patients with histologically positive nodes (Fig. 4) had a higher mean proliferative index than those who were N−, and in addition, there was a trend for patients with four or more positive nodes to have a higher PI than those with three or fewer positive nodes. Patients who had FC analysis done on metastatic lesions had a slightly higher mean PI than those with N+ and a substantially higher PI than those with N− tumors.

Flow Cytometry Data and Prognosis

To determine the role of FC characteristics and prognosis we have initially focused our efforts on N− patients with primary operable disease. The large majority of these patients are not treated with systemic adjuvant therapy, making analysis of disease-free survival and overall survival less likely to be confounded by treatment variables. In these initial studies patients who received adjuvant radiation were included.

Table 3. S-phase, PI and ploidy vs age, tumor size, grade and stage

	S-phase		Proliferative index		Ploidy status	
	n	Mean ± SD	*n*	Mean ± SD	*n*	% Aneuploid
Age						
< 50	43	16.1 ± 7	43	24.4 ± 8.4	50	50
≧ 50	94	14.7 ± 9	94	22.3 ± 10.4	113	50
Tumor size						
T_1 (< 2 cm)	5	11.8 ± 7.9	5	21.0 ± 6.7	5	20
T_2 (2-5 cm)	26	14.1 ± 7.4	26	23.2 ± 9.3	28	54
T_3 (> 5 cm)	10	14.1 ± 6.1	10	23.7 ± 8.2	10	50
Tumor grade[a]						
Well	5	12.0 ± 8.7	5	18.0 ± 8.3	5	20
Moderate	35	12.9 ± 6.2	35	21.8 ± 7.2	36	47
Poor	13	18.6 ± 6.4	13	29.4 ± 8.4	14	57
Stage						
Node negative	55	13.7 ± 6.8	55	21.1 ± 8.7	63	48
Node positive	44	16.0 ± 8.3	44	24.5 ± 9.4	55	55
1-3	14	15.3 ± 8.5	14	22.8 ± 9.2	21	52
≧ 4	30	16.3 ± 8.3	30	25.2 ± 10.0	33	58
Metastatic tissue	17	18.0 ± 14.8	17	26.6 ± 13.8	18	44
Primary (N unknown)	57	15.1 ± 7.4	57	22.3 ± 9.5	74	58

[a] National Surgical Adjuvant Breast and Bowel Project criteria [see 12].

A prospective evaluation of the prognostic role of FC-derived data from patients with N− breast cancer who had frozen tissue available for analysis is under way. All patients had steroid receptor evaluation and questionnaires were sent to referring physicians for follow-up data. Patients who received adjuvant chemotherapy or hormonal therapy were excluded. Patient entry began in August 1978 and was completed in June 1984, and all patients have had at least 18 months of follow-up. There have been 16 recurrences, 10 in patients with aneuploid, and 6 in patients with diploid tumors. S-phase activity for recurrent and nonrecurrent patients were similar. Further follow-up is needed to determine if FC characteristics will prove to be independent predictors of recurrence, but as yet there have been no major differences in frequency or time to recurrence based on FC data.

Because of the difficulties in obtaining long-term follow-up in prospectively studied patients a second study was performed utilizing paraffin-embedded blocks obtained from the primary lesion of women with N− breast cancer. A total of 73 consecutive patients who had surgery before 1984 were identified by our tumor registry. Patients who had received adjuvant postoperative systemic therapy or who did not have axillary dissection or sampling were excluded, leaving 59 evaluable for study. There was no obvious difference in age, number of nodes sampled, tumor size, or tumor grade in recurrent versus relapsed patients. The percentage of patients with aneuploid tumors was similar for each group. More-

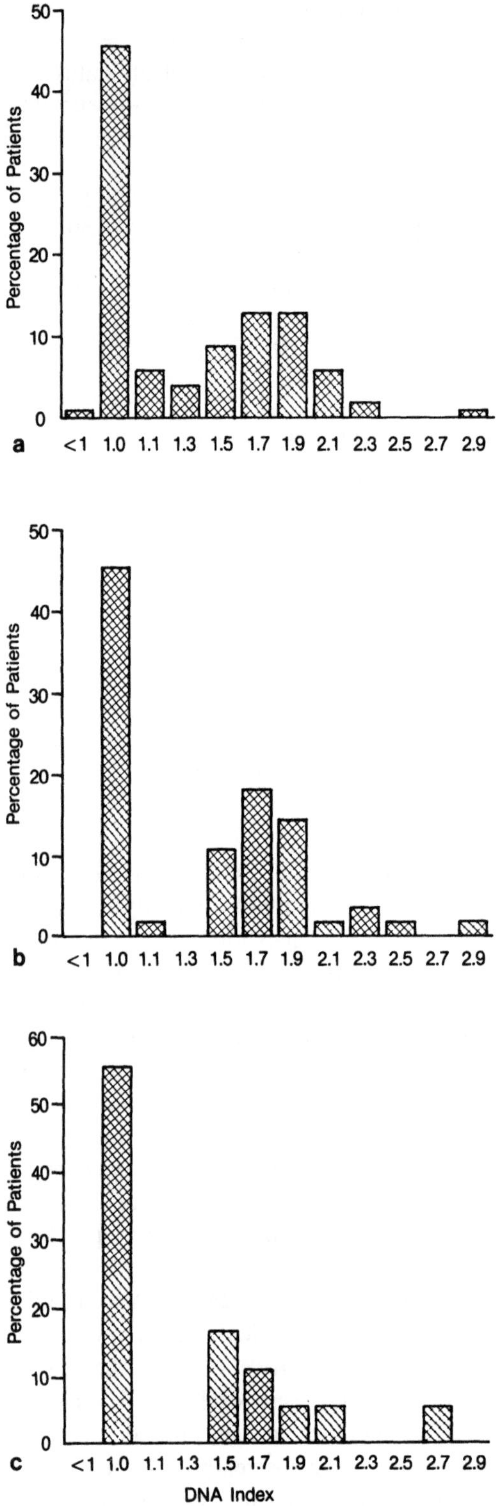

Fig. 4a-c. DNA index distribution. **a** 101 N– patients, **b** 55 N+ patients, **c** 18 patients with metastatic lesions over, there was no relationship of time to progression or survival and ploidy status. Cell kinetic analyses were done on 13 patients with recurrence and 16 without recurrence and showed no difference in mean S-phase activity (16.6% versus 13.8%, respectively). Time to relapse was similar for patients whose S-phase activity was either above or below the median value. However, we found a significant improvement in overall survival ($P=0.02$) for patients whose S-phase activity was below the median value.

Literature Review

Flow Cytometry Characteristics and Selected Clinical Variables

Several investigators have compared FC-derived DNA content and cell kinetic activity with selected patient variables such as age, tumor size, extent of lymph node involvement, histologic grade, and hormone receptor status. A significant relationship of ploidy status and patient age has been found by some investigators [41], but not others [20, 24]. Menopausal status has not been related to ploidy status in two trials [20, 43], but has in one [19]. S-phase activity has been found to be significantly higher for premenopausal patients or women below 50 in one trial [24], but not in two others [19, 20]. These data indicate that age is not clearly related to FC parameters and that a large range of cell kinetic and ploidy activity is found within pre- and postmenopausal patient groups.

Tumor size and ploidy have not been consistently related; several authors, however, have noted a significant association of larger tumors with a higher percentage of aneuploid activity [11, 43] while others have not [18, 19, 20, 24]. Likewise, cell kinetic activity does not appear to be highly correlated with tumor size [18, 24]. A significant association between aneuploidy and the number of positive nodes ($P<0.05$) was noted in Hedley's study of 490 N+ patients [19]. However, in another large trial of 638 patients, there was no correlation of aneuploidy and extent of nodal involvement [11]. In several other small series there was no correlation of aneuploidy and lymph node status [22, 24, 31]. Similarly, in three trials that included a total of 552 patients, no relationship of S-phase activity and lymph node status could be demonstrated [19, 24, 26].

Histologic grade was significantly correlated with aneuploidy in one large trial [19]. In addition, several other studies found that an increased frequency of aneuploidy correlated with moderate and poorly differentiated tumors and higher nuclear grade [20, 31, 33, 43]. Also, a significant correlation between poorly differentiated tumors and increased percentage of cells in S-phase was found in three trials [19, 20, 31]. Our data did not reveal a significant relationship between histologic grade and ploidy, but a significant correlation was noted for poorly differentiated tumors and increased PI [24].

There appears to be a clear relationship between ER status and aneuploidy. Several investigators have noted a significant correlation between tumors which are ER+ and diploid DNA status [19, 22, 24, 33]. Nevertheless, in one large trial of 168 patients, no such relationship was found [26]. A similar correlation has been found for PR activity where diploidy was much commoner in PR+ tumors [19, 21, 24]. S-phase activity has also been found to be significantly related to steroid receptor activity [21, 22, 24, 26]; receptor-positive tumors are more likely to be diploid. However, in one large trial no relationship was found [19]. Significant relationships of high proliferature activity and lack of PR have been noted by two authors [24, 26], but not by another [19]. In addition, our data show significant differences in S-phase activity for patients whose tumors are ER+ and PR+ as opposed to those whose tumors are ER− and PR− negative. Nevertheless, there is wide variability in ploidy and S-phase activity within different ER/PR subgroups.

Aneuploidy and Prognosis

Early investigators quantitated cellular DNA content by Feulgen staining and an integrating microspectrophotometer, a slow and tedious procedure. The results indicated that patients with aneuploid tumors had a poorer survival than those with diploid tumors [2]. The introduction of FC allowed for rapid DNA analysis; 332 tumors analyzed by both Feulgen and FC methods showed similar results for cellular DNA content [40]. There are now numerous reports relating aneuploidy and prognosis for many different cancers [16], with breast cancer a frequently studied tumor type [1, 6, 7, 9, 11, 18, 19, 21, 34, 36].

The relationship of ploidy and survival is presented in Table 4. Coulson et al. studied 74 patients and demonstrated that survival was shorter for patients with aneuploidy, especially in N− or stage II patients [7]. This trial did not include the results of treatment, which may have affected the conclusions. Ewers et al. studied 540 patients and showed a twofold higher recurrence rate for patients with aneuploid tumors compared with diploid tumors [11]; treatment and other prognostic factors were not discussed and follow-up was very short (16 months). In Hedley's study of 490 patients, aneuploidy was a significant variable only when analyzed independently; in the Cox regression model it had no independent relationship to prognosis [19]. Retsky showed aneuploidy to be a significant prognostic variable, but histologic grade was not included in his analysis [36]. Owainati and colleagues with FC data obtained from paraffin-fixed tissues showed that ploidy was significantly related to relapse-free survival (RFS) and overall survival (OS) at 8 months, but not at 30 months [34]. Klintenberg et al. [21] could not document independent prognostic impact for ploidy in 210 patients with primary breast cancer, while Kallioniemi et al. [20] did find ploidy significantly related to RFS, but not OS; this latter study was not analyzed by multivariate techniques. More recently, Dressler has shown aneuploidy to be a significant covariable, suggesting shorter RFS in women with N− breast cancer [10]. Aneuploidy proved to be an independent prognostic variable in her study ($P = 0.02$).

Cell Kinetic Parameters and Prognosis

Prior to the wide availability of FC technology, tumor kinetic studies were mainly performed with tritiated thymidine techniques. Patients with primary operable

Table 4. Flow cytometry-ploidy and proliferative index vs prognosis

Author	*n*	Method	Stage	Ploidy (DNA index) RFS	Ploidy (DNA index) OS	S-phase (or PI) RFS	S-phase (or PI) OS	Comment
Kallioniemi et al. [20]	93	PET	I, II, III	$p=0.05$	NS	$p=0.005$	$p=0.001$	Not corrected for covariables
Thorud et al. [43]	59	FT	I, II	NS	—	—	—	Small sample; 4-5 year follow-up; NAT
Hedley et al. [19]	490	PET	II (N+)	NS	NS	$p<0.07$	NS	TV
Ewers et al. [11]	540	FT	I, II, III	related	—	—	—	No statistics presented; TV
Coulson et al. [7]	74	FT	I, II, III	—	$p<0.05$	—	$p<0.05$	NTD
Retsky et al. [36]	500[a]	PET	II	significant	—	—	—	No grade in model. TV
Cornelisse et al. [6]	566	FT, PET	primary stage	$p<0.02$	$p<0.05$	—	—	Ploidy additional prognostic factor in Cox Model; NTD
Owainati et al. [34]	354	PET	A, B, C,[b]	NS	NS	—	—	Significant <30 months Then NS; NAT
Klintenberg et al. [21]	210	FT, FE	I, II, III	NS	—	$p=0.02$	—	Significant in Cox Model, grade not included; TV
Dressler et al. [10]	395	TP	I, II (N−)	$p=0.02$	—	$p<0.05$	—	Significant in Cox model
Kute and Muss (unpublished data)	59	PET	I, II, III (N−)	NS	NS	NS	$p=0.02$	Retrospective study
Kute and Muss (unpublished data)	101	FT	I, II, III (N−)	NS	NS	NS	NS	Prospective study

FT, frozen or fresh tissue; PET, paraffin embedded tissue; FE, Feulgen staining; TP, tumor powders used for FC; N+, node positive; N−, node negative; RFS, relapse-free survival; OS, overall survival; NS, not significant; dash (−), not reported; TV, post-operative treatment varied among patients; NAT, no adjuvant treatment; NTD, no treatment data.

[a] Numerical model based on clinical data.

[b] Primary operable, comparable to Stage I, II, III.

breast cancer and high labeling indices (LI) generally had a significantly higher relapse rate [29, 38, 37, 39, 44]. In an extensive multivariate analysis, Meyer et al. showed that LI was a powerful and independent prognostic factor, even after adjustment for age, stage, histologic grade, receptor and lymph node status [28].

More recently, investigators have explored the relationship between S-phase activity and recurrence frequency as determined from FC studies (Table 4). Since FC measurements of cell kinetic activity correlate closely with results obtained from thymidine labeling [27], similar relationships would be expected. Kallioniemi et al. [20] and Coulson et al. [7] studied small numbers of patients and showed a significant relationship of higher S-phase activity and shortened relapse-free survival. These two small studies included patients with different stages and treatments and were not analyzed with regression techniques. Hedley et al. [19] studied 490 N+ patients with FC techniques done on paraffin-embedded tissues. Proliferative activity could be measured on 285 of these patients and was a significant covariable when analyzed independently; it was not a significant covariable when analyzed by the Cox regression model. In contrast, Klintenberg et al. showed S-phase activity to be a significant independent variable in predicting RFS in 210 patients with primary breast cancer, but histologic grade and treatment were not used in their regression analysis [21]. Most recently, Dressler and colleagues studied 395 women with N− breast cancer [10]; S-phase activity was a significant independent covariable.

Conclusions

The relationship of FC measurements to other clinical and biologic covariables can be summarized as follows:

1. Menopausal status and age have no clear relationship to frequency of aneuploidy or S-phase activity.
2. Aneuploidy and high S-phase activity (or PI) correlate significantly with hormone receptor status. Receptor-rich tumors are much more likely to be diploid and of low proliferative activity. Because of the wide distributions of S-phase and ploidy values within receptor subgroups, FC information cannot substitute for direct measurement of receptor status.
3. High histologic grade (poorly differentiated) tumors have higher frequencies of aneuploidy and higher S-phase (proliferative) activity.
4. There is no clear relationship of FC data to tumor size or lymph node status.
5. Aneuploidy and S-phase activity are not clearly related to relapse-free or overall survival in primary breast cancer. The data currently available are conflicting and are confounded by many studies which have small patient numbers, variability of patient treatment, and lack of appropriate regression analyses necessary to determine the effect of covariables on relapse-free and overall survival. In N− patients, however, FC analysis may be of prognostic value.

A relatively unexplored area of FC may relate to its ability to predict response to treatment. Clinical trials have shown that malignancies with the shortest doubling times are the most likely to be cured with chemotherapy [32]. In addition, high histologic grade (which is related to increased S-phase activity) has been shown to be a favorable prognostic characteristic in one large trial of breast cancer patients given adjuvant chemotherapy following surgery [13]. Studies are now under way to determine if FC data, specifically cell kinetic studies and aneuploidy, may help predict response to adjuvant treatment (T.E., Kute and H.B. Muss, 1987 in preparation). In addition, others are exploring the relationship of FC characteristics, and response to chemotherapy or endocrine therapy in patients with metastatic disease [25, 30].

FC represents an exciting technical tool, capable of providing important biologic information from human tissues. It is possible that further investigations will define a clear role for this technique in the management of patients with breast malignancy. Presently, most trials have not conclusively shown that this technology provides independent information clearly related to prognosis, although recent data from N− patients have been encouraging. Only large trials of patients treated in a standardized manner will clarify the role of FC in patient management. Such trials should include evaluation of all pertinent variables that may relate to prognosis, including age, menopausal status, tumor size, extent of nodal involvement, histologic grade, receptor status and treatment. In addition, all such trials require meticulous statistical evaluation with regression analysis [8] to verify and identify major prognostic parameters.

References

1. Adami HO, Killander D (1984) Prediction of survival in breast cancer – a review. Acta Chir Scand 519: 25-34
2. Auer G, Eriksson E, Azavedo E, Caspersson T, Wallgren A (1984) Prognostic significance of nuclear DNA content in mammary adenocarcinoma in humans. Cancer Res 44: 394-396
3. Azzopardi JP, Chepick OF, Hartmann WH, Jafarey NA, Llombart-Bosch A, Ozzello L, Rilke F, Sassano N, Sobin LH, Sommers SC, Stalsberg H, Sugar J, Williams HO (1982) The World Health Organization histological typing of breast tumors – second edition. Am J Clin Pathol 78: 806-816
4. Baisch H, Goehde W, Linden WA (1985) Analysis of PCP-data to determine the fraction of cells in the various phases of cell cycle. Radiat Environ Biophys 12: 31-39
5. Barlogie B, Raber MN, Schumann J, Johnson TS, Drewinko B, Swartzendruber DE, Gohde W, Andreeff M, Freireich EJ (1983) Flow cytometry in clinical cancer research. Cancer Res 43: 3982-3997
6. Cornelisse CJ, Moolenaar AJ, Kooyman HJ (1985) Aneuploidy and survival in 566 breast cancer cases. International Conference on Analytical Cytometry XI. Hilton Head, SC, Abst. 340
7. Coulson PB, Thornthwaite JT, Woolley TW, Sugarbaker EV, Seckinger D, (1984) Prognostic indicators including DNA histogram type, receptor content, and staging related to human breast cancer patient survival. Cancer Res 44: 4187-4196
8. Cox DR: (1972) Regression models and life tables (with discussion). J R Stat Soc B 34: 187-220

9. Deshpande N, Mitchell I, Allen D, Morris R (1983) DNA content of carcinomas and prognosis in human breast cancer. Int J Cancer 32: 693-696
10. Dressler L, Clark G, Owens M, Pounds G, Oldaker T, McGuire W (1987) DNA flow cytometry predicts for relapse in node negative breast cancer patients. Proc Am Soc Clin Oncol 6:57 (Abst)
11. Ewers SB, Langstrom E, Baldetorp B, Killander D (1984) Flow cytometric DNA analysis in primary breast carcinomas and clinicopathological correlations. Cytometry 5: 408-419
12. Fisher ER, Gregorio RM, Fisher B (1985) The pathology of invasive breast cancer. Cancer 36: 1-85
13. Fisher B, Fisher ER, Redmond C (1986) Ten-year results from the National Surgical Adjuvant Breast and Bowel Project (NSABP) clinical trial evaluating the use of L-phenylalanine mustard (L-PAM) in the management of primary breast cancer. J Clin Oncol 4: 929-941
14. Fried J (1976) Method for the quantitative evaluation of data from flow microfluorometry. Comput Biomed Res 9: 263-276
15. Fried J, Perez AG, Clarkson BD (1976) Flow cytometric analysis of cell cycle distribution using propidium iodide. J Cell Biol 71: 172-181
16. Friedlander ML, Hedley DW, Taylor IW (1984) Clinical and biological significance of aneuploidy in human tumors – a review. J Clin Pathol 37: 961-974
17. Hedley DW, Friedlander ML, Taylor IW (1983) Method for analysis of cellular DNA content of paraffin-embedded pathological material using flow cytometry. J Histochem Cytochem 31: 1333-1335
18. Hedley DW, Friedlander ML, Taylor IW (1985) Application of DNA flow cytometry to paraffin-embedded archival material for the study of aneuploidy and its clinical significance. Cytometry 6: 327-333
19. Hedley DW, Rugg CA, Gelber RD (1987) Association of DNA index and S-phase fraction with prognosis of nodes positive early breast cancer. Cancer Res 47: 4729-4735
20. Kallioniemi O-P, Hietanen T, Mattila J, Lehtinen M, Lauslahti K, Koivula T (1987) Aneuploid DNA content and high S-phase fraction of tumour cells are related to poor prognosis in patients with primary breast cancer. Eur J Cancer Clin Oncol 23: 277-282
21. Klintenberg C, Stal O, Nordenskjold B, Wallgren A, Arvidsson S, Skoog L (1986) Proliferative index, cytosol estrogen receptor and axillary node status as prognostic predictors in human mammary carcinoma. Breast Cancer Res Treat (Suppl) 7: 99-106
22. Klintenberg C, Wallgren A, Bjelkenkrantz K, Carstenssen J, Humla S, Nordenskjold B, Skoog L et al (1985) DNA distribution, cytosol estrogen receptors and axillary nodes as prognostic predictors in breast cancer. Acta Radiol (Oncol) 24: 253-258
23. Kute TE, Huske MS, Shore A, Rhyne AL (1980) Improvements in steroid receptor assays including rapid computer analysis of data. Anal Biochem 103: 272-279
24. Kute, TE, Muss HB, Hopkins M, Marshall R, Case D, Kammire L (1985) Relationship of flow cytometry results to clinical and steroid receptor status in human breast cancer. Breast Cancer Res Treat 6: 113-121
25. Masters JR, Camplejohn RS, Millis RR, Rubens RD (1987) Histological grade, elastosis, DNA ploidy and the response to chemotherapy of breast cancer. Br J Cancer 55: 455-457
26. McDivitt RW, Stone KR, Craig RB, Palmer JO, Meyer JS, Bauer WC (1986) A proposed classification of breast cancer based on kinetic information. Cancer 57: 269-276
27. McDivitt RW, Stone KR, Meyer JS (1984) A method for dissociation of viable human breast cancer cells that produces flow cytometric information similar to that obtained by thymidine labeling. Cancer Res 44: 2628-2633

28. Meyer JS, Friedman E, McCrate M, Baur WC (1983) Prediction of early course of breast cancer by thymidine labeling. Cancer 51: 1879-1886
29. Meyer JS, Lee JY (1980) Relationship of S-phase fraction of breast carcinoma in relapse to duration of remission, estrogen receptor content, therapeutic responsiveness, and duration of survival. Cancer Res 40: 1890-1896
30. Mitchell I, Deshpande N, Millis R, Rubins R (1985) Deoxyribonucleic acid (DNA) content of primary carcinoma and response to endocrine or cytotoxic drug therapies in patients with advanced breast cancer. Eur J Surg Oncol 11: 251-256
31. Moran RE, Black MM, Alpert L, Straus MJ (1984) Correlation of cell-cycle kinetics, hormone receptors, histopathology, and nodal status in human breast cancer. Cancer 54: 1586-1590
32. Muss HB (1984) Principles of cancer chemotherapy; In: Deppe G (ed) Chemotherapy of gynecologic malignancy. Liss, New York, pp 1-30
33. Olszewki W, Darzynkiewicz Z, Rosen PP, Schwartz MD, Meleamed MR (1981) Flow cytometry of breast carcinoma: 1. Relation of DNA ploidy level to histology and estrogen receptor. Cancer 48: 980-984
34. Owainati AA, Robins RA, Hinton C, Ellis IO, Dowle CS, Ferry B, Elston CW, Blamey RW, Baldwin RW (1987) Tumour aneuploidy, prognostic parameters and survival in primary breast cancer. Br J Cancer 55: 449-454
35. Proceedings of the NIH development conference on adjuvant chemotherapy and endocrine therapy for breast cancer. (1986) NCI Monogr 1: 1-4
36. Retsky MW, Swartzendruber DE, Wardell RH: (1985) Predicting the disease free survival of breast cancer patients using DNA index and a stochastic numerical model of breast cancer growth. International Conference on Analytical Cytometry XI. Hilton Head, SC, abst 343
37. Silverberg E (1987) Cancer statistics. CA 37: 2-19
38. Silvestrini R, Daidone MG, Costa A, Sanfilippo O (1985) Cell kinetics and in vitro chemosensitivity as a tool for improved management of patients. Eur J Cancer Clin Oncol 21: 371-378
39. Silvestrini R, Daidone G, Gasporini G (1985) Cell kinetics as a prognostic marker in node-negative breast cancer. Cancer 56: 1982-1987
40. Stal O, Klintenberg C, Franzen G, Risberg B, Arvidsson S, Bjelken-Krantz K, Skoog L, Nordenskjold B (1986) A comparison of static cytofluorometry and flow cytometry for the estimation of ploidy and DNA-replication in human breast cancer. Breast Cancer Res Treat 7: 15-22
41. Taylor IW, Musgrove EA, Friedlander ML, Foo MS, Hedley DW (1983) The influence of age on the DNA ploidy levels of breast cancer. Eur J Cancer Clin Oncol 19: 623-628
42. Thornthwaite JT, Sugarbaker EV, Temple WJ (1980) Preparation of tissue for DNA flow cytometric analysis. Cytometry 1: 229-237
43. Thorud E, Fossa SD, Vaage S, Kaalhus O, Knudsen OS, Bremer O, Shoaib MC (1986) Primary breast cancer: Flow cytometric DNA pattern in relation to clinical and histopathologic characteristics. Cancer 57: 808-811
44. Tubiana M, Pejovic MJ, Renaud A, Contesso G, Chavaudra N, Gioanni J, Malaise EP (1981) Kinetic parameters and the course of the disease in breast cancer. Cancer 47: 937-943

The Role of Fine-Needle Aspiration in Determining the Risk of Breast Cancer

J. Le Riche, J. Atiba, J. Ragaz, and G. De Jong

Cancer Control Agency of British Columbia, Vancouver, British Columbia, Canada

Introduction

In this report we will review the role of fine-needle aspiration (FNA) in the primary diagnosis and follow-up of breast cancer. We will present some of our own results on flow cytometry performed from fine-needle aspirates, and will focus on the practicality of a more uniform adoption of FNA in the handling of breast neoplasia.

There are several advantages of FNA over conventionally performed open biopsy as a primary diagnostic method. Firstly, the diagnosis can be made immediately, at the first presentation of the lump, with no delays. The reduction of the waiting time may allow more selective investigations and an earlier introduction of therapeutic maneuvers (surgery, preoperative chemotherapy, etc.), in addition to alleviating the patients' anxiety while waiting for confirmation of the pathology.

Whether a reduction of the waiting time will render a therapeutic advantage in human breast cancer is yet to be shown, but on theoretical grounds, diagnostic delays are considered adverse [32]. In tumors with a low doubling time, delays of even several days will result in a meaningful expansion of the tumor burden. The adverse effect of a delayed diagnosis may be more appreciated in view of data on tumor resistance [32] indicating that the emergence of the first resistant cell and its subsequent replication is an instantaneous phenomenon occurring very early in the history of the tumor.

The other aspect of tumor biology where FNA may be of importance when compared to an incisional open biopsy involves tumor kinetics. As the tumor enlarges, it follows the Gompertzian type of growth pattern, with an exponential increase in its doubling time. There are experimental data which show that noncytoreductive surgery will decrease the doubling time with an increase of the cell division rate [80]. The postsurgical acceleration of residual tumor has been documented in many animal tumors [23, 26, 33, 35, 80], with some evidence of an adverse effect on the lifespan [23, 80], or the therapeutic advantage of preoperative chemotherapy [15, 80]. The mechanism for the kinetic alterations after noncurative cytoreduction has not been fully clarified, but outgrowing of the blood supply by larger tumors, with resultant necrosis of their central part, is a possible factor, as is a sensitive interplay of inhibitory and stimulating growth factors [6, 23, 86]. Tissue trauma and immune changes in connection with anesthesia and surgery have been linked with the acceleration of tumor dissemination [72]. After conventionally

Ragaz/Ariel (Eds.), High-Risk Breast Cancer

performed open biopsy of breast cancer, some residual disease is left, either at the incisional margins (incisional biopsy) or spread systemically (micrometastases). Hence, in most cases, open biopsy is an example of noncurative surgery. It is expected that FNA, by causing less tissue trauma and by reason of the virtual absence of cytoreduction, will have lesser kinetic effects. Confirmatory open biopsy (frozen section) permitting more refined assessment of histology and grade is still considered necessary.

At present, FNA is used successfully not only at the time of the initial diagnosis, but also during the follow-up of newly metastasized accessible lesions (cytology). The diagnostic use of FNA may be greatly enhanced by the introduction of techniques which permit risk assessment by DNA flow-cytometric analysis [2, 34], estrophilin/estrogen receptor determinations, estimation of chemotherapeutic uptake and response [3], and, most recently, oncogenic assessment. There are plans at our institution, as reported here, to perform these varied assessments from the same fine-needle aspirate more uniformly. The following is a review of some aspects of such an approach.

Role of FNA in Pathologic Diagnosis

During the first half of the twentieth century, FNA of palpable tumors was introduced in both North America and many countries in Europe. The technique became widely accepted in Sweden several decades ago [84], and by 1970 had been adopted by most Western European countries [8, 11, 17, 27, 31, 73, 96, 97]. Although FNA had become a routine procedure in isolated institutions in the USA as early as 1926 [34, 59], the technique aroused very little interest in North America until recently. In 1975, a group from Sweden visited centers in the eastern states of the USA demonstrating FNA. The response, although cautious at first, was good, and the technique is now being increasingly employed in many centers in North America. In connection with our work on preoperative adjuvant chemotherapy, our group has popularized FNA as a primary diagnostic method for breast carcinoma [70].

Fine-needle aspiration biopsy is already widely employed in the diagnosis of breast masses. As in all other areas, a benign cytology result should never be accepted in the face of any clinical or radiological indications that breast carcioma may be present but should always be followed by repeat aspiration or surgical biopsy. Cytological confirmation of a clinical impression of benign disease should always be monitored by clinical reassessment 1 month and 3 months later [10, 74]. This clinical follow-up is essential to detect false negatives, the rate of which is variously reported as 2%-24% [74, 83].

The lowest false-negative rates (2%-3% of cases) are recorded in centers experienced in the technique [74].

A report of malignancy permits specific preoperative patient counseling and allows for preoperative metastatic screening on an outpatient basis. Advances in mammography and xeroradiography have allowed the detection of small, frequently deeply seated lesions. The mammographic false-positive rate of approximately 5% may be reduced by the use of a mammographically or xeroradiographically directed FNA biopsy with or without fine-wire localization [40].

Aspiration cytology, by confirming primary local disease, may obviate surgical intervention with or without preoperative chemotherapy [14], or, by aspiration of distant metastases, may confirm stage IV disease.

Role of FNA in Determining Receptor Status

Whilst the expansion of FNA cytology services has tended to reduce the need for surgical intervention in obtaining an open biopsy, the proven significance of estrogen and progesterone receptor status has made it mandatory that such biochemical assessments be made on resected tissue [13, 42, 46, 56]. It is not surprising, therefore, that efforts have been made to perform receptor assessments on aspirated material. Before the isolation of estrogen receptor (ER) protein and the development of antibodies to this antigen, attempts were made to assess ER status and progesterone receptor status by measuring the ability of cells to incorporate estradiol-17β and hydroxyprogesterone hemisuccinate-BSA-tetramethylrhodamine [28, 61, 78]. Whilst some authors have reported a correlation between the histochemical and biochemical analyses, there is no real evidence to support the hypothesis that the histochemical techniques employed identify the same binding sites as do biochemical methods [30, 41, 66, 80].

The isolation of ER protein and the development of antibody to this protein has opened further avenues for investigation. Monoclonal anti-ER antibody has been used to assess the nuclear ER content of cells obtained by FNA, using both immunoperoxidase and fluorescence techniques [42, 56, 95]. The correlation between positive staining and the intensity of staining with biochemically determined cytosol ER values can be demonstrated, although there appears to be no correlation between cytosol ER values and the percentage of nuclei showing positive staining. The immunoperoxidase method permits qualitative and semiquantitative assessment of individual nuclei obtained in a cheap and atraumatic fashion, prepared in a relatively simple manner.

The functional heterogeneity of the majority of breast tumors suggests that a fully quantitative assay will be difficult to attain using the immunoperoxidase technique. Tagging of the anti-ER antibody with fluorescent material and assessment by fluorescence microscopy similarly permits qualitative and semiquantitative analysis but also raises the prospect of measuring receptor status and nuclear DNA of individual cells simultaneously within individual cells using a flow cytometer. The preparatory techniques involved are simple and could easily be performed on a routine basis. Unfortunately, the capital equipment costs are high and at present the fluoresceinated antibody is too expensive to use on a routine basis.

During the period January 1, 1985 to December 31 1986, all FNA biopsy specimens of primary or metastatic breast carcinoma seen at our institute were assessed for estradiol-17β using standard immunoperoxidase techniques. We found no correlation between the results of these measurements and the results of prior or subsequent biochemical assessment of ER values, except in those cases showing very high ER values. In such cases, the intensity of immunoperoxidase staining was great. The remaining cases showed inconsistent staining and the presence of scattered strongly positive cells bore no relationship to the biochemical values.

FNA and Tumor Markers

The ability of carcinoma of the breast to elaborate and to release into the circulation a variety of tumor markers has been examined using paraffin-embedded and frozen tissue samples [44, 49, 91]. Whilst there is general agreement concerning the frequency of expression of various antigens, there is no agreement concerning the significance of the expression of such antigens as prognostic indicators. All of the immunohistochemical techniques employed to demonstrate the expression of these varied antigens may be adapted for use with FNA biopsy specimens. However, the results of such procedures are frequently difficult to interpret. FNA biopsy specimens always contain a background of serum. If antigens are not only elaborated but also released into the circulation, the serum background staining, combined with the background contamination resulting from the inevitable disruption of some cytoplasmic membranes during smearing, makes the interpretation of anything less than highly intensely staining cells less precise.

Role of FNA in Determination of Oncogenes

In recent years, it has become established that amplification, alteration, and increased expression of a variety of cellular oncogenes is common in human cancers [24, 36, 43, 51, 85, 90, 93, 94]. More significantly, it has been claimed that such amplification, alteration, and/or over-expression may indicate poor prognosis [90]. In 1985, the first such association between N-*Myc* amplification, stage, and prognosis was reported in human neuroblastoma [76]. A similar association has been demonstrated between C-*Myc* and small cell anaplastic carcinoma of the lung [28, 51] and between the HER-#2/neu oncogene and breast cancer [82]. The substrates used in the assessment of oncogenes and their protein products has been obtained from either frozen or paraffin-embedded tissue. Oncogene assessments have been made on the basis of incorporation of monoclonal antibodies for use in either peroxidase-antiperoxidase or ABC immunoperoxidase systems [36], or in association with fluorescent dyes for direct visualization or flow-cytometric detection. These techniques may be adapted for use with FNA biopsy specimens, sufficient DNA for evaluation being easily obtained.

FNA and Flow-Cytometric Determination of DNA Content and Proliferative Activity

The search for new parameters which may have prognostic and, by implication, therapeutic significance has led to many investigations into the total DNA content and proliferative activity of a wide variety of tumors.

Total DNA Content

For several decades it has been possible to determine total DNA content by microdensitometry [81] and cytophotometry image analysis [1, 2, 9, 77, 87]. These studies have shown that abnormal DNA content is common in solid tumors and that such abnormalities are frequently correlated with poor prognosis. More recently, it has become possible to assess DNA content by flow cytometry, utilizing vital and nonvital staining.

Many studies of DNA content in breast carcinoma have been performed on fresh frozen tissue [12, 62, 63, 67, 69, 73], and it is beginning to be appreciated that FNA biopsy specimens are eminently suited to this technique [7, 71]. Because stage, grade, and ER status are very powerful prognostic indicators, many cases must be accrued within each category before the assessment of total DNA content as an independent indicator will be possible. The lack of predictability of carcinoma of the breast with respect to the timing of recurrence and the propensity of this disease for later recurrence mandates a very long follow-up period before the results of such evaluations can be assessed. The very significant work of Hedley et al. [37-39], describing the technique for assessment of the DNA content of cells embedded in paraffin wax, has made it possible to make such determinations retrospectively.

Proliferative Activity

High mitotic activity, as determined by enumeration of mitotic figures by light microscopy, has for many years been associated with bad prognosis. Similar importance has been demonstrated for the thymidine-labeling index and the bromodeoxyuridine-labeling index [55, 79]. These techniques have most commonly been used to evaluate fresh tissue but their applicability to FNA biopsy specimens has been amply documented [77].

Several studies have now demonstrated that the tumor-labeling index (TLI) stands as an independent prognostic factor when a variety of characteristics are subjected to multivariate analysis [55, 79]. The most recent attempts to delineate proliferative activity in breast tumors involve flow-cytometric analysis. That there is true correlation between TLI and S phase fraction, as determined by flow cytometry, has also been confirmed [55]. Unfortunately, the interpretation of the S phase fraction is not as simple as the DNA content assessment. Variations in methods of histogram analysis may produce very varied results [19, 21]. Fixation and preparation techniques may produce significant changes in the S phase fraction. Reliable cell-kinetic information can be obtained in less than 50% of histograms produced by the evaluation of material embedded in paraffin blocks. The ever-present problems of sampling error and contamination with normal diploid cells adds to the difficulties of accurate evaluation.

British Columbia Results of Flow-Cytometry Analysis from FNA

Over the past 3 years, we have routinely subjected the majority of FNA biopsy specimens of primary and metastatic breast carcinoma at our institute to flow-cytometric analysis. In this analysis, the technical aspects of the methodology and early results correlating the DNA index with different patterns of metastases are presented.

Methods

Sample Preparation

Samples from fine-needle aspirates were collected in 15 ml normasol and stored at 4°C. The storage time was never longer than 7 days. The staining was derived from Clevenger's technique. Cells were washed in PBS and then fixed with 10 ml 0.5% paraformaldehyde (Fisher, Fair Lawn, NJ) in PBS for 10 min. The cell suspension was centrifuged for 10 min. at 200 *g*, then resuspended in 0.1% Triton X-100 (Sigma, St. Louis, Mo) in PBS for 3 min and recentrifuged. Cells were then treated with 1 mg/ml RNase A (Sigma, St. Louis, Mo) in PBS for 30 min. After centrifugation, the cells were resuspended in 1 ml 50 μg/ml propidium iodide (Sigma, St. Louis, Mo) in 1% sodium citrate for at least 60 min. All procedures were performed on ice except the RNase treatment, which was carried out at 37°C.

Flow-Cytometry Preparation Technique

All samples were filtered through a 48-μm nylon-mesh filter prior to analysis and maintained on ice during flow-cytometry analysis. All smaples were analyzed using an EPICS V flow cytometer (Coulter Electronics, Inc. Hialeah, Fl) with a 488-nm argon ion laser (Coherent Laser Products, Palo Alto, Calif). Red fluorescence was monitored through a 515 long-pass interference, a 515 long-pass absorption, and a 590 long-pass absorption filter. Instrument calibration was performed daily with the aid of DNA Check fluorescent microspheres (lot no. 3003, Coulter Electronics). Ten to twenty thousand sample events were acquired on a single-parameter 256-channel integrated fluorescence histogram. To help identify the diploid population, human lymphocytes were analyzed prior to sample analysis and after every fifth sample run. The photomultiplier-tube high voltage was adjusted to maintain the lymphocytoid diploid peak in channel 40. The DNA histograms obtained were analyzed for DNA index and cell-cycle distribution with the STAT and PARA 1 software supplied by Coulter Electronics.

Sample Collection

Three separate passes were made into each lesion. A small amount of each aspirate was expressed onto a glass slide and smeared. The cells remaining in the barrel of the needles were washed into a single tube containing buffered saline and refrigerated immediately. This material was then prepared for DNA analysis by the Taylor's technique [89]. This technique has some very obvious disadvantages. Sampling error, inherent in all FNAs is reduced as much as possible by sampling three different areas. It is difficult to obtain sufficient numbers of cells from scirrhous tumors, and in general, the total number of cells available for assessment is smaller than when cells are obtained from fresh, frozen, or paraffin-embedded material.

There are, however, advantages to using this technique. It is simple, relatively painless, rapid, and economical. The fact that part of the specimen being evaluated can be seen on a glass slide permits an estimate of normal cell contamination and thus allows confidence levels to be set for identification of diploid tumors and assessment of the S phase fraction.

It is to be hoped that the development of multiparametric analysis, using, for example, one of the monoclonal antibodies to breast carcinoma described by Johnston [44], will further resolve the difficulties.

Results

During the period from June 1985 to December 1987, a total of 198 primary and metastatic breast carcinomas were sampled by FNA. The resulting specimens were examined by conventional cytologic methods and by flow-cytometric DNA

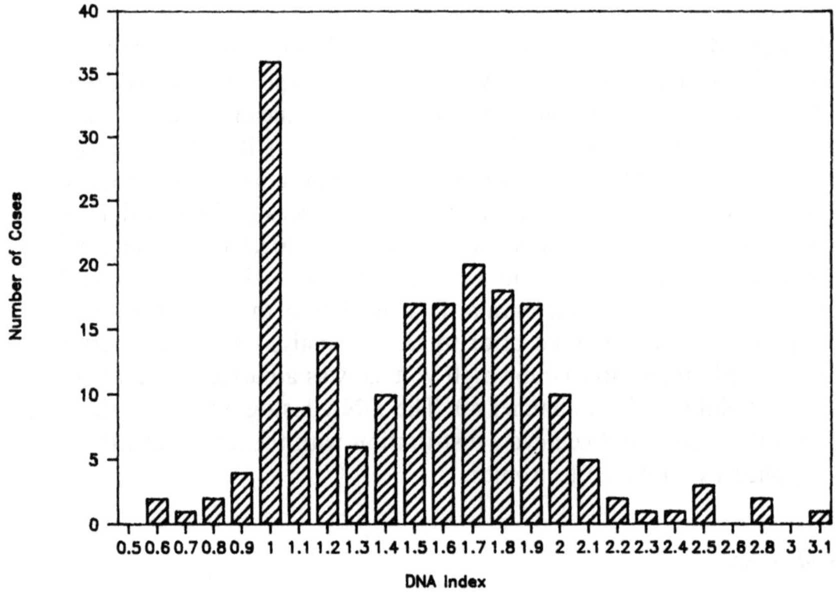

Fig. 1. DNA content of 198 primary and metastatic breast carcinomas. Median DNA index 1.5

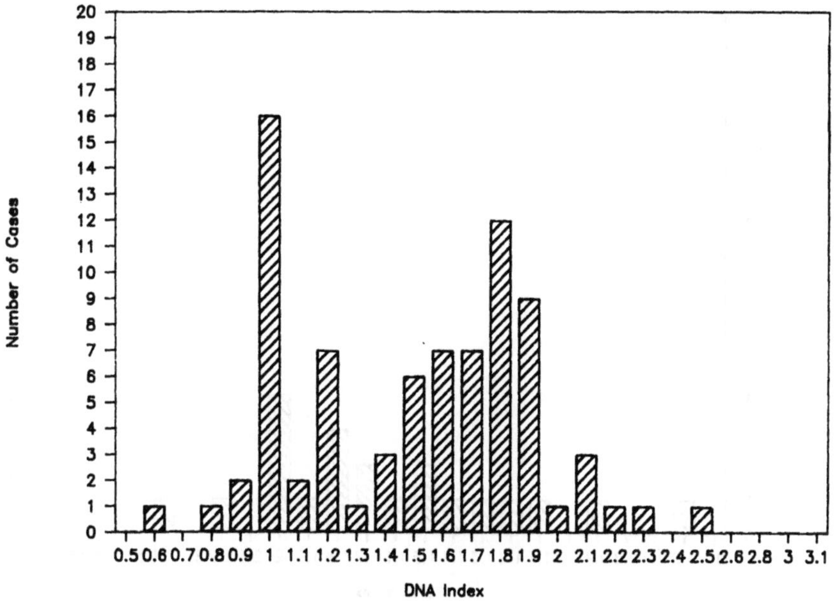

Fig. 2. DNA content of 81 primary breast carcinomas. Median DNA index 1.5

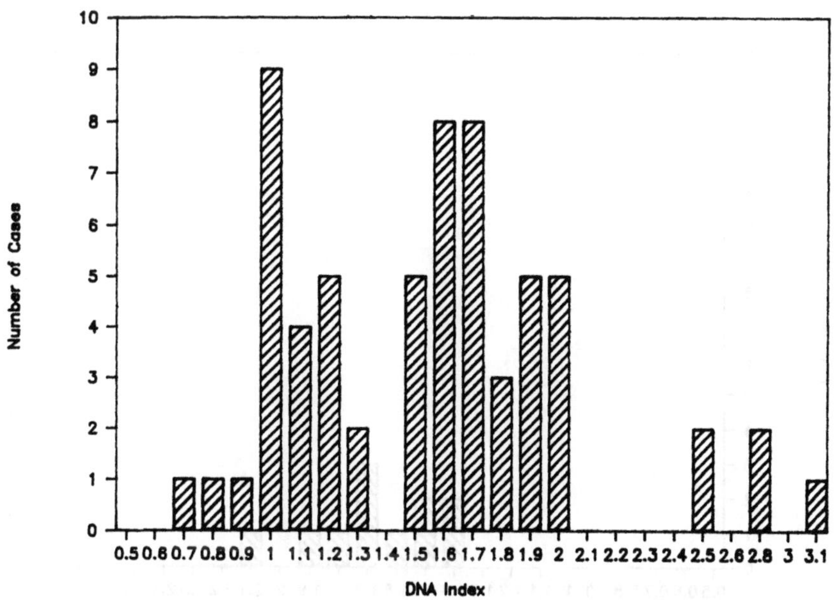

Fig. 3. DNA content of 63 breast carcinomas metastatic to lymph node only. Median DNA index 1.6

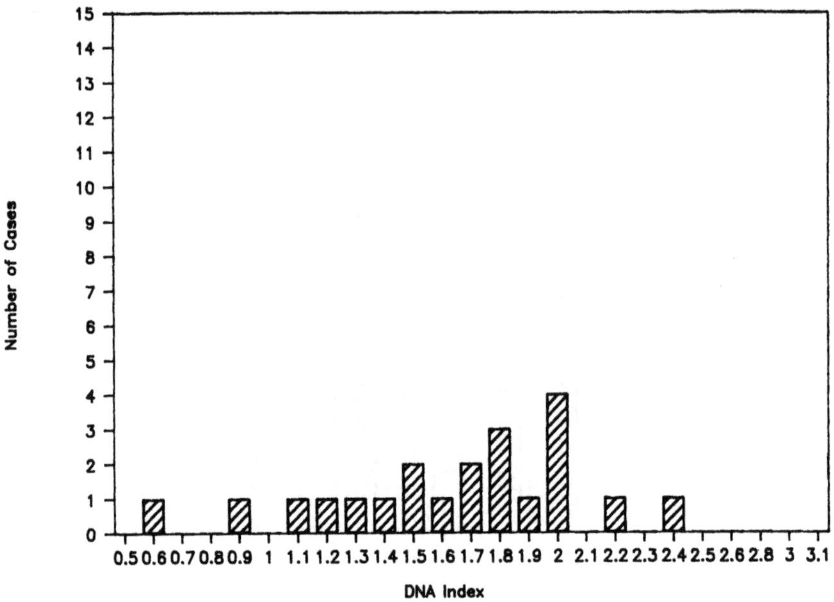

Fig. 4. DNA content of 21 breast carcinomas with metastases to soft tissues other than chest wall. Median DNA index 1.7

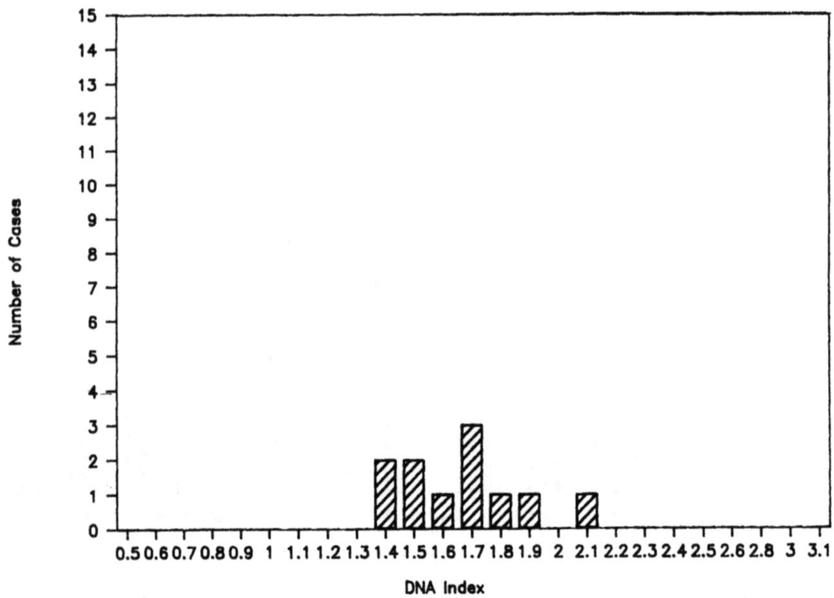

Fig. 5. DNA content of 11 visceral metastases of breast carcinomas. Median DNA index 1.7

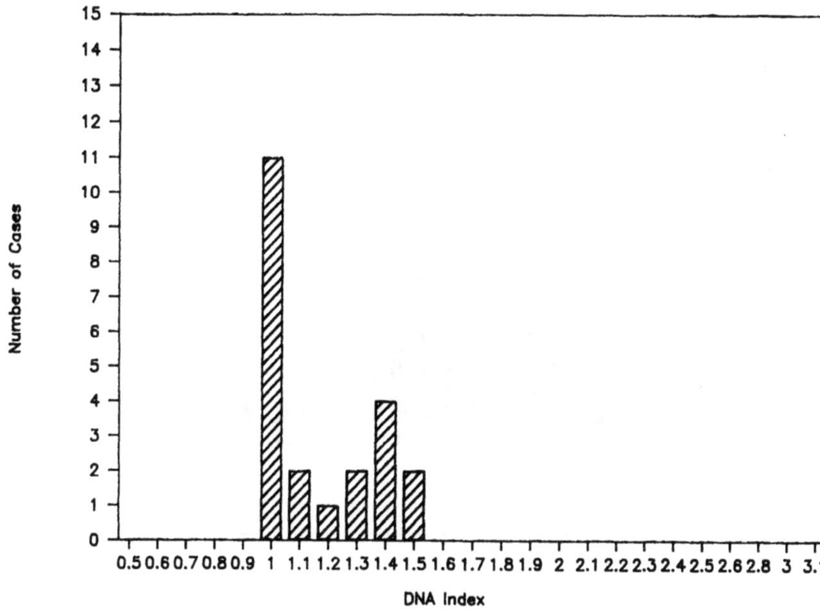

Fig. 6. DNA content of 22 breast carcinoma recurrences in the region of a mastectomy scar. Median DNA index 1.05

analysis. Eighty-one were from primary lesions with no recognizable metastases at the time of aspiration. Sixty-two samples came from patients who had developed metastatic disease in regional nodes after therapy, and 21 patients showed involvement of bone and soft tissue only. Twelve of the samples were from patients with visceral involvement, the metastases being confined to a single system. The remaining 22 patients had developed recurrent intradermal nodules on the anterior chest wall in the region of a previous mastectomy site. The results of DNA analysis of these lesions are itemized in Figs. 1-6.

Discussion of the British Columbia Study on Flow Cytometry Determination from FNA

Our results show a higher incidence (60%) of non-DNA diploid tumors than has been recorded in most other series [18, 21, 57]. This reflects a higher proportion of cases of advanced local disease among our patient population at a secondary referral center. The distribution of the DNA index amongst the DNA aneuploid tumors in our series is similar to that recorded by others. In general, the DNA index distribution among tumors metastastic to lymph nodes only is similar to that encountered in the primary tumors, apart from the expected decrease in the relative numbers of DNA diploid lesions. Those tumors which recurred as intradermal lesions involving the skin of the chest wall showed a preponderance of DNA diploid lesions. Those tumors which displayed DNA aneuploidy all fell within the diploid

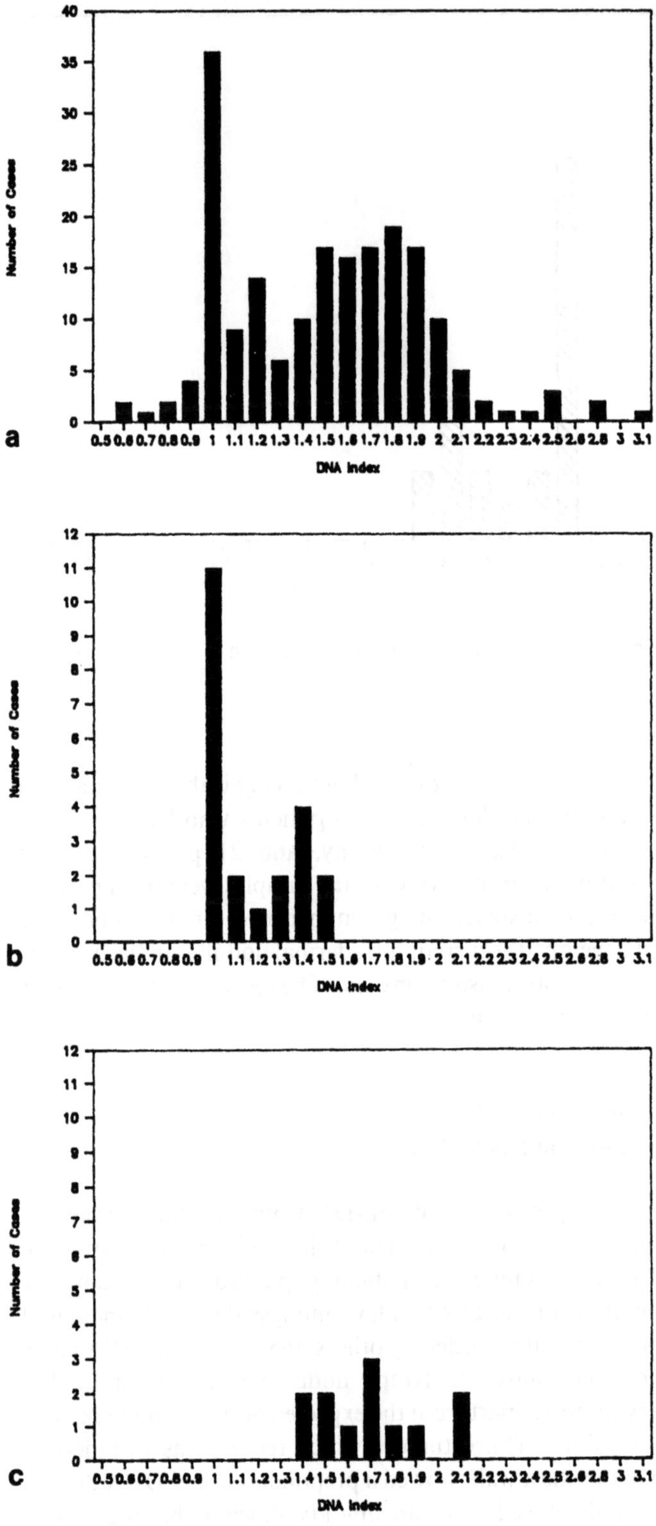

Fig. 7. a DNA content of 198 primary and metastatic breast carcinomas. **b** DNA content of 22 breast carcinoma recurrences in the region of a mastectomy scar. **c** DNA content of 12 breast carcinomas metastatic to liver or lung

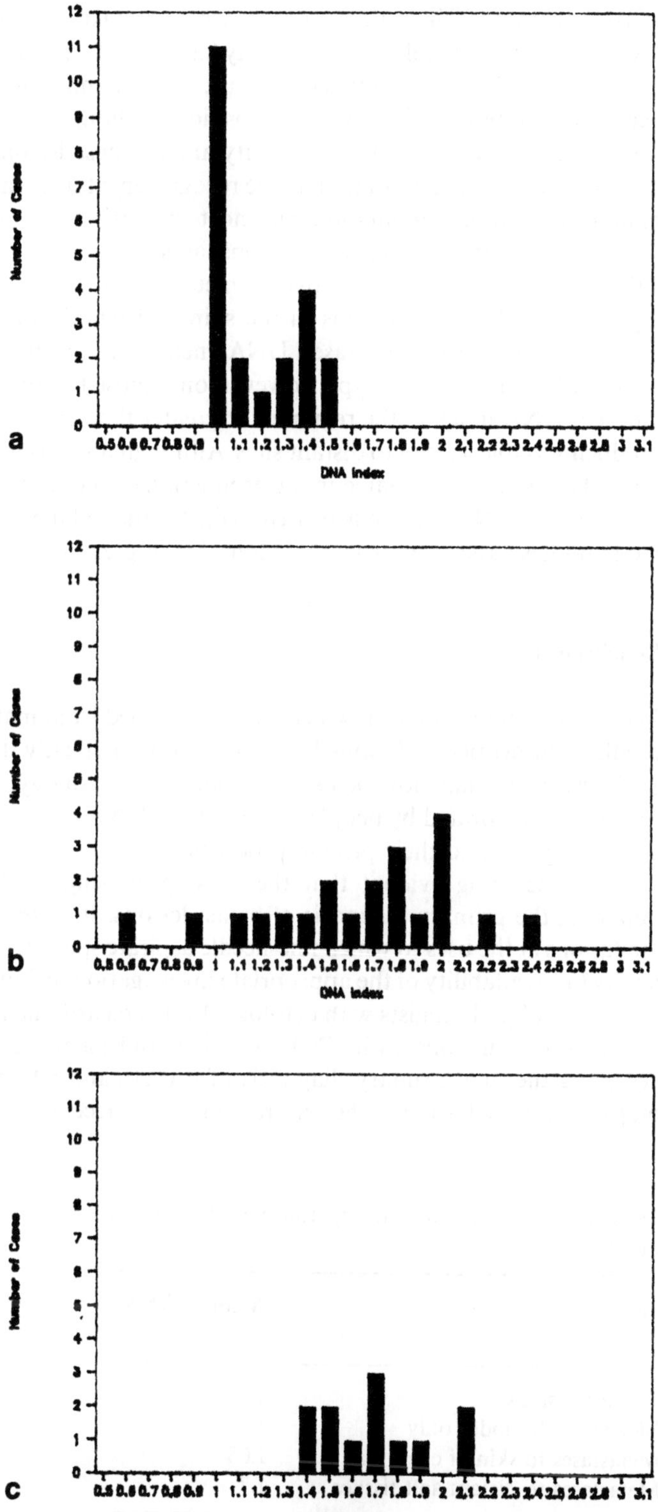

Fig. 8. a DNA content of 22 breast carcinoma recurrences in the region of mastectomy scar. **b** DNA content of 21 breast carcinoma metastases to skeletal muscle, bone, and soft tissue. **c** DNA content of 12 breast carcinoma metastatic to liver and lung

to triploid range, whilst those tumors which metastasized to lung and liver were invariably DNA aneuploid, the majority falling in the range of triploid to tetraploid. Lesions identified in subcutaneous tissue, muscle, and bone outside the chest wall occupied a somewhat intermediate position. Although all were nondiploid, there was a wide range of DNA abnormality among these lesions.

These results suggest that there are recognizable tumor factors which – alone or, more probably, in combination with host-site variations – mitigate for or against the development of metastatic lesions at specific sites. DNA diploid tumors, although demonstrating a low overall metastatic potential, are capable of producing viable proliferative lesions in the skin and lymph nodes, but less frequently produce blood-borne metastases. DNA aneuploid tumors appear to be capable of colonization of any tissue type; however, only those tumors with major abnormalities (i.e., DNA index in the region of or greater than triploid) may be successful in producing viable lesions to distant sites. Although it seems likely that both host and tumor factors are interrelated in the production of viable metastatic lesions, the fact that the total DNA content is related to the location of metastastic growth supports the hypothesis that tumor factors alone are of great significance.

Conclusions

The amount of information which can be obtained from material aspirated by fine needle from neoplastic lesions has increased dramatically during the past decade. Such specimens may now be used, in addition to cytology, to identify a variety of substances elaborated by neoplastic cells, total DNA content, S phase fraction, and also oncogenes and their protein products.

It is becoming evident that the most promising application of FNA is in obtaining the primary diagnosis of breast lesions. It seems that in the future, the limitations in the uses to which fine-needle aspirate specimens can be put will be set not by the availability of the appropriate investigation technique, but by the overall experience of pathologists with cytology. In this regard, the interest and experience of practising surgeons with FNA sampling, and particularly their confidence in accepting the final primary diagnosis of breast cancer from FNA without open biopsy, will determine the more uniform acceptance of this technique.

Table 1. DNA index of primary and metastatic breast carcinomas

Site	Median DNA index
Primary lesions	1.5
Metastases to nodes only	1.6
Metastases to skin of chest wall	1.05
Metastases to distant soft tissues	1.7

The false-negative and -positive results will clearly differ in different institutions, but there are indications, that with time and experience, diagnostic errors can be minimized. It is still believed that confirmatory open biopsy at the time of definitive diagnosis will be required. It is also expected that a refinement of techniques other than cytology, as discussed in this report, will allow the utilization of FNA to obtain sufficient information for risk assessment at the time of diagnosis. Such information will be essential, as different therapeutic approaches are likely to be needed for different risk categories.

The second main role of FNA is in the follow-up of metastatic lesions, where the confirmation of recurrence, as well as the information on kinetics and drug uptake, DNA content, etc., may be of assistance.

In summary, FNA is emerging as a very useful diagnostic method, and its popularization is likely to improve the quality of care of patients with malignancies.

References

1. Auer GU, Casperson TD, Wallgren AS (1980) DNA content and survival in mammary carcinoma. Analyt Quant Cytol Histol 2: 161-165
2. Auer GU, Eriksson E, Azavedo E, Wallgren A (1984) Prognostic significance of nuclear DNA content in mammary adenocarcinomas in humans. Cancer Res 44: 394-396
3. Auer GU, Fallenius AG, Erhardt KY et al. (1984) Progression of mammary adenocarcinomas as reflected by nuclear DNA content. Cytometry 5: 420-425
4. Barlogie B, Johnston DA, Smallwood et al. (1982) Prognostic implications of ploidy and proliferative activity in human solid tumours. Cancer Cytogenet 6: 17-28
5. Barlogie B, Raber MN, Schumann J et al. (1983) Flow cytometry in clinical research. Cancer Res 43: 3982-3997
6. Bates SE, McManawy ME, Lippman ME, et al. (1986) Characterization of estrogen responsive transforming activity in human breast cancer cell lines. Cancer Res 46: 1707-1713
7. Bichel P, Frederiksen P, Kjaer T, Thommesen P, Vindelov LL (1987) Flow microfluorometry and transrectal fine needle biopsy in the classification of human prostatic carcinoma. Cancer 46: 1206-1211
8. Bonneau H, Sommer D (1960) De the G etude critique de la cytologie tumorale par ponction a l'aiguille fine. Presse Med 68: 909
9. Boon ME, Auer GU, van Kaam H, Schwinghammer H (1984) Classifying breast carcinomas with DNA measurements and morphometry. Cytometry 5: 469-472
10. Brifford M, Gentile A, Herbert H (1987) Cytopuncture in the follow-up of breast carcinoma. Acta Cytol 26(2): 195
11. Castelain G, Castelain C (1953) Possibilites et limites du cyto-diagnostic extemporane. Presse Med 61: 1020
12. Chassevent A, Daver A, Bertrand G et al. (1984) Comparative flow DNA analysis of different cell suspensions in breast carcinoma. Cytometry 5: 263-267
13. Clark GM, McGuire WL, Hubay CA, Pearson OH, Marshall JS (1983) Prognostic receptors as a prognostic factor in stage II breast carcinoma. N Engl J Med 309: 1343-1347
14. Cohen C, Sharkey FE, Shulman G et al. (1987) Tumor-associated antigens in breast carcinomas – prognostic significance. Cancer 60: 1294-1298

15. Corbett TH, Griswold DP Jr, Roberts BJ et al. (1981) Cytotoxic adjuvant therapy and the experimental model. In: Stoll BA (ed) Systemic control of breast cancer. Heinemann, London, pp 204-243
16. Cornelisse CJ, van de Velde CJ, Caspers RJ et al. (1987) DNA ploidy and survival in breast cancer patients. Cytometry 8: 224-234
17. Cornillot M, Verhaeghe M, Cappelaere P, Clay A (1971) Place de la cytologie par ponction dans le diagnostic des tumeurs du sein. Lille Med 16: 1027
18. Coulson PB, Thornwaite JT, Wooley TW et al. (1984) Prognostic indicators including DNA histogram type, receptor content, and staging related to human breast cancer patient survival. Cancer Res 44: 4187-4196
19. Dean P, Gray J, Dolbeare F (1983) The analysis and interpretation of DNA distributed measured by flow cytometry. Cytometry 5: 188
20. Dressler LG, Owens M, Seamer L, McGuire WL (1986) Identifying breast cancer patients for adjuvant therapy by DNA flow cytometry and steroid receptors: a 100 patient study. Proc Am Soc Clin Oncol 5: 61
21. Dressler LG, Seamer L, Owens MA, Clark GM, McGuire WL (1987) Evaluation of a modeling system for S-phase estimation in breast cancer by flow cytometry. Cancer Res 47: 5294-5302
22. Dressler LG, Owens M, Seamer L, Dowle CS et al. (1987) Prognostic significance of the DNA content of human breast cancer. Br J Surg 74: 133-136
23. De Wyss WD (1972) Studies correlating the growth rate of the tumor and its metastases and providing evidence for tumor-related systemic growth-retarding factors. Cancer Res 32: 374-379
24. Escot C, Theillet C, Lidereau R et al. (1986) Genetic alteration of the C-*myc* photo-oncogene (MYC) in human primary breast carcinomas. Proc Natl Acad Sci USA 83: 4834-4838
25. Ewers S-B, Langstrom E, Baldertorp B et al. (1984) Flow-cytometric DNA analysis in primary breast carcinomas and clinicopathological correlations. Cytometry 5: 408-419
26. Fisher B, Gunduz N, Saffer EA (1983) Influence of the interval between primary tumor removal and chemotherapy on kinetics and growth of metastases. Cancer Res 43: 1488-1492
27. Fogher L (1954) Etude de la cytologie des tumeurs du sein chez la femme. Memoire d'assistant etranger. Paris 104: 29
28. Funa K, Steinholtz L, Nov E, Bergh J. Increased expression of N-*myc* in human small cell lung cancer biopsies predicts lack of response to chemotherapy and poor prognosis. Am J Clin Pathol 88: 2:216
29. Furnival CM, Chong KC, Watson LR, Visona A (1983) Fluorescent cytochemical oestrogen receptor assay: is it valid in breast cancer? Br J Surg 70: 457-459
30. Garancis JC, Miller LS, Tomita JT et al. (1983) Immunoperoxidase localization of estrogen receptors in human breast carcinoma. Cancer Detect Prev 6: 235-239
31. Godwin JT (1956) Aspiration biopsy: technique and application. Ann NY Acad Sci 63: 1348
32. Goldie JH, Coldman AJ (1979) A mathematical model for relating the drug sensitivity of tumors to their spontaneous mutation rate. Cancer Treat Rep 63: 1727-1733
33. Gorelik E, Segal S, Feldman M (1978) Growth of the local tumor exerts a specific inhibitory effect on progression of lung metastases. Int J Cancer 21: 617-625
34. Greenebaum E, Koss L, Shearman A et al. (1984) Comparison of needle aspiration and solid biopsy techniques in the flow cytometric study of DNA distributions of surgically resected tumors. Am J Clin Pathol 82: 559-564
35. Gunduz N, Fisher B, Saffer EA (1979) Effect of surgical removal on the growth and kinetics of residual tumor. Cancer Res 32: 374-379

36. Hand PH, Thor A, Wundertich D, Muraro R, Caruso A, Schlom J (1984) Monoclonal antibodies of predefined specificity detect activated gene expression in human mammary and colon carcinomas. Proc Natl Acad Sci USA 81: 5227-5231
37. Hedley DW, Friedlander ML, Taylor IW et al. (1983) Method for analysis of cellular DNA content of paraffin-embedded pathological material using flow cytometry. J Histochem Cytochem 31: 1333-1335
38. Hedley DW, Friedlander ML, Taylor IW (1985) Application of DNA flow cytometry to paraffin-embedded archival material for the study of aneuploidy and its clinical significance. Cytometry 6: 327-333
39. Hedley DW, Rugg C, Gleber RD (1987) Association of DNA index and S-phase fraction with prognosis of nodes positive for early breast cancer. Cancer Res 47
40. Hennig K, Johansson H, Rimsten A, Stenkvist B (1975) X-ray and fine needle biopsy in diagnosis of non-palpable breast lesions. Acta Cytol 19: 1-7
41. Janssens JPH, Pylyser K, Bekaert J et al. (1985) Biochemical and histochemical analysis of steroid hormone binding sites in human primary breast cancer. Cancer 55: 2600-2611
42. Jensen EV, de Sombre ER (1973) Estrogen-receptor interaction. Science 182: 126-134
43. Johnson BE, Ihde DC, Makuch RW et al. (1987) Myc family oncogene amplification in tumor cell lines established from small cell lung cancer patients and its relationship to clinical status and course. J Clin Invest 79: 1629-1634
44. Johnston WW (1987) Applications of monoclonal antibodies in clinical cytology. Acta Cytol 31:5:537
45. Kaman EJ, Smeuldens AW, Verbeek PW et al. (1984) Image processing for mitoses in sections of breast cancer: a feasibility study. Cytometry 5: 244-249
46. Knight WA, Gregory EJ, Livingstone RB, McGuire WL (1977) Estrogen receptor as an independent prognostic factor for early recurrence in breast carcinoma. Cancer Res 37: 4669-4671
47. Kuhajcha FP, Offutt LE, Mendelsohn G (1983) The distribution of carcino-embryonic antigen in breast carcinoma. Cancer 52: 1257-1264
48. Kute TE, Muss HB, Hopkins M, et al. (1985) Relationship of flow cytometry results to clinical and steroid receptor status in human breast cancer. Breast Cancer Res Treat 6: 113-121
49. Lee AK, Rosen PP, Delellis RA, et al. (1985) Tumour marker expression in breast carcinomas and relationship to prognosis. An immunohistochemical study. Am J Clin Pathol 84: 687-696
50. Lelle RJ, Heidenreich W, Stauch G, et al. (1987) The correlation of growth fractions with histologic grading and lymph node status in human mammary carcinoma. Cancer 59: 83-88
51. Little CD, Nau MM, Carney DN, Gazdae AF, Minna JD (1983) Amplification and expression of C-*myc* oncogenes in human lung cancer cell lines. Nature 306: 194
52. Lozouski MS, Mishriki Y, Chao S et al. (1987) Estrogen receptor determination in fine needle aspirates of the breast. Acta Cytol 31: 557-562
53. Lundy J (1980) Anaesthesia in surgery: a double-edged sword for the caner patient. J Surg Oncol 14: 61-65
54. McDivitt RW, Stone KR, Meyer JS (1984) A method for dissociation of viable human breast cancer cells that produces flow cytometric kinetic information similar to that obtained by thymidine labeling. Cancer Res 44: 2628-2633
55. McDivitt RW, Stone KR, Craig RB, et al. (1986) A proposed classification of breast cancer based on kinetic information. Derived from a comparison of risk factors in 168 primary operable breast cancers. Cancer 57: 269-276

56. McGuire WL (1980) Steroid hormone receptors in breast cancer treatment strategy. Recent Prog Horm Res 36: 135-156
57. McGuire WL, Meyers JS, Barlogie B et al. (1985) Impact of flow cytometry on predicting recurrence and survival in breast cancer patients. Breast Cancer Res Treat 5: 117-128
58. McGurrin JF, Doria MI, Dawson PJ, et al. (1987) Assessment of tumour cell kinetics by immunohistochemistry in carcinoma of the breast. Cancer 59: 1744-1750
59. Martin HE, Ellis EB (1930) Biopsy by needle puncture and aspiration. Ann Surg 92: 169
60. Martin HE, Ellis EB (1934) Aspiration biopsy. Surg Gynecol Obstet 59: 578
61. Masood S, Johnson H (1987) Value of imprint cytology in cytochemical detection of steroid hormone receptors in breast cancer. Am J Clin Pathol 87: 30-36
62. Mauro F, Teodori L, Schumann J, Gohde W (1986) Flow cytometry as a tool for the prognostic assessment of human neoplasia. Int J Radiat Oncol Biol Phys 12: 625-636
63. Olszewski W, Darzynkiewicz Z, Rosen PP et al. (1981) Flow cytometry of breast carcinoma I. Cancer 48: 980-984
64. Olszweski W, Darzynkiewicz Z, Rosen PP et al. (1981) Flow cytometry of breast carcinoma II. Cancer 48: 985-988
65. Opfermann M, Brugal G, Vassilakos P (1987) Cytometry of breast carcinoma: significance of ploidy balance and proliferation index. Cytometry 8: 217-224
66. Pertschuk LP, Eisenberg KB, Carter AC et al. (1985) Heterogeneity of estrogen binding sites in breast cancer: morphologic demonstration and relationship to endocrine response. Breast Cancer Res Treat 5: 137-147
67. Podhajcer OL, Bravo AI, Sorin I et al. (1986) Determination of DNA synthesis, estrogen receptors, and carcinoembryonic antigen in isolated cellular subpopulations of human breast cancer. Cancer 58: 720-729
68. Prey MU, Meyer JS, Stone KR, McDivitt RW (1985) Heterogeneity of breast carcinomas determined by flow cytometric analysis. J Surg Oncol 29: 35-39
69. Raber MN, Barlogie B, Latreille J, Bedrossian C, Fritscho H, Blumenschein G (1983) Ploidy, proliferative activity and estrogen receptor content in human breast cancer. Cytometry 3: 1-36
70. Ragaz J (1986) Preoperative (neoadjuvant) chemotherapy for breast cancer: outline of the British Columbia trial. In: Preoperative (neoadjuvant) chemotherapy, Ragaz J, Band PR, Goldie JH (eds) Springer, Berlin Heidelberg New York, pp 85-95
71. Ronstrom L, Tribukait B, Esposti P-L (1981) DNA pattern and cytological findings in fine-needle aspirates of untreated prostatic tumours. A flow-cytofluorometric study. Prostate 2: 79-88
72. Saba TM (1972) Effect of surgical trauma on the clearance and localization of blood-borne particulate matter. Surgery 71: 675
73. Saphir O (1952) Early diagnosis of breast lesions. JAMA 150: 859
74. Schondorf H (1978) Aspiration cytology of the breast. Saunders, Philadelphia
75. Schwartz MR, Randolf RL, Panko WB (1985) Carcinoembryonic antigen and steroid receptors in the cytosol of carcinoma of the breast. Cancer 55: 2464-2471
76. Seeger RC, Brodeur GM, Sather H et al. (1985) Association of multiple copies of the N-*myc* oncogene with rapid progression of neuroblastomas. N Engl J Med 313: 1111-1116
77. Seppelt U, Sprenger E (1984) Nuclear DNA cytophotometry in prostate carcinoma. Cytometry 5: 258-262
78. Silversward C, Humla S (1980) Estrogen receptor analysis on needle aspirates from human mammary carcinoma. Acta Cytol 24: 1: 54-57
79. Silvestrini R, Diadone MG, Gasparini G (1985) Cell kinetics as a prognostic marker in node-negative breast cancer. Cancer 56: 1982-1987

80. Simpson-Herren L, Sanford AH, Holmquist JP (1976) Effects of surgery on the cell kinetics of residual tumor. Cancer Treat Rep 60: 1749-1760
81. Sincock AM (1986) Semiautomated measurement of rapidly hydrolyzed DNA in the diagnosis of mammary carcinoma. Cancer 57: 1-5
82. Slamon DJ, Clark GM, Wong SG, Levin W, Ullrich, A, McGuire W (1987) Human breast cancer: correlation of relapse and survival with amplification of HER-Z/neu oncogene. Science 235: 177
83. Smith IH, Fisher JH, Lott JS, et al. (1959) The cytologic diagnosis of solid tumors by small needle aspiration and influence on cancer clinical practice. Can Med Assoc J 80: 855-860
84. Soderstron N (1952) Puncture of goiters for aspiration biopsy. Acta Med Scand 144: 237-244
85. Spandidos DA, Agnantis NJ. Human malignant tumours of the breast, as compared to their respective normal tissue, have elevated expression of the Harvey ras oncogene. Anticancer Res 4: 269-272
86. Sporn MB, Roberts AB (1985) Autocrine growth factors in cancer. Nature 313: 745-747
87. Stal O, Klintenberg C, Franzen G et al. (1986) A comparison of static cytofluorometry and flow cytometry for the estimation of ploidy and DNA replication in human breast cancer. Breast Cancer Res Treat 7: 15-22
88. Sumida C, Magdelenat H, Pasqualini JR et al. (1985) Cytosol and nuclear estrogen receptors (occupied and unoccupied sites) and progesterone receptors in human breast cancer. Breast Cancer Res Treat 5: 165-169
89. Taylor IW (1980) A rapid single step staining technique for DNA analysis by flow microfluorometry. J Histochem Cytochem 28: 1021-1024
90. Theillet C, Lidereau R, Escot C, et al. (1986) Loss of a C-H-ras-1 Allele and aggressive human primary breast carcinomas. Cancer Res 46: 4776-4781
91. Tosi P, Baak JP, Luzi P, et al. (1987) Correlation between immunohistochemically determined oestrogen receptor content using monoclonal antibodies, and qualitative and quantitative tissue features in ductal breast cancer. Histopathology 11: 741-751
92. Walker R, Cample JR (1986) DNA flow cytometry of human breast carcinomas and its relationship to transferring and epidermal growth factor receptors. J Pathol 150: 37-42
93. Watson JV (1986) Oncogenes, cancer and analytical cytology. Cytometry 7: 400-410
94. Watson JV, Stewart J, Evan GI, Ritson A, Sikora K (1986) The clinical significance of flow cytometric *C-myc* oncoprotein quantitation in testicular cancer. Br J Cancer 53: 331-337
95. Weintraub J, Weintraub D, Redaud M, Vassilakos P (1987) Evaluation of estrogen receptors by immunocytochemistry on fine needle aspiration biopsy specimens from breast tissue. Cancer 60: 1163-1172
96. Zajdela A, Ghossein NA, Pilleron JP, Ennuyer (1975) The value of aspiration cytology in the diagnosis of breast cancer. Cancer 35: 499-506
97. Zajicek J (1965) Sampling of cells from human tumours by aspiration biopsy for diagnosis. Cancer 1: 253

Tumor Kinetics

Measurements of Cellular Proliferation and DNA in Breast Carcinoma

John Strauch Meyer

Chief Pathologist and Director of Laboratories, St. Luke's Hospital,
232 South Woods Mill Road, Chesterfield, MO 63017, USA

Introduction

Risk assessment in breast carcinoma patients has traditionally been approached through an evaluation of the clinical or pathologic stage and histologic variables. The number of metastasis-bearing axillary lymph nodes, the size and local extent and presence or absence of distant spread of the carcinoma determine the stage, and each has accepted prognostic significance. Useful histologic variables include the histologic grade (degree of gland or tubule formation), nuclear grade, mitotic index, characteristics of the border of the tumor, presence or absence of necrosis or lymph- and blood-vascular invasion and characteristics of the cellular or interstitial tissue's response to the carcinoma. Mitotic frequency has been included as a component of nuclear grade by some authors. Of these variables, the histologic and nuclear grade have been most useful and have repeatedly shown power to predict outcome independent of stage [14, 27, 37, 38, 89, 101]. On the other hand, they have repeatedly proven difficult to reproduce from one observer to another [30, 45, 116]. To make them reproducible, quantitative measurement is needed. This can be accomplished by quantitative microscopy or image analysis [7, 60, 103].

More recently, other stage-independent quantifiable prognostic features have been defined. The most studied have been estrogen receptor (ER) [59] and progesterone receptor (PR) [19]. The prognostic properties of the steroidal receptors are discussed elsewhere in this volume, and the relationships between receptor content and proliferative indices will be covered later in this chapter.

Radiolabeling with tritiated thymidine ([^{3}H] TdR) made proliferative measurements practical in breast carcinoma [122]. Mitotic counts are impractical in breast carcinomas because of their usually low magnitudes and difficulty in discriminating mitotic figures from nuclear changes associated with cell death (apoptosis). [^{3}H] TdR labels S-phase nuclei, thereby marking cells that are engaged in replication of nuclear DNA, a prerequisite for cellular division. Since cells in the S-phase have DNA contents intermediate between the resting (G_1) and premitotic (G_2) levels, they can also be distinguished by DNA measurements. This can be accomplished by static microdensitometry or microfluorimetry after appropriate stoichiometric staining of DNA or by the newer technology of flow cytometry. We will devote our attention chiefly to thymidine labeling and flow cytometry.

Ragaz/Ariel (Eds.), High-Risk Breast Cancer

Tumor Growth and Cellular Proliferation

A tumor is composed of neoplastic and non-neoplastic cells of the host tissues. The relative cellularity of breast carcinomas measured by point count varies from approximately 3% to 90% with a mean near 30% [85]. Most of the volume of most carcinomas is non-neoplastic. The neoplastic cells represent a compartment with certain rates of cell proliferation and cell death. The cell death rate is usually high, and in some carcinomas probably approaches 100% [72, 113, 114, 115]. Therefore, growth rate may not be closely related to proliferative index of breast carcinoma, although a low order of correlation appears to exist [72]. The opportunity to measure volume doubling time under unperturbed circumstances arises chiefly by accident, and these measurements are usually made in retrospect. Evidence of rapid growth predicts early relapse [16], but direct measurement of growth requires a delay in treatment of the patient.

Studies of growth rates of tumors, since the time of the stimulating paper by Collins and associates [20], led to more general appreciation of the population dynamics of neoplasms. With each successive doubling beginning with a single neoplastic cell, the increment of growth increases. Thus, approximately 20 doublings are necessary to reach a diameter of 1 mm if the neoplasm consists entirely of neoplastic cells, and 30 doublings to reach 1 cm (Table 1). Since only another 10 doublings yield a mass of 1 kg, it is clear that much of the course of a neoplasm has transpired before it is clinically discoverable. Even several doublings early in the life history of a neoplasm can go completely unnoticed, but late in the history a single doubling may look like explosive growth. Whether the doublings require the same time early as late (constant versus variable doubling time) is controversial for human tumors.

Where V is the volume at a given time, V_0 is the volume at some prior time, the elapsed time is t, the growth constant of acceleration is k_1, that of deceleration is k_2, and e is the base of natural logarithms, Eq. 1 describes simple exponential growth and Eq. 2 describes gompertzian (double exponential) growth.

$$V = V_0 e^{k_1 t} \tag{1}$$

$$V = V_0 e^{(k_1/k_2)(1 - e^{-k_2 t})} \tag{2}$$

Table 1. Idealized growth of spherical tumor. (After [111])

Diameter (mm)	No. of cells	No. of antecedent binary divisions
1	5×10^5	19
2	4×10^6	22
6	1.2×10^8	27
10	5×10^8	29
100	5×10^{11}	39

Extensive work with neoplasms in laboratory animals has established that the growth curve is usually gompertzian [63, 107] which implies a slowing down of the growth rate and lengthening of the doubling time with age (Fig. 1).

The various experimental tumors that show distinct gompertzian growth patterns have short doubling times. When the doubling times are longer, as in most breast carcinomas, very long times are required to reach plateau, or it is reached at very high tumor volumes. Thus, the three gompertzian growth curves in Figs. 2 and 3 form plateaus off the scale, although they are different from the simple exponential curve. Note that deceleration occurs early in the gompertzian plots so that the times required to reach 1 cm^3 would be distinctly longer than for simple exponential growth. The deceleration of growth noted subsequently would permit the long-term survival often noted for breast carcinoma patients. Note also that with simple exponential growth, 90% or more of the life history of the tumor must be subclinical, whereas with gompertzian growth the absolute and relative durations of the clinical phase are prolonged. The gompertzian model seems to represent the clinically observable growth pattern more realistically than the exponential model, but this does not mean that breast carcinoma growth is really gompertzian. Skehan tested 18 equations to model in vivo tumor growth and found that all but one provided a best fit to at least one of 248 data bases, thereby demonstrating that no model was generally applicable [128]. Rates of cell proliferation of breast carcinomas usually remain constant over time [81], and a small but significant positive

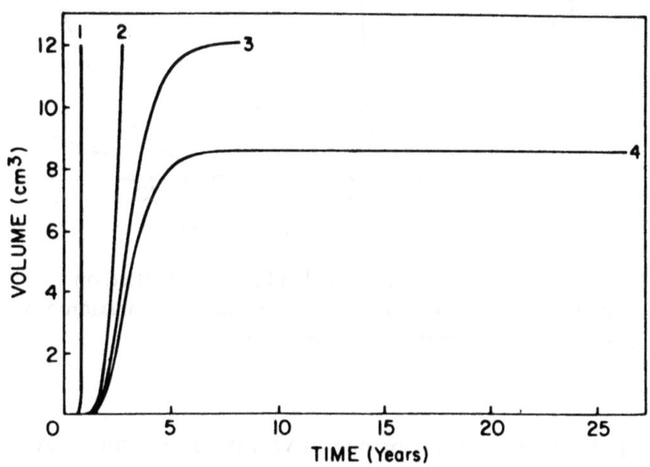

Fig. 1. Simple exponential growth and gompertzian growth compared. The growth constant k_1 was selected to represent the potential doubling time (10 days), assuming no cell loss, equivalent to the median TLI for primary breast carcinomas (5.5%), $k_1 = 0.0693$/year. *Curve 1*, a simple exponential function, is governed by k_1. *Curves 2-4* are gompertzian and are governed by both k_1 and k_2. For curve 2 $k_2 = 0.0030$/year. The gompertzian characteristics of curve 4 are fully developed with a plateau at 8.6 cm^3, whereas curves 2 and 3 plateau at volumes off scale, 36.3 cm^3 at about 8 year for curve 2 and only 12.1 cm^3 at about 8 year for curve 3. Note the striking differences produced by only slight variation in k_2, and that the time to plateau increases only slightly as the final volume increases greatly

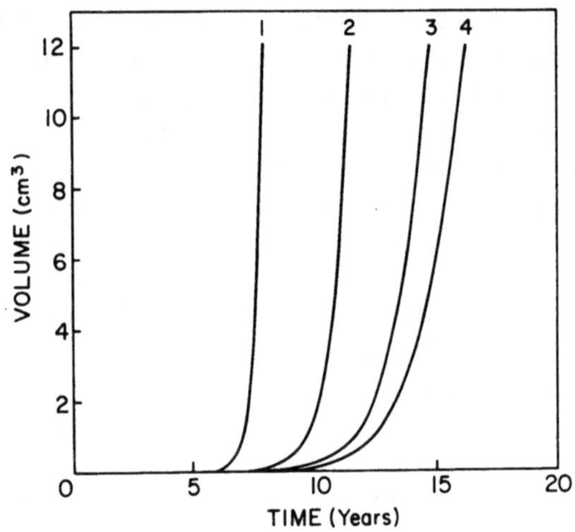

Fig. 2. Similar to Fig. 1, but with k_1 derived from the median observed actual doubling time for metastatic breast carcinomas (91 days), $k_1 = 0.00762$/year. *Curve 1* is for simple exponential growth, and *curve 2-4* are for gompertzian growth with the same k_1 and with $k_2 = 0.00019$/year, 0.00261/year, and 0.00028/year for curves 2, 3 and 4, respectively. Curve 2 plateaus at about 150 year and 883 000 l! Curve 3 plateaus at 140 year and 16.1 l, and curve 4 at 110 year and 2.22 l

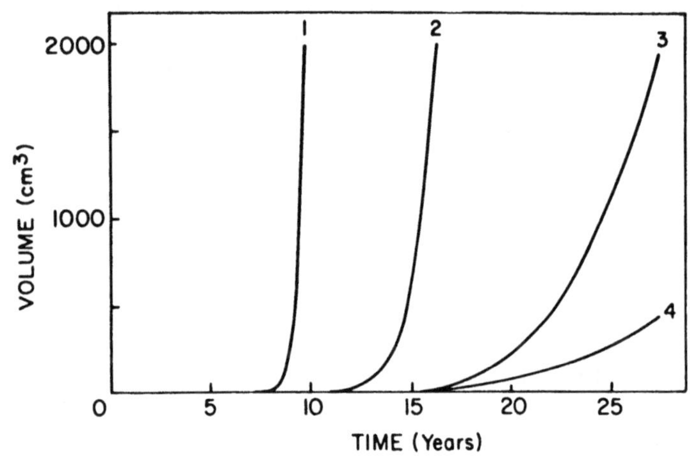

Fig. 3. The same functions plotted in Fig. 2 are plotted on a scale allowing their behavior to be appreciated as larger volumes are reached. The maximum volume shown would almost invariably be greater than the lethal limit

relationship between proliferative rate and tumor size has been observed [83]. These findings do not support the concept of deceleratory growth. Furthermore, breast carcinomas can be separated into several kinetic groups [73, 83]. A given model for growth could apply to one, but not to another, and we have no good evidence that any particular model accurately describes the growth of any type of breast carcinoma over its life history.

A survey of breast carcinoma doubling time studies in 1980 revealed three substantial studies of primary tumors (total of 101 patients) and five of metastatic tumors (total of 378 patients) [72]. The tumors were measured by caliper or in radiographic images. The mean doubling time for primary tumors from this survey was 231 days, with means of individual studies ranging from 109 to 327 days. The mean doubling time for metastatic tumors was 91 days, with means of individual studies ranging from 17 to 199 days. The extreme ranges are no doubt outside these limits, but cannot be assessed accurately because of large errors of measurement that are likely to occur in individual cases. Subsequently, von Fournier and associates published a study of 147 primary carcinomas by serial mammography and noted a range of 44-1869 days with a mean of 212 days for the doubling time [124]. This mean doubling time implies an average time of 4 years for a 2-mm tumor to grow to 10 mm. The mean doubling time was short in patients under age 50, particularly if they had axillary lymph nodal metastases. Evidence of rapid growth prior to primary therapy, which Boyd and co-workers referred to as "transition" events, has been associated with early death from breast carcinoma [16].

Cell Kinetics Measurements: Methodology

The cell cycle has been divided into four discrete segments (Fig. 4). The M-phase, as indicated in the figure, actually includes only metaphase, anaphase, and small adjacent portions of prophase and telophase, the phases of mitosis that are recognizable in ordinary microscopic preparations. Although useful, the concept of four *discrete* phases may not be strictly correct. Recent observations using high resolution microscopy show that early prophase overlaps G_2 and even late S, and late telophase extends into G_1 [33]. The cell cycle measurements for which practical methods exist are summarized in (Table 2).

Mitotic Index

Mitotic frequency has been used as a component of grading systems for breast carcinoma in conjunction with other nuclear features and assessment of differ-

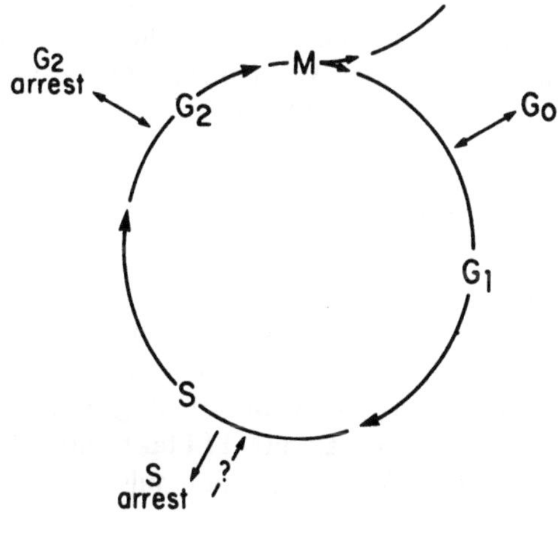

Fig. 4. The cell cycle. G_1 and G_2 are apparent gaps in activity that separate the S-phase (DNA synthesis) from the M-phase (mitosis). Cells can enter and leave the cell cycle in G_1 and G_2. They can leave, but probably not re-enter in M (colchicine-induced mitotic arrest, for example) or S (S-phase arrest associated with local vascular insufficiency within tumors)

Table 2. Various cell cycle and DNA measurements

Measurement	Method	Comment
M-phase	Mitotic count	Impractical for many breast carcinomas because of very low mitotic index
	Monoclonal antibody	Practical; fresh frozen tissue
S-phase	Thymidine labeling	Practical for clinical use; fresh tissue required
	Bromodeoxyuridine labeling	Similar to thymidine, but more rapid
	Microdensitometry	Possible, but too slow; best results on smears
	Flow cytometry	Practical, but occasionally gives misleading results; fresh or frozen tissue
G_1-phase	Flow cytometry	Practical
	Microdensitometry	Too slow
G_2-phase	Flow cytometry	Practical
S-phase duration	Double labeling	Practical with [^{3}H] thymidine + bromodeoxyuridine
	FLM curve analysis	Impractical; requires multiple biopsies
Growth fraction	Primer-dependent DNA polymerase (PDP)	Difficult
	Monoclonal antibody	Practical; fresh or frozen tissue required
DNA index	Microdensitometry	Time-consuming, best results on smears
	Flow cytometry	Practical with fresh, frozen, or paraffin-embedded tissue

entiation [14]. Actual counting of mitotic figures has been accomplished by determination of the frequency per high power field because of the scarcity of mitoses in most breast carcinomas [7, 67]. The neoplastic cells of breast carcinomas are associated with variable amounts of reactive stroma and inflammatory cells so that the high power field method lacks specificity. Nonetheless, multivariate analysis of the data of Baak and associates showed the mitotic count to be one of only three independent predictors of survival of breast carcinoma patients in multivariate analysis [7]. The other predictors were lymph nodal status and size of the primary tumor. Wallgren and Zajicek also found the mitotic index to be a major predictor of survival [126].

DNA Labeling Procedures

These procedures have the advantage of yielding indices sufficiently high to permit accurate measurements of neoplastic cells. Clinical and pathologic correlations have been accomplished with the thymidine labeling index (TLI). The bromodeoxyuridine labeling index (BrUdRLI) gives results essentially similar to TLI and offers the advantage of rapidity. TLI takes more than 1 week because of the time required for exposure of photographic emulsion to mark the labeled cells in autoradiographs

(Figs. 5, 6). BrUdR-labeled cells are detectable histochemically by use of monoclonal antibodies against BrUdR in DNA (Figs. 5, 6), and the results can be available within 48 h. Correlation between the two labeling methods, thymidine and bromodeoxyuridine, is good (Fig. 7). In either case, viable tissues is required. Tissue can be held at room temperature for up to 2 h [73] and in the refrigerator at approximately 4°C for 24 h (J.S. Meyer and J.L. Craver 1984, unpublished work) without affecting the labeling index. To effect labeling, thin slices (0.5-1 mm) are cut freehand and placed in Hanks' balanced salt solution prior to incubation with the DNA precursor under hyperbaric oxygen [75]. Addition of 5-fluoro-2'-deoxyuridine (FUdR) in a concentration of 10 μM enhances uptake of labeled thymidine [78] or bromodeoxyuridine [31] by blocking endogenous synthesis of thymidylate from deoxyuridine as catalyzed by thymidine synthase [54]. The autoradiographs (TLI) or histochemical preparations (BrUdRLI) are comparable to ordinary tissue sections in histologic detail so that the cells of interest can be identified and evaluated without inclusion of extraneous inflammatory or stromal cells. Tissues can be disaggregated prior to labeling, but relationships useful in identifying cells are thereby lost and the labeling indices may be reduced because of damage to cells by the disaggregating procedure [24].

As with any measurement, effects of sampling must be considered for the TLI. Smallwood and co-workers expressed concern about sampling variation [110].

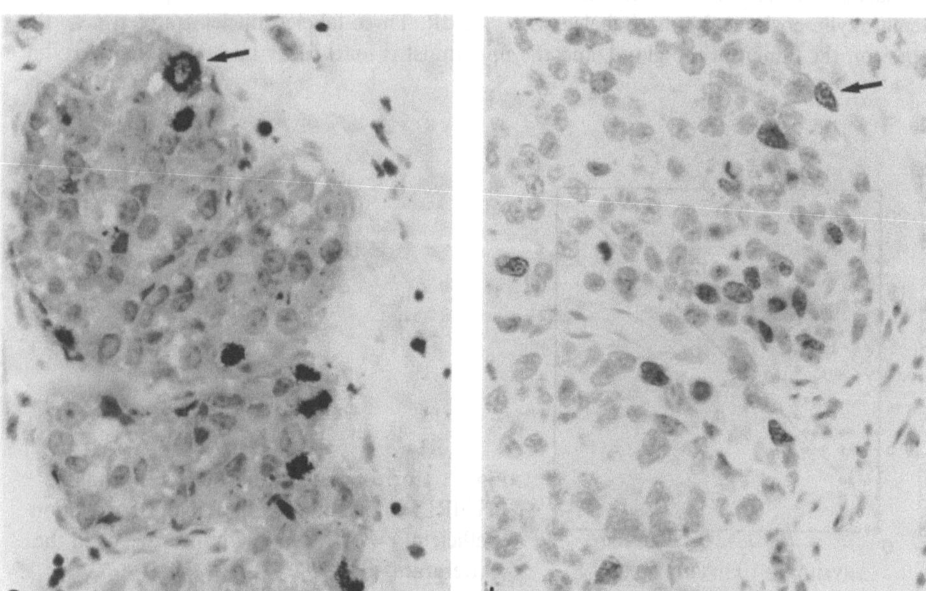

Fig. 5a, b. Breast carcinoma with high labeling indices, TLI = 22%. **a** Labeled with [^{3}H] thymidine. The S-phase nuclei are covered by silver grains and their nuclei appear black. The uppermost labeled nucleus is marked by an *arrow*. Hematoxylin-eosin, × 540. **b** Labeled with BrUdR. Contrast between labeled and unlabeled nuclei is less, but nuclear detail is preserved. The uppermost labeled nucleus is marked by an *arrow*. Hematoxylin, × 540

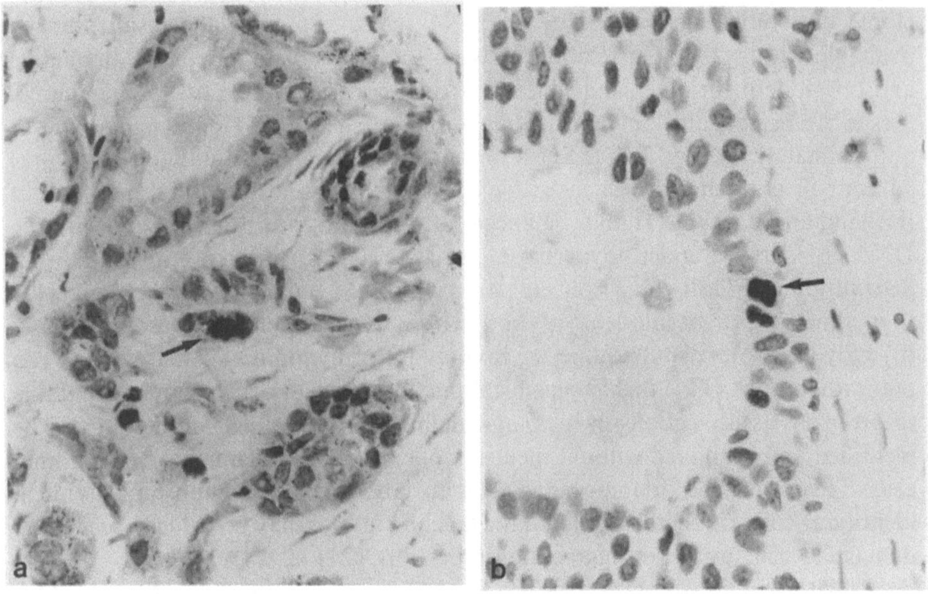

Fig. 6a, b. Breast carcinoma with low labeling indices, TLI = 4.3%. **a** Labeled with [^{3}H] thymidine. Only one labeled nucleus is present (*arrow*). Scattered grains over cytoplasm of neoplastic cells are ascribable to transmethylation of the labeled methyl group of thymidine. Hematoxylin-eosin, × 540. **b** Labeled with BrUdR. Three labeled nuclei are seen near the center on the lumen of the gland, and the uppermost is marked by an *arrow*. Hematoxylin, × 540

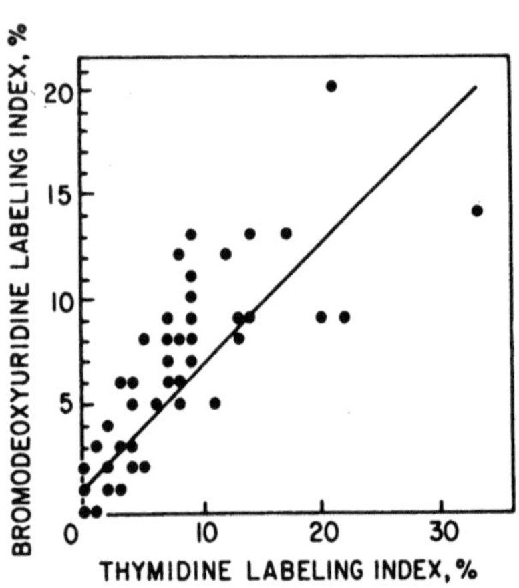

Fig. 7. Correspondence between TLI and BrUdRLI in 56 tumors. Spearman's correlation coefficient, $r = 0.81$. No far outliers occur in the scattergram

Their procedure for thymidine labeling or perhaps their selection of tumors yielded a narrow range of TLI, 0.37%-5.6% in 18 carcinomas, with the upper limit of the range scarcely at the median value for our laboratory. When TLIs are low, the relative variation of repeat samplings is large. In our study of 38 paired samples from the primary carcinoma, we noted by linear correlation analysis $r = 0.90$, and for 68 primary carcinomas versus their axillary metastases $r = 0.89$ for log TLI. Substantial correlation was also observed between the TLIs of 18 primary carcinomas and their recurrent or metastatic lesions ($r = 0.75$). Our range of TLI values extended from 0.05% to 35%, median 5.5% [81, 83]. In a study of 40 breast carcinomas, Costa and associates also obtained a significant correlation between TLI of the primary tumor and of the axillary metastasis ($r = 0.52$) [23]. We believe that TLI is a reliable measurement in breast carcinoma that is not much influenced by variation in sampling.

The uptake of [^{3}H] TdR can also be measured by homogenizing the tissue and measuring the specific activity of DNA in a scintillation counter. This method is unsuitable for kinetic studies because breast carcinoma cells cannot be distinguished from other cells that contribute DNA. Furthermore, variations in specific activity can occur without corresponding variations in TLI. This has been observed on stimulation of cultured breast carcinoma cells with estradiol, and could reflect induction of thymidine kinase with resultant enhanced transport of [^{3}H] TdR into the cells [56]. Without autoradiographic control, such a change could be misinterpreted as a proliferative response.

Estimation of % S-Phase by Static Microdensitometry or Microfluorimetry of DNA

This method requires availability of whole nuclei. It can be done on smears or cytospin preparations on glass slides. Tissue sections are less satisfactory because G_2 nuclei cleaved by the sectioning process will give spuriously low DNA readings, but DNA-aneuploidy can be distinguished nonetheless [129]. DNA can be stained stochiometrically by the Feulgen method, in which case specific ultraviolet absorption is measured [17], or alternatively, with DNA-specific fluorescent dyes to allow measurement of emitted light [112]. Excellent resolution is now obtainable, but probably not so good as with flow cytometry [1, 112]. The ability to identify and select individual cells for measurement is an important advantage. Extraneous cells, for example lymphocytes and other inflammatory cells, can be excluded to some extent, particularly in aneuploid carcinomas [112]. This advantage is counterbalanced by the expenditure of time.

Estimation of % S-Phase by Flow Cytometry of DNA

This method has the advantage of automation, and thousands of cells can be evaluated rapidly. It requires preparation of a suspension of single cells or nuclei in which inflammatory and stromal cells are unavoidably included along with the neoplastic cells of interest. The DNA is stained with a fluorescent dye, and the fluorescence of each cell is evaluated electronically as the cells flow singly through a high intensity beam of appropriate wavelength for excitation of the dye [102]. The continuum of fluorescence intensity is divided into intervals called channels so that a doubling of the channel number is equivalent to a doubling of the fluorescence.

Thus, if the G_1/G_0 cells were placed at channel 100, the G_2/M cells would be at channel 200. A histogram plotting fluorescent intensity against number of cells is generated by a computer (Fig. 8).

Elimination of non-neoplastic cells from the flow cytometric histogram would be desirable. Dual parameter measurements utilizing protein content, cell volume, or staining for antigens specific to neoplastic cells may prove useful. Up to now, no notable improvement in flow cytometric analysis of breast carcinoma has been achieved by these means. The effect of contamination by host stromal cells is likely to be most troublesome when the neoplastic cells have diploid or nearly diploid DNA content (Fig. 8).

If the tumor has a high % S-phase, but many lymphocytes are present, the % S-phase will appear to be lower than it is [77]. When the neoplastic cells have hyperdiploid DNA contents, interference by diploid host cells can usually be avoided in the analysis of the histogram (Fig. 8). However, not all of the neoplastic cells may be hyperdiploid; some may be diploid [96], and the latter cells would be lost to the analysis.

Comparison of the TLI with % S-phase of breast carcinomas measured by flow cytometric quantitation of DNA has yielded correlation coefficients in the range $r = 0.12$-0.43 for diploid carcinomas, whereas for aneuploid carcinomas the correlations have been better, in the range $r = 0.59$-0.73 [77, 82]. When breast carcinomas of both ploidy types, diploid and aneuploid, are included together, the correlation

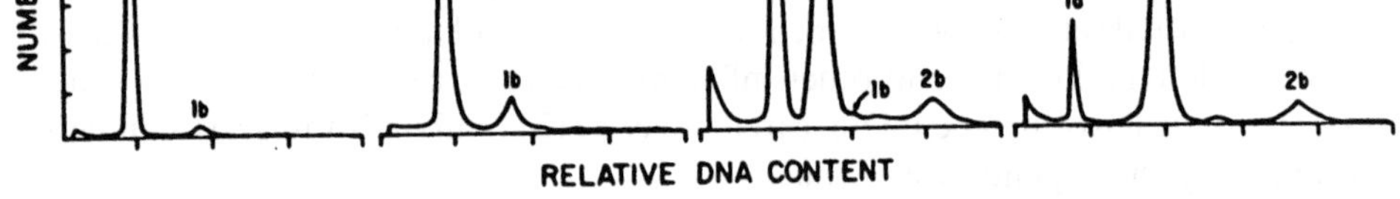

Fig. 8. a Flow cytometric histogram of diploid breast carcinoma with low proliferative index, % S-phase = 3%. Coefficient of variation of G_1/G_0 population (peak 1a) = 3.2%. Peak 1b represents the G_2/M cells. DNA index = 1.0. **b** Flow cytometric histogram of diploid breast carcinoma (with higher % S-phase = 8.5%). Note that the number of S-phase events keeps the region between the two peaks above the baseline. DNA index = 1.0. **c** Flow cytometric histogram of aneuploid (hyperdiploid) breast carcinoma with a high proliferative index, % S-phase = 14%. G_1/G_0 and G_2/M peaks of the diploid population are marked 1a and 1b, respectively, and those of the aneuploid population are marked 2a and 2b. DNA index = 1.65. **d** Flow cytometric histogram of aneuploid (hypertetraploid) breast carcinoma, showing that aneuploidy is not always associated with high % S-phase, here only 4%. Peaks are labeled as in previous histogram. The diploid G_2/M peak is buried in the aneuploid G_1/M peak. DNA index = 2.5

coefficients are comparable to those for hyperdiploid carcinomas alone because the diploid carcinomas tend to have low TLI.

Comparison of flow cytometric % S-phase with TLI has shown that both the method of analysis of the histogram and the method of preparation of the specimen are important in obtaining accurate estimates of % S-phase. The analysis has to take into account whether or not the rate of DNA synthesis varies during the S-phase, a question not yet clearly answered. If DNA synthesis began at a relatively slow rate, peaked in mid S-phase, and then slowed down again [26, 98], a considerable proportion of S-phase events would fall within the G_1/G_0 and G_2/M peaks in the DNA histogram rather than in the S-phase plateau. Algorithms have been devised that take this into account when calculating % S-phase from DNA histograms [29, 40, 41]. These algorithms perform very well for DNA histograms of cultured cells with high % S-phase [8, 98]. If the rate of DNA synthesis remained constant throughout the S-phase, a rectangular model would be appropriate [9]. Rectangular models also perform well for cultured cells [8]. In our experience, the highest correlations between TLI and % S-phase by flow cytometry in breast carcinoma have been achieved with a mathematically simple rectangular or parallelogram estimate of % S-phase based on the minimum height of the interval between G_1/G_0 and G_2/M [67, 131]. This analysis assumes no large number of S-phase cells to be present within the G_1/G_0 and G_2/M peaks, and it is not confounded by skews in these peaks resulting from other causes. Methods of preparation that reduce debris in the histograms also increase the accuracy of % S phase measurement [69, 130]. Fluorescent debris tends to increase apparent % S-phase.

Haag has defined the debris curve by an exponential function, and debris can now be subtracted mathematically from DNA histograms [47, 48]. When this is done, % S-phase tends to approximate the TLI. Otherwise, % S-phase derived from flow cytometry is 1.5-2 times the TLI measured in the same set of tumors [47, 77, 82, 130, 131]. The contribution of debris to the S-phase region of DNA histograms can be 90% or more of the total events, and can result in gross overestimation of % S-phase [47, 48, 131]. It is now clear that debris subtraction is necessary when evaluating % S-phase of human mammary carcinomas.

Measurement of % S-Phase by Flow Cytometric Analysis After Labeling with BrUdR

By staining with monoclonal anti-BrUdR, S-phase cells that have incorporated BrUdR can be identified by flow cytometry [28, 127]. This is a means of increasing the accuracy of flow cytometric % S-phase , but it is not currently practical for use in the majority of breast carcinoma patients. Labeling of S-phase cells can be accomplished by infusion of BrUdR shortly before excision of tissue, but would probably not be acceptable when the diagnosis of carcinoma is uncertain. In vitro BrUdR-labeled tissue could be dissociated for flow cytometry, but the practicality of this approach has not been tested, and the problem of identifying neoplastic cells would remain unsolved.

Measurement of Growth Fraction

The growth fraction was defined by Mendelsohn [71] as the fraction of cells in the mitotic cycle. A cell is considered to be in cycle if it is progressing toward mitosis. If it is not so progressing, it is considered to be in the G_0 fraction (see Fig. 1). Growth fractions of neoplasms can vary within wide limits from 10% or less, to virtually 100% [43, 65, 70, 72]. The term "growth fraction" should not be used loosely to indicate TLI or % S-phase. TLI or % S-phase will always be less than the growth fraction, for the cycling cells that comprise the growth fraction are in all parts of the cell cycle, G_1, G_2, and M, in addition to S. The growth fraction can be estimated by labeling procedures, but the cells must be exposed to the label for an interval equal to the longest cell cycle time of the population to ensure that all cycling cells are labeled. Methods available for clinical application include the primer-dependent DNA polymerase labeling method of Schiffer and associates [100] and a monoclonal antibody, Ki-67 [44], that may recognize a DNA polymerase epitope. The labeling method utilizes labeled nucleotide triphosphates to which viable cells are exposed prior to autoradiography to detect labeling. Only light labeling is achieved by this method, and autoradiographic results often are not clear-cut. The Ki-67 antibody produces clear-cut results. All cycling cells are marked. Frozen sections of unfixed tissue are required; the method does not work on fixed, paraffin-embedded material. The antigen is easily eluted unless the frozen sections are fixed in organic solvents.

The DNA Index: Methodology

The DNA index is the DNA content of a G_1/G_0 population of interest relative to the DNA content of normal G_1/G_0 cells. It can be measured by static microdensitometry, microfluorimetry, or by flow cytometry. Usually it is expressed as a multiple of 1 (Fig. 8). Static and flow cytometric measurements of DNA are insufficiently precise to detect minor quantitative changes associated with translocations, gene amplifications in homogeneously staining regions, and double minute chromosomes. The DNA index does correlate well with the modal chromosome number [10, 121].

Classical Cell Kinetics Studies in Breast Carcinoma

Cell kinetics implies motion of cells through the cell cycle. Motion can be measured only by making observations at intervals, and not by one observation at a point in time such as a mitotic index, TLI, or % S-phase. The classic approach to cell kinetics measurements is the fraction of labeled mitosis (FLM) curve [114]. An FLM curve is constructed by counting labeled mitotic figures after a single dose of tritiated thymidine. Ideally several peaks should result, and the interval between successive peaks is equivalent to the mean cell cycle time. In practice with human tumors, the curve is so greatly dampened by variability in transit times of individual cells that only one distinct peak can be appreciated. Nonetheless, analysis of FLM curves can provide estimates of cell cycle duration T_c, and G_1, S, G_2, and M transit times. These estimates must be interpreted with caution because FLM curves are much more influenced by rapidly cycling populations of cells than slowly cycling populations in tumors that are heterogeneous for cell cycle transit time. The prerequisites for obtaining FLM curves preclude their routine application, and only a few have been done for breast carcinomas. The results indicate that S-phase transit (T_s) is approximately 18 h, G_2 approximately 4 h, G_1 highly variable, and M (essentially metaphase and anaphase only) less than 1 h [72]. T_s can also be estimated by double labeling. This procedure depends on differentiation of one precursor [^{3}H]-thymidine) from another ([^{14}C] thymidine) by differential autoradiography, or by use of a radiolabeled precursor in conjunction with a precursor which is detectable histochemically (BrUdR, for example). Studies by double labeling have given similar (99) or slightly shorter estimates of T_s in the range of 12-16 h [18].

Another way to gain insight into the dynamics of cellular proliferation is to give [^{3}H] TdR at short intervals or as a continuous infusion with assessment of the percentage of labeled mitoses at intervals. This will allow an approximation of the length of G_1 and estimation of the growth fraction. Data obtained by Post and coworkers [95] using this method indicate that breast carcinomas with low TLIs have prolonged or highly variable G_1 durations. This conclusion was based on the failure of the FLM to approximate 100% after continuous administration of [^{3}H] TdR. In one patient, fewer than 20% of mitoses were labeled after 72 h of continuous exposure to the precursor. Straus and associates administered [^{3}H] TdR repeatedly to a patient with multiple chest wall recurrent tumors and an initial TLI of 22%, and obtained a maximum TLI of only 40% after 5 days [117]. Another way to interpret these findings is that a large G_0 compartment is feeding cells into G_1, and at the same time is being replenished by cells entering G_0 from G_1.

The measured doubling times of breast carcinomas consistently exceed potential doubling times computed from labeling index data [72]. Malaise and coworkers estimated cell loss of approximately two-thirds from TLI data [66]. Higher TLIs subsequently obtained by others [42, 83, 117, 118] indicate even greater cell loss.

Results of Measurements with Widespread Clinical Applicability

The TLI, DNA index, and % S-phase by DNA measurement have been used to characterize groups of patients in several institutions. Both TLI and % S-phase distributions are consistently positively skewed and have been described as lognormal [83, 99] (Fig. 9) or exponential [42, 104]. The TLI values were higher when incubations with tritiated thymidine were carried out under hyperbaric oxygen in the presence of thymidylate synthase inhibition [78]. In a series of 757 primary infiltrating breast carcinomas, the median TLI was 5.2%, mean 7.1%, and the range 0% (one case) to 35% [83]. Without hyperbaric oxygen and thymidylate synthase inhibition, results were lower [104, 105, 122]. With enzymatic dissociation

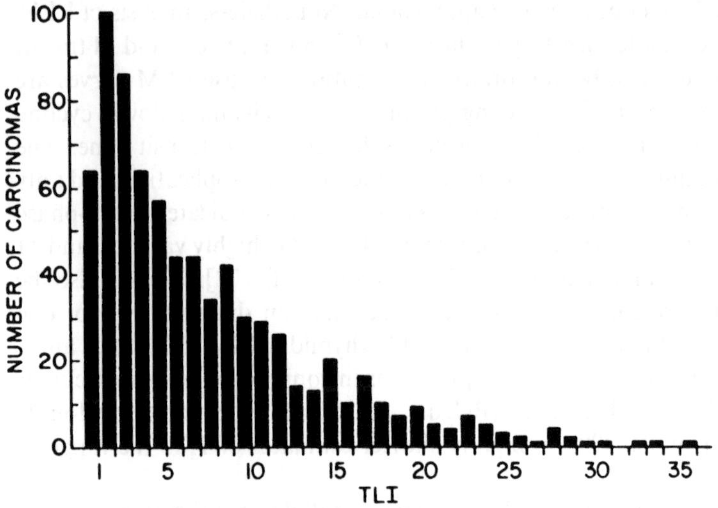

Fig. 9. Frequency distribution of TLI in 757 primary infiltrating breast carcinomas measured with hyperbaric oxygen and inhibition of thymidylate synthase [83]

to reduce debris levels [69] or with subtraction of fluorescent debris [32, 47], median % S-phase by flow cytometry was similar to the results of optimal thymidine labeling. When mechanical dissociation was used without subtraction of debris, median % S-phase was one and one-half times or twice as high as median TLI [52, 61, 62, 77, 92].

DNA ploidy measurements by microdensitometry, microfluorimetry, and flow cytometry have demonstrated aneuploidy or tetraploidy in 50%-92% of breast carcinomas, whereas 8%-50% had diploid DNA content. A consensus figure would be approximately 60%-70% aneuploidy by current methods of static or flow cytometric DNA analysis. The majority of aneuploid breast carcinomas have DNA contents between the diploid and tetraploid levels ($1 < \text{DNA index} < 2$), some are hypertetraploid (DNA index > 2), and very few are hypodiploid (DNA index < 1).

Two studies of the growth fraction in a total of 187 primary invasive breast carcinomas based on labeling with the Ki-67 antibody showed means of 15% and 20% and a range of 3%-60% (65, 70). By primer-dependent DNA polymerase assay in 88 primary invasive carcinomas, the mean was 29% and the range 8%-100% [99].

Relationships Between Cell Kinetics or DNA Index and Other Prognostic Factors

Fairly strong relationships exist between the TLI and DNA content of breast carcinoma and other prognostic variables (Tables 3, 4). In general, a proportional relationship has been found between, on one hand, the size of the breast carcinoma, the histologic and nuclear grades, inflammatory findings and other indications of rapid progression at the primary site and, on the other hand, TLI. An inverse relationship has been observed for age, controversial as a prognostic variable [55, 88], ER and PR contents on one hand and TLI on the other hand. No significant relationship has been noted between TLI and the number of axillary lymph nodes or the presence or absence of distant metastases at time of initial diagnosis of breast carcinoma. For aneuploidy versus diploidy, the findings generally parallel those of TLI wherein aneuploidy is equated to high TLI. We can now consider each of several prognostic variables in relationship to kinetic and DNA measurements.

Age

Age is inversely related to TLI, but the relationship is a weak one and is statistically significant only when large numbers of patients are considered [12, 83, 104].

Table 3. Correlates of TLI[a]

Source	No.	Age	Size	Nodes	Metastases	Histology	ER	PR
Milan (42)	541	−	+	0			−	
Villejuif (122)	98		+	0				
St. Louis (83)	757	−	+	0	+	+	−	−
Valhalla (117, 118)	32			0			−	

[a] Negative correlation is indicated by −; positive correlation by +; no correlation by 0. When no data were presented, the space is left blank.

Table 4. Correlates of DNA index[a]

Source	No.	Age	Size	Nodes	Metastases	Histology	ER	PR
Leiden (22)	565		0	0			−	
Sydney (52, 119)	473	+		+			+	
Winston-Salem (62)	226	0	0	Tr+			−	−
Lund (35)	638	0	+	Tr+				
Oslo (120)	59	Tr+	0	0			0	
Houston (11)	43	0	0	0		0	0	
Aarhus (13)	46					+	−	
Tampere (57)	92	0	Tr+	Tr+			Tr−	−
New York (91)	92					+	−	
Stockholm (58)	210						0	
Nedlands (49)	80			+			+	
St. Louis (68)	168	0				+	+	

[a] + indicates a significant positive relationship; Tr+ a positive relationship of borderline significance; − a significant negative relationship; Tr− a negative relationship of borderline significance; 0 no relationship; blank space indicates no data presented.

Essentially any TLI within the entire observed range, from nearly 0% to 35%-40%, can occur at any age, but low TLIs are unusual in young patients and are much commoner after age 60 years (Fig. 10). This may relate to the proliferative status of the mammary epithelium at the time of carcinogenesis, since the lobular epithelial proliferative index declines with age [46, 76]. Aneuploidy was more frequent in postmenopausal than in premenopausal patients, but % S-phase tended to be higher in premenopausal patients, in agreement with thymidine labeling studies [52].

Size of Primary Tumor

The size of the primary tumor is significantly related to TLI, with an upward trend in TLI with increasing size up to 8 cm. The correlation between size and TLI, however, is low ($r = 0.17$, log TLI versus diameter). Therefore, the two variables are only weakly related, and a wide range of TLIs is found for any size of tumor [83]. Gentili and co-workers, however, found a significant relationship only in the premenopausal patients with negative lymph nodes [42]. The DNA index did not relate to size of the tumor [22].

Histologic Type of Tumor

Thymidine labeling [74, 83] and flow cytometric studies [34, 68, 87, 92] show that the proliferative rates of adenocystic carcinomas, mucinous carcinomas with small nuclei, tubular and probably papillary carcinomas are consistently low. These carcinomas all have distinctively good prognosis. Most infiltrating lobular carci-

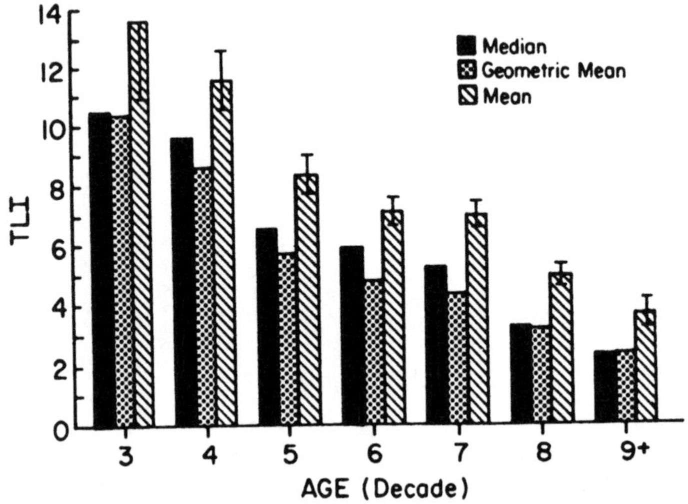

Fig. 10. Relationship between TLI and age of patient [83]

nomas also have low TLIs, although they have high metastatic rates. Medullary carcinomas consistently have high TLIs despite their low tendency toward metastasis. These and other special forms comprise only 20% of breast carcinomas. The remaining tumors, termed not otherwise specified (NOS) [37] or infiltrating duct carcinoma, show a wide spectrum of TLI or flow cytometric % S-phase. Not unexpectedly, in view of the relationship between TLI and diploidy versus aneuploidy, breast carcinomas with low TLIs are usually diploid, whereas medullary carcinomas are usually aneuploid [34, 68, 87].

Stage of Tumor

TLI relates only weakly to the number of axillary lymph nodal metastases. Even with 757 carcinomas analyzed, the trend toward higher TLI with more metastatic nodes failed to reach statistical significance ($P = 0.06$) [83]. Other studies have also shown the same trend, but without statistical significance [42, 100, 122]. The flow cytometric % S-phase showed the same trend as the TLI, but no stronger [52].

By either Feulgen microdensitometry [39] or flow cytometry [52], tumors with aneuploid DNA content are associated with a higher clinical stage than diploid tumors, but the relationship is not a strong one. In 565 primary breast cancers, Cornelisse and co-workers [22] found no correlation between DNA index and stage.

Estrogen and Progesterone Receptors

Although attempts to relate ER and PR status to histologic characteristics of breast carcinomas have yielded variable results, TLI has consistently shown an inverse relationship to ER content [21, 86, 104, 105, 118]. The relationship in our experience was stepwise for PR, but all or none for ER. The weakly ER-positive carcinomas had TLIs as high as the carcinomas which were strongly ER-positive. Despite impressive *P* values for the inverse correlations, the correlation coefficients have been low ($r = 0.19$-0.4) [83]. In fact, one cannot predict either the receptor content from the TLI or vice versa with any confidence in an individual case. Tumors with either high or low receptor values can have either high or low TLIs. The relationships therefore have only scientific interest rather than practical clinical value. Microdensitometric measurements of DNA in smears of breast carcinomas have shown a relationship between ploidy and ER. Diploid carcinomas were usually ER-positive, whereas aneuploid tumors were usually ER-negative [3, 39].

Several studies have related flow cytometric % S-phase and DNA index to receptor concentrations, with mixed results. Olszewski and co-workers [91, 92] found an inverse relationship for both variables with ER content. Raber and co-workers noted a significant inverse relationship between % S-phase and ER content [97]. Kute and co-workers confirmed this finding for ER and in addition demonstrated that PR-negativity was significantly associated with aneuploidy [62]. They also showed that a high proliferative index, as measured by flow cytometry, significantly predicted for the lack of either receptor. Dressler and co-workers, in a study of 1331 patients, observed a strong inverse relationship between both DNA index and % S-phase and both ER and PR status [32]. Kallioniemi and associates observed a significant tendency for aneuploid tumors to be PR-negative and a trend for them to be ER-negative [57].

The broad range of proliferative indices found in ER-positive carcinomas has led to speculation that the proliferative rate might predict response in this group. In fact, two studies have shown a significant inverse relationship between TLI and hormonal response [80, 94]. Nordenskjold and associates measured TLI of aspirates from breast carcinoma before and after hormonal therapy and noted decrease in TLI only in responders [90].

The DNA Index and Proliferative Index

Aneuploidy has been consistently associated with a tendency toward high TLI [77, 82] or % S-phase [25, 61, 77, 82, 92], but it does not guarantee that % S-phase or TLI will be high in a given tumor. Nor does diploidy guarantee low TLI or % S-phase. We have found no relationship whatsoever in aneuploid tumors between the degree of aneuploidy and the % S-phase or TLI [77].

Prognostic Value of the DNA Index, TLI, and % S-Phase

DNA Index

The first evidence that the DNA content of breast carcinoma cells was related to prognosis came from the microdensitometric studies of Auer and associates and Atkin [2, 4]. These retrospective studies utilized archival breast carcinoma smears. DNA per cell was measured by ultraviolet absorbance after Feulgen staining. In both studies, carcinomas with clear peaks only in the diploid and tetraploid regions of the DNA histogram were associated with few relapses, whereas relapses were common when appreciable numbers of cells had DNA contents intermediate between diploid and tetraploid or beyond the tetraploid zone. A recent study by Opferman and coworkers [93] has confirmed these results, but with the conclusion that the ploidy profile was not a strong enough predictor to be of much value. Auer and Tribukait have shown an excellent correlation between static microdensitometric and flow cytometric DNA measurements in breast carcinoma [6], a finding confirmed by Fallenius and coworkers [36]. Stal and associates have similar findings from comparison of static microfluorimetry with flow cytometry [112]. This indicates that valid results are achieved by either static or flow methods.

Development of a method for flow cytometry of archival paraffin blocks by Hedley and coworkers [50] permitted retrospective study and quickly showed the DNA index to be prognostic [53, 57] (Table 5). Although the DNA index at first appeared to be a promising prognostic marker, a recent comprehensive analysis utilizing archival paraffin-embedded tissue proved it to be a relatively weak

Table 5. Prognostic value of DNA index[a]

Source	No.	General	Stage I	Stage II	Stage III	Stage IV	Metastases	Independence[b]
Leiden (22)	565	+						+
Sydney (52)	490	+		+				0
Miami (25)	74	+						
San Antonio (32)	327		+					+
Stockholm (58)	210	0						

[a] Indicates a significant prognostic relationship: 0 no significant relationship; blank space indicates no data presented.
[b] Independent prognostic relationship by multivariate analysis.

prognostic factor [51, 52]. Klintenberg and associates found the DNA index to be nonprognostic [58]. Our observation that the TLI is not correlated with the DNA index of *aneuploid* tumors [77] may explain the finding of Hedley and Rugg that the DNA index of *aneuploid* tumors did not relate to outcome [52]. Not only was an increasing DNA index in the aneuploid range not associated with declines in relapse-free survival and overall survival, but carcinomas with more than one aneuploid line were no worse than those with a single aneuploid line. These observations suggest that the proliferative index, not the DNA content, is the chief prognostic factor.

When Hedley and Rugg applied multivariate analysis to their data, they found that the DNA index did not predict independently of the axillary nodal status, but % S-phase did [53]. However, % S-phase did not predict independently of the histologic grade. The latter is based on structural characteristics, nuclear features, and the mitotic index, each of which relates strongly to % S-phase or TLI [68, 83]. A variety of prognostic indicators, which include histologic variables, DNA index, and oncogene amplification [109], may all operate through a relationship to the proliferative index.

Recently, Harvey and associates confirmed a strong prognostic relationship for the DNA index determined *microdensitometrically* rather than by flow cytometry [49]. The DNA index was prognostic, independent of tumor size, ER and nodal involvement, and was the strongest prognostic indicator of all these variables. They suggested that microdensitometric measurement of DNA may be superior to flow cytometric measurement because microdensitometry permits selection of neoplastic cells recognized by cytologic criteria, whereas flow cytometry includes all cells.

Tumor Labeling Index (TLI)

The frequency distribution of TLIs of 757 primary infiltrating breast carcinomas is shown in Fig. 9. All measurements were made with hyperbaric oxygen and blockade of thymidylate synthesis so that S-phase cells were well defined by high grain counts in autoradiographs. The median TLI was 5.2%, and the mean was 7.1%. The ranges of 0%-3%, 3.1%-8%, and 8.1%-35.5% divided the population into equal thirds [84]. The TLI has been shown to be a prognostic indicator for breast carcinoma in stage I [42, 79, 84, 106] (Fig. 11), to a lesser extent for stage II breast carcinomas [42, 79, 84], and in breast carcinoma after relapse [80] (Table 6). In the studies by Silvestrini et al. [105] and us [84], the prognostic power of TLI in node-negative or stage I patients was independent of ER content. It was also independent of PR content in the one study in which adequate PR data were

Table 6. Prognostic value of TLI[a]

Source	No.	General	Stage I	Stage II	Relapsed	Independence[b]
Milan (42, 106)	541	+	+	+ −		+
Villejuif (123)	98	+				+
St. Louis (80, 83)	326	+	+	+	+	+
Valhalla (117)	32	+				

[a] Significant prognostic relationship is indicated by +; a trend by + −; no data by blank space.
[b] Independent prognostic relationship by multivariate analysis.

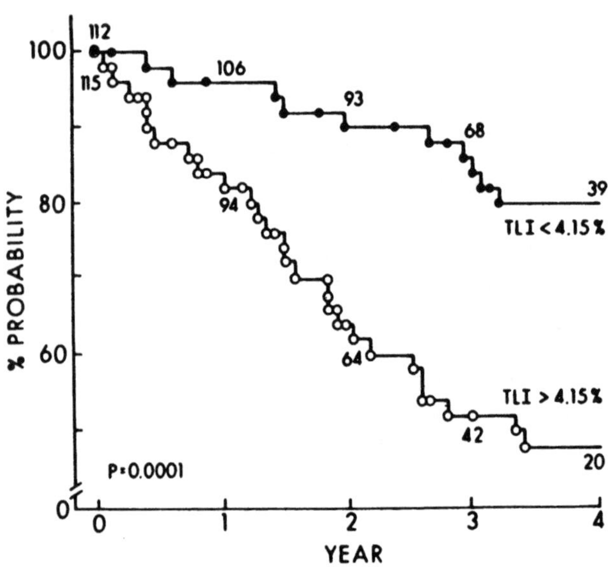

Fig. 11. Relapse-free survival of patients with breast carcinomas, American Joint Committee stage I, relative to TLI. Low TLI predicted a high probability of survival [79]

available [84]. In the node-positive group of breast carcinoma patients, TLI predicts within stage II (Fig. 12). In stage III (massive local tumor volume), we found that TLI did not predict significantly, although a trend exists toward improved relapse-free survival with low TLI (Fig. 13). In contrast to the loss of statistical power with large tumor size, TLI retained predictiveness in the presence of many positive axillary lymph nodes (Fig. 14). Here, as perhaps in the lower stages, the proliferative index does not predict ultimate death or relapse so much as the timing of death or relapse. When many nodes are positive, the natural history appears to include relapse in nearly all patients. Nonetheless, the group with low TLI clearly shows postponement of relapse, and of death once relapse has occurred. An interplay with ER is suspected here, for low TLI is associated with ER-positivity, and the latter with prolongation of survival on hormonal treatment. In patients presenting with stage IV, TLI was also predictive for outcome (Fig. 15).

Role of % S-Phase by Flow Cytometry

Distributions of % S-phase measured by flow cytometry in breast carcinomas vary from one laboratory to another according to methods of flow cytometry and algorithms used to derive % S-phase from the DNA histograms. When corrections for debris were not made, the median % S-phase was usually approximately twice the median TLI measured in the author's laboratory. Various studies have used the median % S-phase as the boundary for prognostic evaluations. Kallioniemi and

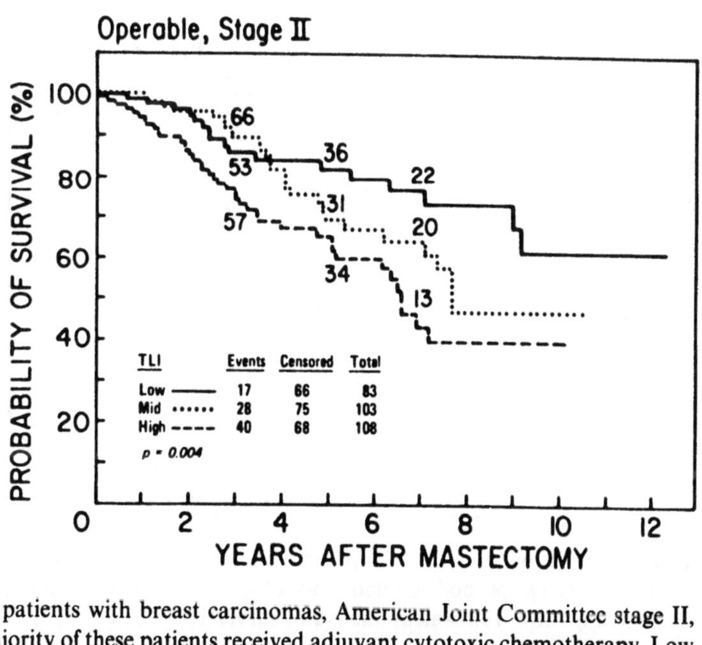

Fig. 12. Survival of patients with breast carcinomas, American Joint Committee stage II, relative to TLI. A majority of these patients received adjuvant cytotoxic chemotherapy. Low or intermediate TLI predicted a relatively high probability of survival

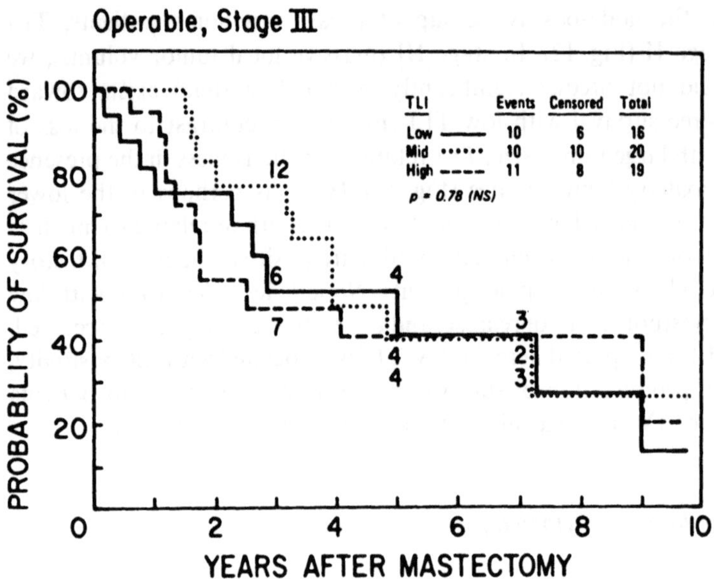

Fig. 13. Survival of patients with breast carcinomas, American Joint Committee stage III, relative to TLI. A majority of these patients received adjuvant cytotoxic chemotherapy. TLI did not predict

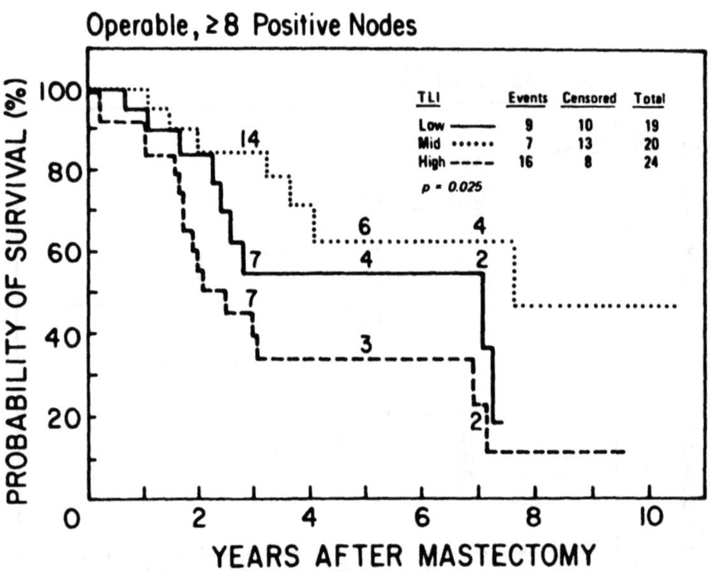

Fig. 14. Survival of patients with operable breast carcinoma with at least eight metastasis-bearing axillary lymph nodes, relative to TLI. Most patients received adjuvant cytotoxic chemotherapy. Low TLI was predictive of survival

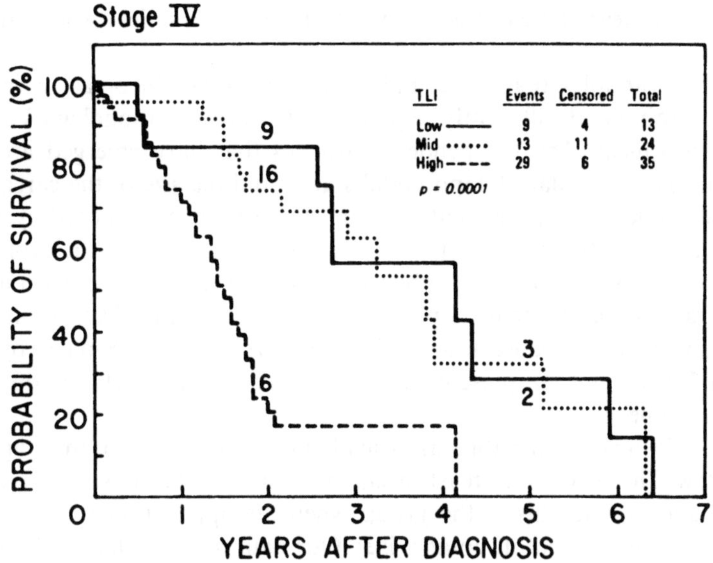

Fig. 15. Survival of stage IV breast carcinoma patients. Those with high TLIs had a significantly reduced probability of survival in comparison with those with intermediate or low TLIs

Table 7. Prognostic value of the % S-phase by flow cytometry[a]

Source	No.	General	Stage				Metastasses	Independence[b]
			I	II	III	IV		
Tampere (57)	59	+						
Sydney (52)	285			+				
San Antonio (32)	215		+				+	
Stockholm (58)	177	+	+	+			+	

[a] Significant prognostic power is indicated by +; no data by blank space.
[b] Independent prognostic relationship by multivariate analysis.

associates observed that % S-phase was a better predictor of survival and relapse-free survival than the DNA index [57]. Hedley and Rugg [52, 53] noted that % S-phase from paraffin-embedded tissue was prognostic in node-positive breast carcinomas. % S-phase determined flow cytometrically from paraffin-embedded tissue was a better predictor of survival and relapse-free survival than the DNA index [57, 58]. Klintenberg and associates [58] found that % S-phase was an independent prognostic entity along with the axillary lymph nodal status and the results of ER assay, whereas the DNA index was ineffective. Dressler and co-workers presented evidence that % S-phase by flow cytometry of frozen tissue was an independent predictor of survival in node-negative patients [32] (Table 7).

Assessment of Risk: Choice of a Method and Practical Application

The variables that relate independently to risk in breast carcinoma have been corroborated sufficiently to permit us to devise a rational working method for risk assessment. The independent variables that have emerged are the proliferative index, the axillary lymph nodal status, and the size of the carcinoma. Since these variables are independently prognostic, risk can be adjusted by setting the level of any of the three. TLI is the most extensively studied of the proliferative indices at present. BrUdRLI will probably give similar results. Ki-67LI, a measure of growth fraction rather than S-phase, may duplicate the TLI results and should be investigated because it can be done on frozen tissue. % S-phase by flow cytometry is effective, but at present can be measured accurately in only about 70% of specimens.

Prognostic variables are usually most effective when the stage of the disease is low. This is true for breast carcinoma, where TLI is most effective in node-negative patients, and this is the group where its application is most appropriate. The question of a cutoff point arises. Our data indicate that TLIs of lower, mid, and upper thirds divide early stage breast carcinoma into groups with significantly different survival and relapse-free survival rates at 3 years, but at 5 years after diagnosis and application of potentially curative therapy, the survival and relapse-free survival rates of the lower third TLI group remain high while those of the mid and upper third groups are similar and significantly lower. Therefore, the cutoff point should probably be somewhere between the point dividing the middle and the lower thirds (3% in our data) and the median (5.6%). The impact of size as a third variable has not been well evaluated, but at some point even with negative nodes and low TLI, the probability for relapse would appear to increase with tumor size. One might then arbitrarily define as high risk tumors those with diameters of 5 cm or more, even if the nodes are negative and TLI low. These would be relatively few, so that by adding the patients with TLI in excess of the median, only slightly more than half of node-negative patients would be placed in the high risk group.

Flow cytometric % S-phase could be substituted for TLI, but this would presuppose that all specimens would be amenable to this measurement. Our experience suggests that % S-phase can be forced from the histogram in over 95% of cases, provided that a simple, rectangular model for computing % S-phase is used. We would recommend, however, that in trials depending on this type of risk definition, both DNA labeling and flow cytometry be carried out. Not only would this ensure that a proliferative index would always be available, but it would allow the two methods to be further evaluated one against the other.

Adjuvant therapy could blunt the prognostic effectiveness of the proliferative index if rapidly proliferative tumors were more likely to be sterilized than slowly proliferative tumors. Our data support this concept. Very few of our stage I patients, in whom TLI was highly prognostic, received adjuvant cytotoxic therapy, but 40% of the stage II and 52% of the stage III patients, in whom TLI was much less prognostic, received adjuvant cytotoxic therapy. In the stage II group, 80% of the treated patients received cyclophosphamide (Cytoxan), methotrexate, and 5-fluorouracil (CMF) [15], and 5% received doxorubicin (Adriamycin). In stage III,

55% of those treated received CMF and 30% received a doxorubicin-based regimen. Thus, chemotherapy may be responsible for the decreased association of early relapse with high TLI in patients with advanced disease.

Inflammatory carcinoma is the most common example of inoperable breast carcinoma without detectable metastases. Here the proliferative index is of almost no value because nearly all of these carcinomas are rapidly proliferative [83]. Since by definition all tumors in this category are large, one can fall back only on the steroid hormonal receptors for possible prognostic variables.

The proliferative index of experimental neoplasias is known to relate to the effectiveness of cytotoxic therapy [64, 108]. It should be investigated in advanced breast carcinoma as a biologic measurement of potential value in selection of therapeutic drugs.

References

1. Allison DC, Ridolpho PF, Anderson S, Bose K (1985) Variations in the [^{3}H] thymidine labeling of S-phase cells in solid mouse tumors. Cancer Res 45:6010-6016
2. Atkin NB (1972) Modal deoxyribonucleic acid value and survival in carcinoma of the breast. Br Med J 1:271-272
3. Auer GU, Caspersson TO, Gustafsson SA, Humla SA, Ljung B-M, Nordenskjold B (1980) Relationship between nuclear DNA distribution and estrogen receptors in human mammary carcinomas. Anal Quant Cytol 2:280-284
4. Auer GU, Caspersson TO, Wallgren AS (1980) DNA content and survival in mammary carcinoma. Anal Quant Cytol 2:161-165
5. Auer G, Eriksson E, Azavedo E, Caspersson T, Wallgren A (1984) Prognostic significance of nuclear DNA content in mammary adenocarcinomas in humans. Cancer Res 44:394-396
6. Auer G, Tribukait B (1980) Comparative single cell and flow DNA analyses in aspiration biopsies from breast carcinomas. Acta Pathol Microbiol Scand 88A: 355-358
7. Baak JPA, Van Dop H, Kurver PHJ, Hermans J (1985) The value of morphometry to classic prognosticators in breast cancer. Cancer 56:374-382
8. Baisch H, Beck H-P, Christensen IJ, Hartmabn NR, Fried J, Dean PN, Jett JH, Johnston DA, White RA, Nicolini C, Zeitz S, Watson JV (1982) A comparison of mathematical methods for the analysis of DNA histograms obtained by flow cytometry. Cell Tissue Kinet 15:235-249
9. Baisch H, Gohde W, Linden WA (1975) Analysis of PCP-data to determine the fraction of cells in the various phases of cell cycle. Radiat Environ Biophys 12:31-39, 1975
10. Barlogie B, Raber MN, Schumann J, Johnson TS, Drewinko B, Swartzendruber DE, Gohde W, Andreef M, Freireich EJ (1983) Flow cytometry in clinical cancer research. Cancer Res 43:3982-3997
11. Bedrossian CWM, Raber M, Barlogie B (1981) Flow cytometry and cytomorphology in primary resectable breast cancer. Anal Quant Cytol 3:112-116
12. Bertuzzi A, Diadone MG, Di Fronzo G, Silvestrini R (1981) Relationship among estrogen receptors, proliferative activity and menopausal status in breast cancer. Breast Cancer Res Treat 1:253-262
13. Bichel P, Poulsen HS, Andersen J (1982) Estrogen receptor content and ploidy of human mammary carcinoma. Cancer 50:1771-1774

14. Black MM, Barclay THC, Hankey BR (1975) Prognosis in breast cancer utilizing histologic characteristics of the primary tumor. Cancer 36:2048-2055
15. Bonadonna G, Brusamolino E, Valagussa P. et al. (1975) Combination chemotherapy as an adjuvant treatment in operable breast cancer. N Engl J Med 294:405-410
16. Boyd NF, Meakin Jw, Hayward JL, Brown TC (1981) Clinical estimation of the growth rate of breast cancer. Cancer 48:1037-1042
17. Caspersson TO (1979) Quantitative tumor cytochemistry. Cancer Res 39:2341-2355
18. Christov K, Todorov V (1981) Cell population kinetics and DNA content of mammary tumours. Cell Tissue Kinet 14:664
19. Clark GM, McGuire WL, Hubay CA, Pearson OH, Marshall JS (1983) Progesterone receptors as a prognostic factor in stage II breast cancer. N Engl J Med 309:1343-1347
20. Collins VP, Loeffler RK, Tivey H (1956) Observations on growth rates of human tumors. Am J Roentgenol Radium Ther 76:988-1000
21. Cook T, George D, Maynard P, Griffiths K (1979) Hormone receptors and cell kinetics in breast cancer. Cancer Treat Rep 63:1190
22. Cornelisse CJ, van de Velde CJH, Caspers RJC, Moolenaar AJ (1987) DNA ploidy and survival in breast cancer patients. Cytometry 8:225-234
23. Costa A, Del Bino L, Ventura L, Silvestrini R (1984) Relationship between cell kinetics of primary tumour and lymph node metastasis of the same patient. Cell Tissue Kinet 17:302-203
24. Costa A, Silvestrini R, Del Bino G, Motta R (1987) Implications of disaggregation procedures on biological representation of human solid tumours. Cell Tissue Kinet 20:171-180
25. Coulson PB, Thornthwaite JT, Woolley TW, Sugarbaker EV, Seckinger D (1984) Prognostic indicator including DNA histogram type, receptor content, and staging related to human breast cancer survival. Cancer Res 44:4187-4196
26. Culpin D, Morris VB (1985) Pattern of DNA synthesis and its effect on the classification of cells by flow cytometry. Cell Tissue Kinet 18: 1-12
27. Davis BW, Gelber RD, Goldhirsch A, Hartmann WH, Locher WG, Reed R, Golouh R, Save-Soderbergh J, Holloway L, Russell I, Rudestam CM (1986) Prognostic significance of tumor grade in clinical trials of adjuvant therapy for breast cancer with axillary lymph node metastasis. Cancer 58: 2662-2670
28. Dean PN, Dolbeare F, Gratzner H, Rice GC, Gray JW (1984) Cell-cycle analysis using a monoclonal antibody to BrdUrd. Cell Tissue Kinet 17: 427-436
29. Dean PN, Jett HJ (1974) Mathematical analysis of DNA distributions derived from flow microfluorometry. J Cell Biol 60: 523-527
30. Delides GS, Garas G, Georgouli G et al (1982) Intralaboratory variations in the grading of breast carcinoma. Arch Pathol Lab Med 106: 126-128
31. Dormer P, Brinkmann W, Born R, Steel GG (1975) Rate and time of DNA synthesis of individual Chinese hamster cells. Cell Tissue Kinet 8: 399-412
32. Dressler L, Clark G, Owens M, Pounds G, Oldaker T, McGuire WL (1987) DNA flow cytometry predicts for relapse in node negative breast cancer patients (abstract). Proc Am Soc Clin Oncol 6: 57
33. El-Alfy M, Leblond CP (1987) Long duration of mitosis and consequences for the cell cycle concept, as seen in the isthmal cells of the mouse pyloric antrum. I. Identification of early and late steps of mitosis II. Duration of mitotic phases and cycle stages, and their relation to one another. Cell Tissue Kinet 20: 205-213, 215-226
34. Erhardt K, Auer G, Folin A, Silfversward C, Skoog L (1986) Comparison between histologic type, estrogen receptor, and nuclear DNA content in mammary carcinoma. Am J Clin Oncol 9: 83-89

35. Ewers SB, Langstrom E, Baldetorp B, Killander D (1984) Flow-cytometric DNA analysis in primary breast carcinomas and clinicopathological correlations. Cytometry 5: 408-419
36. Fallenius AG, Askentsen UG, Skoog LK, Auer GU (1987) The reliability of microspectrophotometric and flow cytometric nuclear DNA measurements in adenocarcinomas of the breast. Cytometry 8: 260-266
37. Fisher ER, Gregorio RM, Fisher B (1975) The pathology of invasive breast cancer. Cancer 36: 1-85
38. Fisher ER, Redmond C, Fisher B (1980) Pathologic findings from the National Surgical Adjuvant Breast Project (protocol no. 4) VI. Discriminants for five-year treatment failure. Cancer 46: 908-918
39. Fossa SD, Marton PF, Knudsen PS, Kaalhus P, Bormer O, Vaage S (1982) Nuclear Feulgen DNA content and nuclear size in human breast carcinoma. Human Pathol 13: 626-630
40. Fried J (1977) Analysis of deoxyribonucleic acid histograms from flow cytometry. J Histochem Cytochem 25: 942-951
41. Fried J, Perez AG, Clarkson B (1980) Quantitative analysis of cell cycle progression of synchronous cells by flow cytometry. Exp Cell Res 126: 63-74
42. Gentili C, Sanfilippo O, Silvestrini R (1981) Cell proliferation in relation to clinical features and relapse in breast cancers. Cancer 48: 974-979
43. Gerdes J, Dallenbach F, Lennert K, Lemke H, Stein H (1984) Growth fractions in malignant non-Hodgkin's lymphomas (NHL) as determined in situ with the monoclonal antibody Ki-67. Hematol Oncol 2: 365-371
44. Gerdes J, Schwab U, Lemke H, Stein H (1983) Production of a mouse monoclonal antibody reactive with a human nuclear antigen associated with cell proliferation. Int J Cancer 31: 13-20
45. Gilchrist KW, Kalish L, Gould VE, Hirschl S, Imbriglia JE, Levy WM, Patchefsky AS, Penner DW, Pickren J, Roth JA, Schinella RA, Schwartz IS, Wheeler JE (1985) Interobserver reproducibility of histopathological features in state II breast cancer. An ECOG study. Breast Cancer Res Treat 5: 3-10
46. Going JJ, Anderson TJ, Battersby S, Macintyre CCA (1988) Proliferative and secretory activity in human breast during natural and artificial menstrual cycles. Am J Pathol 130: 193-204
47. Haag D, Feichter G, Goerttler K, Kaufmann M (1987) Influence of systematic errors on the evaluation of the S phase portions from DNA distributions of solid tumors as shown for 328 breast carcinomas. Cytometry 8: 377-386
48. Haag D, Goerttler K, Tschahargane C (1984) The proliferative index (PI) of human breast cancer as obtained by flow cytometry. Pathol Res Pract 178: 315-322
49. Harvey J, de Klerk N, Berryman I, Sterrett G, Byrne M, Papadimitriou J (1987) Nuclear DNA content and prognosis in human breast cancer: a static cytophotometric study. Breast Cancer Res Treat 9: 101-109
50. Hedley DW, Friedlander ML, Taylor IW, Rug CA, Musgrove EA (1983) Method for analysis of cellular DNA content of paraffin-embedded pathological material using flow cytometry. J Histochem Cytochem 31: 1333-1335
51. Hedley D, Leary J, Rugg C (1986) Suggestion that aneuploidy results from rather than is the cause of tumor progression. Personal Commmunication
52. Hedley DW, Rugg CA, Gelber RD (1987) Association of DNA index and S-phase fraction with prognosis of nodes positive early breast cancer. Cancer Res 47: 4729-4735
53. Hedley DW, Rugg CA, Alun BP, Taylor IW (1984) Influence of cellular DNA content on disease-free survival of stage II breast cancer patients. Cancer Res 44: 5395-5398

54. Heidelberger C (1982) Pyrimidine and pyrimidine nucleoside antimetabolites. In: Holland JF, Frei E III (eds) Cancer medicine. Lea and Febiger, Philadelphia, pp 801-824
55. Host H, Lund E (1986) Age as a prognostic factor in breast cancer. Cancer 57: 2217-2221
56. Jozan S, Gay G, Marques B, Mirouze A, David JF (1985) Oestradiol is effective in stimulating ^{3}H-thymidine incorporation but not on proliferation of breast cancer cultured cells. Cell Tissue Kinet 18: 457-464
57. Kallioniemi O-P, Hietanen T, Mattila J, Lehtinen M, Lauslahti K, Koivula T (1987) Aneuploid DNA content and high S-phase fraction of tumour cells are related to poor prognosis in patients with primary breast cancer. Eur J Cancer Clin Oncol 23: 277-282
58. Klintenberg C, Stal O, Nordenskjold B, Wallgren A, Arvidsson S, Skoog L (1986) Proliferative index, cytosol estrogen receptor and axillary node status as prognostic predictors in human mammary carcinoma. Breast Cancer Res Treat 7 (Suppl): 99-106
59. Knight W III, Livingston RB, Gregory EJ, McGuire WL (1977) Estrogen receptor as an independent prognostic factor for recurrence in breast cancer. Cancer Res 37: 4669-4671
60. Kuenen-Boumeester V, Hop WCJ, Blonk DI, Boon ME (1984) Prognostic scoring using cytomorphometry and lymph node status of patients with breast carcinoma. Eur J Cancer Clin Oncol 29: 337-345
61. Kute TE, Muss HB, Anderson D, Crumb K, Miller B, Burns D, Dube LA (1981) Relationship of steroid receptor, cell kinetics and clinical status in patients with breast cancer. Cancer Res 41: 3524-3529
62. Kute TE, Muss HB, Hopkins M, Marshall R, Case D, Kammire L (1985) Relationship of flow cytometry results to clinical and steroid receptor status in human breast cancer. Breast Cancer Res Treat 6: 113-121
63. Laird, AK (1964) Dynamics of tumor growth. Br J Cancer 18: 490-502
64. Laster WR Jr, Mayo JG, Simpson-Herren L, Griswold DP Jr, Lloyd HH, Schabel FM Jr, Skipper HE (1969) Success and failure in the treatment of solid tumors. II. Kinetic parameters and "cell curve" of moderately advanced carcinoma 755. Cancer Chemother Rep 53: 169-188
65. Lelle RJ, Heidenreich W, Stauch G, Gerdes J (1987) The correlation of growth fractions with histologic grading and lymph node status in human mammary carcinoma. Cancer 59: 83-88
66. Malaise E-P, Chauvel P, Chavaudra N, Pierquin B (1973) La cinetique des cancers du sein. Gas Med Fr 80: 5391-5400
67. McDivitt RW, Stone KR, Craig RB, Meyer JS (1985) A comparison of human breast cancer cell kinetics measured by flow cytometry and thymidine labeling. Lab Invest 52: 287-319
68. McDivitt RW, Stone KR, Craig RB, Palmer JO, Meyer JS, Bauer WC (1986) A proposed classification of breast cancer based on kinetic information. Cancer 57: 269-276
69. McDivitt RW, Stone KR, Meyer JS (1984) A method for dissociation of viable human breast cancer cells that produces flow cytometric kinetic information similar to that obtained by thymidine labeling. Cancer Res 44: 2628-2633
70. McGurrin J, Doria MI Jr, Dawson PJ, Karrison T, Stein H, Franklin WA (1987) Assessment of tumor cell kinetics by immunohistochemistry in carcinoma of breast. Cancer 59: 1744-1750
71. Mendelsohn ML (1962) Autoradiographic analysis of cell proliferation in spontaneous breast cancer of C3h mouse. III. The growth fraction. J Natl Cancer Inst 28: 1015-1029

72. Meyer JS (1981) Growth and cell kinetic measurements in human tumors. Pathol Annu 16(2): 53-81
73. Meyer JS, Bauer WC (1976) Tritiated thymidine labeling index of benign and malignant human breast epithelium. J Surg Oncol 8: 165-181, 1976
74. Meyer JS, Bauer WC, Rao BR (1978) Subpopulations of breast carcinoma defined by S-phase fraction, morphology, and estrogen receptor content. Lab Invest 39: 225-235
75. Meyer JS, Connor RE (1977) In vitro labeling of solid tissues with tritiated thymidine for autoradiographic detection of S-phase nuclei. Stain Technol 52: 185-195
76. Meyer JS, Connor RE (1982) Proliferation in fibrocystic disease and postmenopausal breast ducts measured by thymidine labeling. Cancer 50:746-751
77. Meyer JS, Coplin MD (1988) Thymidine labeling index, flow cytometric %S and DNA index in human tumors: comparisons and correlations. Am J Clin Pathol 87: 586-595
78. Meyer JS, Facher R (1977) Thymidine labeling index of human breast carcinoma. Enhancement of in vitro labeling by 5-fluoro and 5-fluoro-2′-deoxyuridine. Cancer 39: 2524-2532
79. Meyer JS, Friedman E, McCrate MM, Bauer WC (1983) Prediction of early course of breast carcinoma by thymidine labeling. Cancer 51: 1879-1886
80. Meyer JS, Lee JY (1980) Relationships of S-phase fraction of breast carcinoma in relapse to duration of remission, estrogen receptor content, therapeutic responsiveness, and duration of survival. Cancer Res 40: 1890-1896
81. Meyer JS, McDivitt RW (1986) Reliability and stability of the thymidine labeling index of breast carcinoma. Lab Invest 54: 160-164
82. Meyer JS, Micko S, Craver JL, McDivitt RW (1984) DNA flow cytometry of breast carcinoma after acetic-acid fixation. Cell Tissue Kinet 17: 185-197
83. Meyer JKS, Prey MU, Babcock DS, McDivitt RW (1986) Breast carcinoma cell kinetics, morphology, stage and host characteristics. A thymidine labeling study. Lab Invest 54: 41-51
84. Meyer JS, Province M (1988) Proliferative index of breast carcinoma by thymidine labeling: prognostic power independent of stage, estrogen and progesterone receptors Breast Cancer Res Treat 12: 191-204
85. Meyer JS, Schechtman K, Valdes R (1983) Estrogen and progesterone receptor assays on breast carcinoma from mastectomy specimens. Cancer 52: 2139-2143
86. Meyer JS, Rao BR, Stevens SC, White WL (1977) Low incidence of estrogen receptor in breast carcinomas with rapid rates of cellular replication. Cancer 40: 2290-2298
87. Moran R, Black M, Alpert L, Straus MJ (1984) Correlation of cell-cycle kinetics, hormone receptors, histopathology and nodal status in human breast cancer. Cancer 54: 1586-1590
88. Mueller CB, Ames F, Anderson GD (1978) Breast cancer in 3558 women: age as a significant determinant in the rate of dying and causes of death. Surgery 83: 123-132
89. Nealon TF Jr., Nkongho A, Gross C, Ward R, Nealon C, Gillooley JIF (1981) Treatment of early carcinoma of the breast ($T_1N_0N_0$ and $T_2N_0M_0$) on the basis of histologic characteristics. Surgery 89: 279-289
90. Nordenskjold B, Lowhagen T, Westerberg H, Zajicek J (1976) ^{3}H-thymidine incorporation into mammary carcinoma cells obtained by needle aspiration before and during endocrine therapy. Acta Cytol (Baltimore) 20: 137-143
91. Olszewski W, Darzynkiewicz Z, Rosen PP, Schwartz MK, Melamed MR (1981) Flow cytometry of breast carcinoma: I. Relation of DNA ploidy level to histology and estrogen receptor. Cancer 48: 980-984

92. Olszewski W, Darcynkiewicz Z, Rosen PP, Schwartz MK, Melamed MR (1981) Flow cytometry of breast carcinoma: II. Relation of tumor cell cycle distribution to histology and estrogen receptor. Cancer 48: 985-988
93. Opfermann M, Brugal G, Vassilakos P (1987) Significance of ploidy balance and proliferation index. Cytometry 8: 217-224
94. Paradiso A, Lorusso V, Tommasi S, Schittulli F, Maiello E, DeLena M (1988) Relevance of cell kinetics to hormonal response of receptor-positive advanced breast cancer. Breast Cancer Res Treat 11: 31-36
95. Post J, Sklarew Rh, Hoffman J (1977) The proliferative patterns of human breast cancer cells in vivo. Cancer 39: 1500-1507
96. Prey MU, Meyer JS, Stone KR, McDivitt RW (1985) Heterogeneity of breast carcinomas determined by flow cytometric analysis. J Surg Oncol 29: 35-39
97. Raber MN, Barlogie B, Latrielle J, Bedrossian C, Fritsche H, Blumenschein G (1982) Ploidy, proliferative activity and estrogen receptor content in human breast cancer. Cytometry 3: 36-41
98. Scheck LE, Muirhead KA, Horan PK (1980) Evaluation of the S phase distribution of flow cytometric DNA histograms by autoradiography and computer algorithms. Cytometry 1: 109-117
99. Schiffer LM, Braunschweiger PG, Stragand JJ, Poulakos L (1979) The cell kinetics of human mammary cancers. Cancer 43: 1707-1719
100. Schiffer LM, Markoe Am, Nelson JSR (1976) Estimation of tumor growth fraction in murine tumors by the primer-available DNA-dependent DNA polymerase assay. Cancer Res 36: 2415-2418
101. Sears HF, Janus C, Levy W, Hopson R, Creech R, Grotzinger P (1982) Breast cancer without axillary metastases. Are there high-risk biologic subpopulations? Cancer 50: 1820-1827
102. Shapiro HM (1985) Practical flow cytometry. Liss, New York
103. Sharkey FE, Pavlak RJ, Greiner AS (1983) Morphometric analysis of differentiation in human breast carcinoma: tumor grading. Arch Pathol Lab Med 107: 406-410
104. Silvestrini R, Diadone MG, Di Fronzo G (1979) Relationship between proliferative activity and estrogen receptors in breast cancer. Cancer 44: 665-670
105. Silvestrini R, Diadone MG, Di Fronzo G, Morabito A, Valagussa P, Bonadonna G (1986) Prognostic implication of labeling index versus estrogen receptors and tumor size in node-negative breast cancer. Breast Cancer Res Treat 7: 161-169
106. Silvestrini R, Diadone MG, Gasparini G (1985) Cell kinetics as a prognostic marker in node-negative breast cancer. Cancer 56: 1982-1987
107. Simpson-Herren L, Lloyd HH (1970) Kinetic parameters and growth curves for experimental neoplasms. Cancer Chemother Rep 54: 143-174
108. Skipper HE, Schabel FM Jr, Mellett LB, Montgomery JA, Wilkoff LJ, Lloyd HH, Brockman RW (1970) Implications of biochemical, cytokinetic, pharmacologic, and toxicologic relationships in the design of optimal therapeutic schedules. Cancer Chemother Rep 54: 431-450
109. Slamon DJ, Clark GM, Wong SG, Levin WJ, Ullrich A, McGuire WL (1987) Human breast cancer: correlation of relapse and survival with amplification of the HER-2/-*neu* oncogene. Science 235: 177-182
110. Smallwood JA, Cooper A, Taylor I (1983) The errors of thymidine labelling in breast cancer. Clin Oncol 9: 331-335
111. Spratt JS Jr (1965) The rates and patterns of growth of neoplasms of the large intestine and rectum. Surg Clin N Am 45: 103-115
112. Stal O, Klintenberg C, Franzen G, Risberg B, Arvidsson S, Bjelkenkrantz K, Skoog L, Nordenskjold B (1986) Comparison of static cytofluorometry and flow cytometry for

the estimation of ploidy and DNA replication in human breast cancer. Breast Cancer Res Treat 7: 15-22

113. Steel GG (1967) Cell loss as a factor in the growth of human tumours. Eur J Cancer 3: 381-387
114. Steel GG (1977) Growth kinetics of tumours. Clarendon Press, Oxford
115. Steel GG (1982) Cytokinetics of neoplasia, In: Holland JF, Frei E III (eds) Cancer medicine 2nd edn. Lea and Febiger, Philadelphia, pp 177-189
116. Stenkvist B, Bengtsson E, Erikson O, Jarkrans T, Nordin B, Westman-Naeser S (1983) Histopathological systems of breast cancer classification: reproducibility and clinical significance. J Clin Pathol 36: 392-398
117. Straus MJ, Moran RE (1980) The cell cycle kinetics of human breast cancer. Cancer 46: 2634-3639
118. Straus MJ, Moran R, Muller RE, Wotiz HH (1982) Estrogen receptor heterogeneity and the relationship between estrogen receptor and the tritiated thymidine labeling index in human breast cancer. Oncol 39: 197-200
119. Taylor IW, Musgrove EA, Friedlander ML, Mings F, Hedley DW (1983) The influence of age on the DNA ploidy levels of breast tumours. Eur J Cancer Clin Oncol 19: 623-628
120. Thorud E, Fossa SD, Vaage S, Kaalhus O, Knudsen OS, Bormer O, Shoaib MC (1986) Primary breast cancer. Flow cytometric DNA pattern in relation to clinical and histopathologic characteristics. Cancer 57: 808-811
121. Tribukait B (1984) Clinical DNA flow cytometry. Oncol Tumor Pharmacother 1: 211-218
122. Tubiaina M, Chauvel P, Ranaud A, Malaise EP (1975) Vitesse de croissance et histoire naturelle du cancer du sein. Bull Cancer (Paris) 62: 341-358
123. Tubiana M, Pejovic MH, Chavaudra N, Contesso G, Malaise EP (1984) The long-term prognostic significance of the thymidine labelling index in breast cancer. Int J Cancer 33: 441-445
124. von Fournier D, Weber E, Hoeffken W, Bauer M, Kubli F, Barth V (1980) Growth rate of 147 mammary carcinomas. Cancer 45: 2198-2207
125. Wallgren A, Silfversward C, Sklund G (1976) Prognostic factors in breast cancer. Acta Radiol (Ther) 15: 1-16
126. Wallgren A, Zajicek J (1976) The prognostic value of the aspiration biopsy in mammary carcinoma. Acta Cytol 20: 479-485
127. Wilson GD, McNally NJ, Dunphy E, Karcher H, Pfragner R (1985) The labeling index of human and mouse tumours assessed by bromodeoxyuridine staining in vitro and in vivo and flow cytometry. Cytometry 6: 641-647
128. Skehan P (1986) On the normalicy of growth dynamics of neoplasms in vivo: a data base analysis. Growth 50: 496-515
129. Bauer HCF, Kreicbergs A, Tribukait B (1986) DNA microspectrophotometry of bone sarcomas in tissue sections as compared to imprint and flow DNA analysis. Cytometry 7: 544-550
130. Dressler LG, Seamer LC, Owens MA, Clark GM, McGuire WL (1988) DNA flow cytometry and prognostic factors in 1331 frozen breast cancer specimens. Cancer 61: 420-247
131. Dressler LG, Seamer L, Owens MA, Clark GM, McGuire WL (1987) Evaluation of a modeling system for S-phase estimation in breast cancer by flow cytometry. Cancer Res 47: 5294-5502

Tumor Kinetics in Experimental Mammary Carcinoma

L. Simpson-Herren

Southern Research Institute, 2000 Ninth Avenue South, P.O. Box 55305,
Birmingham, AL 35255-5305, USA

Introduction

Cell kinetics describe the dynamic processes involved in growth or regression of tumors in untreated hosts and in hosts perturbed by therapy or other factors. Changes in tumor volume are determined by the cell population kinetics, i.e., the length of the tumor cell cycle and its phases, the growth fraction, the rate of cell loss or cell death, and the volume of noncellular components of the tumor. The observed response of tumors to therapy is determined by all of these factors.

Numerous experimental models of mammary adenocarcinoma have been developed and the kinetic data on these models have been extensively reported and reviewed [30, 82, 99, 114, 116]. This chapter will include selected data on a limited number of tumor systems to describe the dynamic processes in spontaneous, induced, and transplanted experimental mammary adenocarcinomas and the effects of various types of perturbation on these processes. Although no common etiology between any of the tumor models and breast cancer in humans has been objectively shown, the biologic principles described may provide useful guidelines for clinical therapy.

Tumor Growth Kinetics

Growth of experimental tumors has been described by several mathematical models [31], but the Gompertz function that describes exponential growth which is in turn exponentially retarded is most frequently used [75, 76, 78, 111, 128]. When the Gompertz-fitted growth curve is extrapolated back to one cell, it may yield time periods for tumor initiation that are unrealistic for human breast cancer [39]. However, this mathematical function generally fits the measurable growth of tumors and is useful in describing tumor behavior. The Gompertz function was used to describe progressive changes in tumor volume with time for spontaneous or induced tumors, early transplant generations, and long-transplanted tumor lines, as well as tumor metastasis of the mouse and rat [40, 78, 109]. Several examples are shown in Fig. 1. In general, spontaneous or induced tumors grow with a longer mass doubling time and exhibit less retardation of growth than do the transplanted tumors, although exceptions to this have been reported for individual spontaneous

Ragaz/Ariel (Eds.), High-Risk Breast Cancer

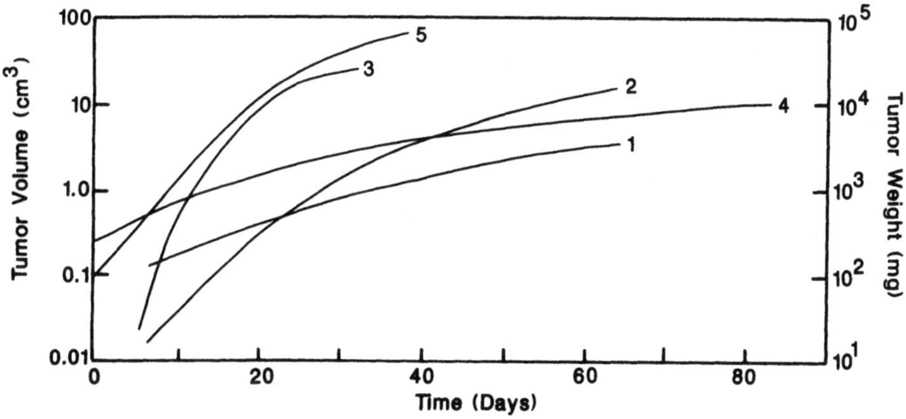

Fig. 1. Gompertz-fitted growth data from mammary adenocarcinomas: *1* C3H spontaneous; *2* C3H syngeneic first-generation transplant; *3* C3H syngeneic long passage transplant; *4* DMBA-induced; *5* Mam Ad 1/C transplanted from a DMBA-induced tumor. *Curves 1, 2,* and *3* redrawn from [78]; *4* and *5* from [110]

tumors and the first-generation transplants into syngeneic hosts [112]. Extended passage of a tumor line is usually associated with increasing growth rate and increasing retardation of growth (seen as an increase in volume doubling time with time postimplant), but exceptions to this have also been reported [6]. In studies of C3H spontaneous and transplanted tumors, McCredie [78] attributed the initial rapid growth rate of transplanted tumors to poor differentiation of the tumor cell population, and the retardation of the transplants to an increase in the relative volume of necrosis (Fig. 2). The latter presumably resulted from deterioration of the vascular supply.

The C3H spontaneous and transplanted tumors generally grow as nodules with expansion of nodules leading to centrinodular necrosis in the transplants [78]. Other transplanted tumors may exhibit a single necrotic core surrounded by a shell of proliferative tissue. Presumably, the centrinodular or central necrosis occurs when the tumor nodule expands from the periphery rather than by invasion of the surrounding tissue.

Whether or not the presence of multiple spontaneous C3H or 7,12-dimethylbenz(*a*)anthracene- (DMBA)-induced mammary adenocarcinoma tumors in a host inhibits the growth of individual tumors is unclear. Inhibition of secondary or metastatic growth by the presence of a primary or local tumor has been shown in mouse, rat, and hamster tumor models [22, 33, 38, 44, 47, 48, 53, 54, 56, 57, 68, 71-73, 84, 86, 89, 113, 120, 130]. In contrast, no interaction between tumors was observed in multiple implants of KHT sarcomas in C3H/Km mice [95] or in small and large implants of B16 melanoma in the same host [116]. Steel suggested that interaction between the tumors used in these studies may have been minimal or absent, owing to the small tumor sizes (<0.5 g). Interaction between a large implant of Lewis lung carcinoma and spontaneous lung metastasis became evident when retardation of

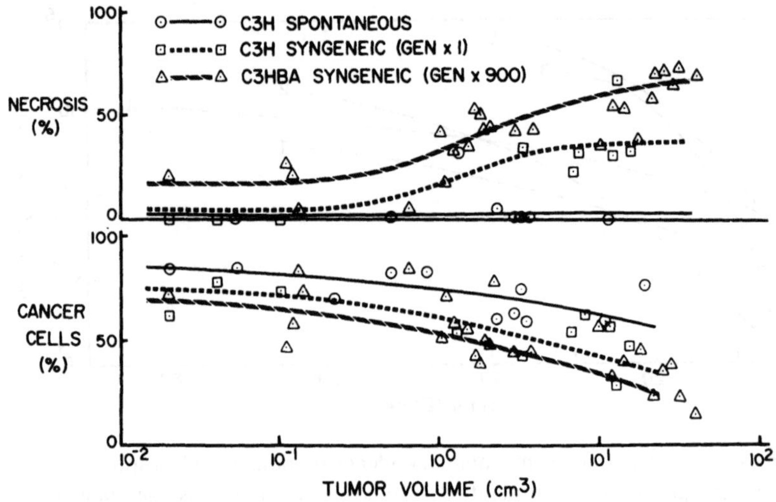

Fig. 2. Change with growth in the relative volume of cancer cells and of necrosis in mouse mammary carcinoma. The lines represent "best fit" curves for the data [78]

growth occurred in the large tumor foci [33]. An immune mechanism for suppression of tumor growth has been indicated in numerous investigations [5, 7, 21, 37, 44, 46, 49-51, 53, 63, 66, 85, 86, 91, 92, 119, 127]. An immune response as a stimulus of early tumor growth has also been described [63, 91, 92], but a specific role of the immune response in unperturbed and perturbed tumors remains elusive.

Cell Population Kinetics of Unperturbed Tumors

Studies of the kinetics of cell division in experimental tumors have provided insight into the dynamic processes that result in tumor growth or regression. While these studies of unperturbed tumors failed to provide a simple basis for converting "ineffective" or "noncurative" therapy into "curative" therapy, the cell population kinetics of perturbed animal tumor models can be extremely useful for rational design of protocols to improve the results that may be obtained with the available therapeutic modalities.

Selected kinetic data on a few experimental tumor models are included in the following discussion to illustrate biologic principles. The cell cycle (T_C) or intermitotic time is usually considered to be the orderly progression of events from the appearance of a new cell through the preparation for DNA synthesis (T_{G_1}), DNA synthesis (T_S), premitosis (T_{G_2}), and mitosis (T_M) where two daughter cells are formed. The thymidine labeling index (TLI) is, by definition, the percentage of cells within the tumor cell population that incorporate tritiated thymidine ([^{3}H] TdR) into DNA during a short or pulse exposure. The tumor growth fraction (GF) may be calculated from the measured kinetic parameters [83] or may be estimated as the primer-template-available, DNA-dependent DNA polymerase index (PDPI)

[102, 103]. This value gives an indication of the fraction of the cell population that is actively engaged in cell proliferation, but does not necessarily have a direct relationship to the viable cell fraction or the fraction of tumor mass.

Tumors of the C3H Mouse Strain

The C3H mouse strain is known to carry the mouse mammary tumor virus (MTV), and the spontaneous mammary tumors that arise in aging female mice are usually considered to be virally induced and hormone unresponsive. In the absence of information to the contrary, the transplanted lines of the C3H tumors are considered to be derived by viral induction.

Bresciani [17] compared cell cycle parameters in normal, hyperplastic, and neoplastic mammary gland cells of the C3H mouse (Table 1). The data indicate that progression to neoplasm, in this system, is accompanied by a decrease (to approximately 50%) in the length of the cell cycle and its phases. The observed values for TLI have a broad range in each of the three tissues studied, but the mean TLI of the tumors is increased about threefold over TLI of normal mammary tissue (Table 1).

An increase in TLI, a decrease in T_C, and a decrease in the tumor doubling time are usually observed when spontaneous or induced tumors are transplanted into syngeneic hosts [26, 81, 112]. With serial passage, the growth rate usually accelerates and marked retardation becomes evident (see Fig. 1). By selection of slowly or rapidly growing tumors as donor tumors at each passage, slow or fast lines can be isolated (Table 2). In the C3H fast and slow lines, the length of the G_1 phase accounted for most of the difference in cell cycle parameters. The growth characteristics of the fast and slow line are not stable and the lines will revert if selective passage is stopped.

The decrease in vascularity associated with the growth of experimental solid tumors [78] may be responsible for the observed changes in cell population kinetics where a prolongation of the cell cycle, a reduction in growth fraction, or possibly both [45, 111] may be observed. Fisher and Gunduz [40] investigated kinetic parameters of transplanted mammary tumors of C3H mice as a function of tumor

Table 1. Kinetic parameters for mammary tissues of C3H mouse [17]

Tissue	TLI (range)	T_{G_1} (h)	T_S (h)	T_C (h)	GF (%)
Normal alveoli	4.9 (2.7-7.6)	~45.7	21.7	~71	
Hyperplastic nodules	9.7 (5.8-18.2)	~26.8	15.9	~46	
Tumors	14.1 (5.7-26.4)	16.5-19.5	11.6	~33	40

Table 2. Kinetic parameters for spontaneous, first-generation transplant and extended transplant generations of the C3H mammary adenocarcinoma

Tumor	TLI (%)	T_{G_1} (h)	T_S (h)	T_C (h)	T_D (h)	GF or PDPI	Reference
Spontaneous	14	19.4 ± 8.7	11.7 ± 5.2	34.6 ± 10.2	204	0.40	79, 83
First-generation transplants	15.9	6.5 ± 4.7	6.5 ± 1.1	15.0 ± 4.8	108	0.37	26
Fourth-generation transplants	35.7 ± 3.9	3.0 ± 2.0	7.2 ± 1.5	12.8		0.50	118
Long passage lines							
S102F		6.5 ± 4.6	7.7 ± 3.4	17.2 ± 5.9		0.55	80, 82
Fast line		6.7 ± 3.0	11.0 ± 5.5	20.1 ± 6.3	88	0.30	80, 82
Slow line		17.3 ± 12.3	12.5 ± 7.2	33.5 ± 14.3	460	0.23	80, 82

Table 3. Kinetic parameters of transplanted C3H mammary tumors as a function of tumor volume and time postimplant

Tumor and host	Time postimplant (days)	Tumor volume (mm^3)	TLI (%)	T_{G_1} (h)	T_S (h)	T_C (h)	T_D (h)	GF	Reference
Transplanted C3H/HeB		34-82	26-30		6.7-7.4	11.3-12.5	34-35	0.47-0.49	40
		523-547	24-37		7.2-7.7	11.8-14.3	35	0.44-0.48	
		1483-1697	21-22		7.3-9.2	13.1-16.6	59-67	0.38-0.40	
		5845-9653	13-18		8.3-11.6	15.1-17.6	178-250	0.21-0.37	
Transplanted HB	7	~ 200		5.2	6.8	14.6	36	0.53	25
C3H/Tif/Bom	21	~ 10000		5.7	7.6	15.3	178	0.46	
	30	~ 14000		10.3	8.4	22.9		0.39	

volume from about 50 mm^3 to more than 5 000 mm^3, and found that TLI decreased to about one-half, T_S increased less than twofold, T_C increased about 50%, and T_D increased from about 35 to about 200 h over this range of tumor size (Table 3). In contrast, studies of a transplantable mammary carcinoma HB in the C3H mouse at three phases of growth described as the exponential phase (7 days postimplant, $\sim 0.2\ cm^3$), the phase of growth retardation (21 days postimplant, $\sim 10\ cm^3$), and the stationary phase (30 days postimplant, $\sim 13.5\ cm^3$) [25] indicated that no significant changes in the cell cycle parameters or in the growth fraction were observed between 7 and 21 days. During this interval, the tumor doubling time increased from 36 to 178 h (Table 3). In these studies the authors specified that the cell cycle parameters and growth fraction were measured on the tumor cell population at the periphery of the tumor and did not reflect a change until growth had essentially ceased.

Induced and Transplantable Mammary Tumors of the Rat

Primary mammary adenocarcinomas of the Sprague-Dawley rat have been induced by administration of DMBA using the technique described by Huggins [60]. The DMBA-induced tumors are hormone responsive during early growth, but the hormone responsiveness decreases with time from administration of the carcinogen and, possibly, with tumor size. Kinetic parameters for the growing DMBA-induced tumors as a function of tumor size, for tumors regressed by ovariectomy and stimulated by administration of estradiol and progesterone, and for small tumors of a long-transplanted line derived from DMBA-induced primary tumors are shown in Table 4 [109, 110]. There was no significant change in the cell cycle parameters of the DMBA-induced tumors with tumor age or size. The cell cycle parameters for the transplanted mammary adenocarcinoma (Mam Ad 1/C) derived from a DMBA-induced tumor were similar to those for the induced tumors, but TLI was more than twice as high. In this system, as in the C3H tumors, the transplanted line grew more rapidly with a shorter T_D (1.8 days for small tumors compared with 7-10 days in the DMBA-induced tumors of similar size), and retardation of growth was evident when tumors were very advanced.

Cell Population Kinetics of Perturbed Tumors

The kinetic parameters measured in untreated tumors describe the dynamics of the cell population until perturbed by surgery, radiation, drug therapy, or other therapeutic or environmental insults. Growth rate of residual tumor may be decreased or, more likely, will be stimulated by perturbation [107, 108, 113].

Table 4. Kinetic parameters for growing DMBA-induced, hormone-stimulated, and transplanted tumor [109, 110]

Tumor system	Tumor size (g)	Mean tumor weight (g)	Mean TLI (%)	T_{G_1} (h)	T_S (h)	T_C (h)	T_D (days)
Growing induced							
Small	1.0	0.43	6.0	5.5	11.4	18.4	7-10
Medium	1.0-3.0	1.75	6.2	5.8	8.5	17.5	10-16
Large	3.0	6.75	6.9	7.1	8.1	12.3	16-49
Regressed by ovariectomy, then stimulated with estrogen and progesterone		0.40	11	13.0	8.5	23.0	4
Mam Ad 1/C transplanted		0.37	15	6.2	7.7	16.4	1.8

Effects of Surgery

As early as 1913, the possibility that surgical excision of a primary tumor might stimulate growth of the residual tumor was recognized and investigated experimentally [120]. "Outbursts" [36] of metastatic growth following surgery or other trauma have been described in the clinical and experimental literature [20, 77, 93]. Efforts to quantitate the effects of surgical excision of the primary tumor on growth rate, size, or number of metastatic foci led to conflicting results [73, 74, 77, 98]. DeWys [33] described a synchronous slowing of the growth rate of primary Lewis lung tumor and metastases; the decreased growth rate of the metastases was reversed by surgical removal of the primary tumor.

The effects of surgical excision of a primary implanted Lewis lung tumor on the cell population kinetics of established lung metastases was described by Simpson-Herren et al. [113]. She reported that TLI of the primary tumor and the spontaneous lung metastases decreased with time postimplant. When the primary tumor was excised on day 14 postimplant, TLI of the residual lung metastases were elevated within 48 h and did not decrease with time postimplant, but remained high until the mice were terminal (day 30 or later) (Fig. 3). The surgical procedure did not significantly change the cell cycle parameters in the residual lung metastases. Sham surgery, in this case blunt dissection of a section of skin similar in size and shape to that removed with a large subcutaneous tumor ($\sim$ 2 cm diameter), but from the side of the mouse opposite to the tumor implant, resulted in elevation of TLI of both primary tumor and lung metastases [113].

The perturbations of cell population kinetics that resulted from surgical reduction of tumor mass were soon confirmed in experimental mammary tumors (Table 5). In a study of C3H mice bearing spontaneous mammary tumors, surgical excision of one tumor increased TLI of the second tumor twofold within 24 h. Bisection of the first tumor increased TLI of the residual tumor and the second tumor threefold [101]. Similar studies in C3H mice bearing doubly transplanted mammary tumors confirmed the stimulation, but the magnitude of the increase was less [55].

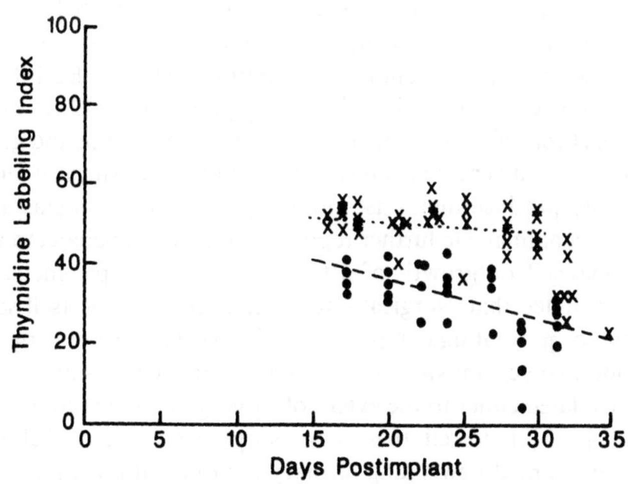

Fig. 3. Thymidine labeling indices of spontaneous Lewis lung metastases for intact mice (*circles*) and following surgical excision of the primary implanted tumors on day 14 (*crosses*). Pooled data [108, 113]

Table 5. Effects of surgical excision of a primary spontaneous or transplantable tumor on labeling of the residual tumor with [^{3}H] TdR or [^{125}I] UdR

Tumor system	TLI			Reference
	0 h	24 h post surgery		
	Tumor 1	Tumor 1 (residual)	Tumor 2	
Spontaneous C3H tumors (double); resect tumor 1	4.5		9.1	101
Spontaneous C3H tumors (double); bisect tumor 1[a]	3.7	11.3	11.7	101
Transplanted C3H tumors (double); surgical excision 1				
Day 14	30		36	55
Day 21	25		35	
Day 28	20		25	

[a] Only a portion of the first tumor was removed.

Gorelik et al. [52] described cell proliferation in lung metastases measured by uptake of ^{125}I-labeled iododeoxyuridine ([^{125}I] UdR) following surgical excision of intrafootpad-inoculated Lewis lung tumors and concluded that the degree of acceleration of growth in the metastases was related to the rate of growth of the primary tumors.

Kinetic analysis of residual tumor demonstrated an increase in GF 18-42 h after surgical removal of a transplanted murine neuroblastoma, but the peak proliferation in bone marrow cells was delayed 24-96 h [88]. Growth curves for lung metastases of transplanted neuroblastoma also indicated more rapid growth following surgical removal of the tumor-bearing leg [90].

Keller [65-67, 69] used the transplantable D-12 rat fibrosarcoma to investigate the effects of surgical intervention on the incidence and growth rate of micrometastases and macrometastases. He concluded that surgical removal of a primary tumor could produce metastases in a model where no metastases were observed in the intact animal. He further reported that partial hepatectomy in a tumor-bearing rat enhanced outgrowth of established macroscopic metastases in other sites, but concluded that "surgical intervention does not of itself seem to constitute a *major* tumor promoting component" [67, 69]. The role of surgical intervention that does not involve removal of the primary tumor remains unclear, but the effect appears to be related either to the extent of surgery or to the tumor model. Simpson-Herren et al. [113] reported that sham surgery enhanced TLI of lung metastases from transplanted Lewis lung primary tumors, but no enhancement of cell proliferation was observed following sham surgery in the spontaneous C3H tumors [100]. Amputation of a non-tumor-bearing extremity, celiotomy, and celiotomy with partial hepatectomy enhanced the incidence of pulmonary metastases from Lewis sarcoma T241 in C57BL/6JN mice, but only celiotomy with partial hepatectomy had an enhancing effect on metastasis of Cloudman S91 melanoma in (C × DBA/2) F_1 hybrids [96]. Schatten and Kramer [99] reported no acceleration of metastatic growth of S91 melanoma or DBA49 tumors as a result of amputation of a non-tumor-bearing leg, anesthesia, or cortisone administration.

In contrast, Shapiro et al. [104] reported acceleration of growth of metastasis from Lewis lung carcinoma and B16 melanoma by four anesthetic drugs. When rats were anesthetized with chloroform or ether, the percentage of animals with lung metastases from intravenously implanted Walker 256 cells was 64% and 55%, respectively, compared with 37% in the control and 46% in those animals given barbital sodium [2].

Effects of Irradiation

The population kinetics of the recurring tumor following radiation therapy have been extensively investigated [18, 27, 58, 59, 105, 106], but the kinetic changes that occur during the immediate posttreatment period are unclear. Tumor regression was apparent within the first day after irradiation of an experimental carcinoma, but did not occur for several days in sarcomas in studies by Denekamp and Thomlinson [27]. When these investigators measured the cell cycle phases and TLI in irradiated tumors at least ten cycles after treatment, no kinetic changes were found in the treated tumors.

Local irradiation of a highly metastatic P388 rat sarcoma was reported to stimulate the growth of lung and lymph node metastases present at the time of treatment [121], but to cause an exponential decrease in dissemination of tumor cells from the irradiated tumor. van Peperzeel [122] observed a period of accelerated growth 3-6 days after X-irradiation of tumors in both humans and experimental animals; an increase in TLI preceded the increase in growth rate. He concluded that for most clinical tumors, daily treatment was nearly optimal, but other schedules might be better in very rapidly growing and very slowly growing tumors.

Development of transplanted C3H mouse mammary tumors was significantly perturbed by irradiation of host tissues both before and after tumor transplantation [1]. This perturbation involved an extended latent period, a slower average growth rate, and greater variability of growth. In contrast, treatment of the mice by injection of radiation-killed tumor cells prior to implantation of a tumor reduced the latent period and increased the growth rate.

Braunschweiger et al. [14] defined the response of the cell kinetic parameters of the T1699 transplantable mouse mammary tumor to radiation. The initial response phase (first 24 h) was characterized by a decrease in TLI, an increase in PDPI, and an increase in length of the S-phase.

The length of the second phase of decreased cell proliferation was dose dependent, followed by a recovery phase with increased TLI, increased PDPI, and return of the S-phase to normal length. The fourth phase of response was characterized by a reestablishment of normal proliferative patterns.

Of particular interest in therapy design was the observation that local irradiation might stimulate the growth of distant metastases. Kaplan [64] reported that irradiation of a primary Bagg-Jackson mammary carcinoma augmented its capacity for dissemination. Further, significantly more mice died with metastases following local irradiation of the 2661 carcinoma than following amputation of the tumor-bearing foot [28]. Using large (2×10^5 cells) and small implants (3×10^4 cells) in the left and right hindlimb to simulate primary and metastatic C3H mammary tumors, Fisher et al. [42, 43] demonstrated an increase in TLI and a decrease in the estrogen receptor index (ERI) of the "metastatic" foci following irradiation of the primary tumor. The effect on each index was of a lesser magnitude than was observed following surgical removal of the primary tumor. Irradiation of the primary tumor 1, 3, or 5 days prior to surgical excision of the tumor eliminated the increase in TLI and the decrease in ERI that was observed in the secondary tumor foci in the surgery-only controls. Crile and Deodhar [24] reported that radiation destruction of Lewis (T241) fibrosarcoma in the footpads of C57/BL6 mice controlled distant metastatic appearance better than surgical amputation of the tumor-bearing foot.

Effects of Chemotherapy

The kinetic perturbations that result from administration of antineoplastic agents in vivo may be obscured by the presence of drug-damaged cells with limited proliferative capacity. Cells lethally damaged by alkylating agents or the nitrosoureas may continue through several cycles of DNA synthesis prior to death and lysis [3, 4]. Thus, kinetic data obtained during the early post-treatment period may be questionable.

Extensive data from empirically designed therapeutic protocols have demonstrated the importance of treatment schedules. Rational design of treatment schedules based on knowledge of the recovery kinetics of residual tumor have proved successful experimentally, but are difficult to apply clinically because the interval between treatment and recovery is dependent on tumor, drug, and dose.

Using flow cytometric and autoradiographic techniques to analyze Adriamycin-perturbed C3H mouse mammary tumors (S102F), Dethlefsen et al. [32] found that a dose of 10 mg/kg Adriamycin did not induce tumor regression, but inhibited growth for 4-5 days. They reported that TLI of treated tumors was 29% of the control at 96 h after Adriamycin administration, and there was no increase in degenerate index. He concluded that the inhibition of tumor growth was due to extended cell cycle delay rather than cell killing. A dose of 5 mg/kg Adriamycin to rats bearing the 13762 mammary tumor resulted in growth inhibition of at least 3 days and recovery of cell proliferation between days 4 and 7 [11]. Sequential chemotherapy with cyclophosphamide was most effective when it coincided with recovery of proliferative activity.

When single doses of cyclophosphamide were administered to mice bearing C3H spontaneous mammary adenocarcinomas, or rats bearing the 13762 transplantable mammary tumors, increases in TLI or PDPI occurred within the first

24 h and coincided with periods of increased sensitivity to Adriamycin [10]. Similar studies with the T1699 transplantable mouse mammary tumor indicated that recovery of proliferative activity occurred 3 days after Adriamycin treatment (5 mg/kg) and 6-7 days after cyclophosphamide treatment (100 mg/kg) [12].

Following administration of single doses of cyclophosphamide (60 mg/kg, i.p.) to C3HeB mice bearing transplanted C3H mammary tumors, depression of both TLI and GF were evident within the first day and were maximal in TLI at 3 days (41% of control) and in GF at 5 days (54% of control) [40]. By day 7, both parameters were returning to normal. Successive doses of cyclophosphamide given every 7 days failed to intensify the depression of TLI and GF, resulted in a lesser effect with each successive dose, and produced only a reduction in growth rate. When immunotherapy (*Corynebacterium parvum*) was administered 4 days after the cyclophosphamide rather than 3 days before or simultaneously, the depression of TLI and GF was more profound, the recovery less complete, and the tumors regressed. Cyclophosphamide (240 mg/kg) administered 3 days after surgical removal of transplanted C3H mammary tumors, when TLI was highest, had a more favorable effect than if given 7 days after surgery, when TLI had returned to normal [41]. When given prior to surgery, cyclophosphamide prevented the increase in TLI of residual tumor usually observed after surgery, and prolonged survival. If a small dose of cyclophosphamide (60 mg/kg) was given on the day of surgery, the increase in TLI of residual tumor at 24 h was greater than in the surgery-only control [41]. By the third and fourth day, TLI of residual tumor was lower than TLI of the surgery-only control, but was similar to TLI prior to treatment.

Relevant to growth of cells that survive initial treatment with chemotherapy are the observations on lung colony formation from KHT cells injected intravenously into mice 1 day following treatment with various cytotoxic drugs given at approximately two-thirds the $LD_{50/30}$ [19]. The number of lung colonies was increased 81-fold over the saline-treated control following cyclophosphamide (200 mg/kg), 6.6-fold following actinomycin D (0.27 mg/kg), and 3.6 fold following mithramycin treatment (1 mg/kg). Adriamycin (10 mg/kg), methotrexate (50 mg/kg), 5-fluorouracil (140 mg/kg), cytosine arabinoside 2500 mg/kg), and bleomycin (6 units/kg) had minimal or no effect on lung colony incidence. Further, Vollmer and Conley [124] reported that cyclophosphamide caused a dramatic increase in the number of lung tumor nodules from intravenous or intra-arterial injection of KHT cells in C3H/HcW mice, but were unable to document tumor promotion in brain, heart, kidney, adrenal, or ovary. These data suggest that noncurative therapy with cyclophosphamide may result in a higher incidence of metastases, owing to increased survival of residual tumor cells.

Effects of Hyperthermia

The incidence of metastasis of a transplantable C3H mouse mammary adenocarcinoma was dramatically increased following application of heat to a local tumor for a period of time adequate to eradicate the local tumor [125]. Enhanced dissemination of Yoshida sarcoma in rats as a result of local heating that failed to destroy the tumor completely was reported [34, 35]. Metastasis formation from Lewis lung carcinoma did not appear to be promoted by local heating, but was promoted by total body hyperthermia of mice [129].

Effects of Environmental Factors

Factors other than scheduled therapy may perturb the cell kinetics of tumors. Nutritional deprivation significantly reduced the tumor volume and markedly suppressed TLI and PDPI of the T1699 transplantable mammary tumor and the C3H/HeJ spontaneous mammary tumor [117]. Refeeding promptly restored proliferative activity. Increased incidence of spontaneous tumors, increased incidence of metastases, or accelerated growth of tumor or metastases have been attributed to experimental burns [87], to mechanical trauma [8], to stress produced by environmental isolation or crowding [94], and to inescapable shock [115, 123].

Effects of Immunologic Perturbation

Janik and Steel [61, 62] studied the kinetic changes in four transplantable tumor systems that resulted from perturbation of the host. Immunologic perturbation was accomplished by transfer of tumors into another host strain (e.g., implantation of a mouse tumor into rats), by immunization with radiation-killed tumor cells, by inoculation of tumor cell numbers below the doses required to induce tumors, or by treatment with Freund's complete adjuvant. In two instances where tumor growth was essentially arrested by the perturbation there was no significant change in duration of the cell cycle, but a reduction in the proportion of actively proliferating cells.

Treatment of mice with anti-mouse lymphocyte serum resulted in a marked increase in the growth rate of the EMT6/M/AC tumor at all tumor volumes [126]. In contrast, the length of the cell cycle and its phases were not significantly changed and the growth fraction was reduced. Thus, in spite of a decrease in the rate of cell production, the growth rate of the tumor increased. These investigators attributed this change to a marked decrease in the rate of cell loss.

Effects of Hormonal Changes

The C3H spontaneous and transplanted mammary adenocarcinomas are generally unresponsive to changes in the endocrine status of the host or to administration of estrogen and progesterone. However, the DMBA-induced mammary adenocarcinoma in the Sprague-Dawley rat is responsive to the hormonal status of the host during the initial phases of growth and has been utilized to investigate the cell kinetic changes that occur.

Combs et al. [23] reported that the proliferating fraction of DMBA-induced tumors varied systematically with the estrus cycle, the lowest fraction in proestrus and the highest fraction in early diestrus. Ovariectomy of rats bearing growing DMBA-induced tumors resulted in a decrease in TLI to near 0 by day 14 after surgery [108, 113]. Regressed tumors that recurred were no longer hormone responsive. Daily administration of estradiol and progesterone to intact rats with growing tumors, or to rats bearing tumors regressed by ovariectomy, resulted in an increase in TLI (Fig. 4).

Braunschweiger et al. demonstrated that administration of methylprednisolone or dexamethasone following surgery [16] or chemotherapy [9, 13, 15] produced a stasis in proliferative recovery of residual tumor. Bone marrow recovery following chemotherapy was not delayed by the corticosteroids, thus providing a rationale for minimizing marrow toxicity and maximizing antitumor effects of subsequent chemotherapy.

Treatment of C3H/HeJ spontaneous mammary tumors with methylprednisolone resulted in a temporary stasis of tumor growth with little or no regression in

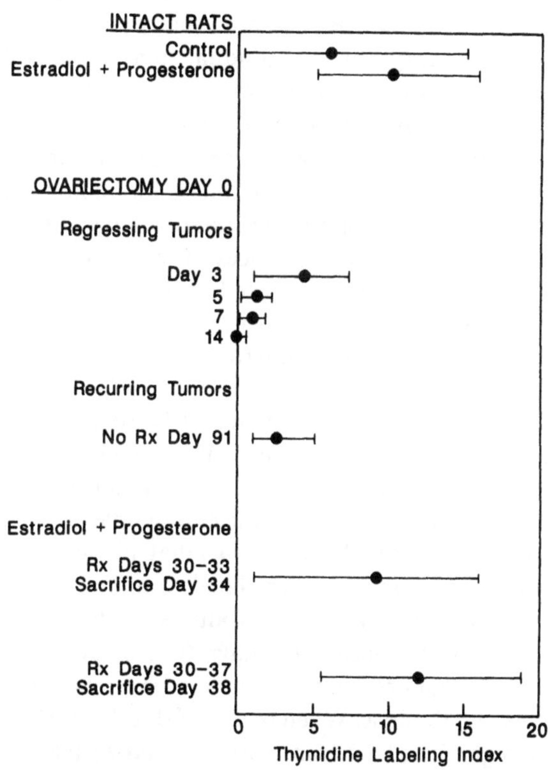

Fig. 4. Thymidine labeling indices for DMBA-induced tumors in intact rats (control), and following administration of estradiol and progesterone. In the remaining groups, ovariectomy was performed on day 0 and TLI was measured in regressing tumors on days 3, 5, 7, and 14. Tumors that were studied on day 91 recurred without treatment and were hormone unresponsive. Two groups of rats bearing tumors that regressed after ovariectomy were given 17-β-estradiol (2 μg per rat per day) and progesterone (8 mg per rat per day) for 4 or 8 days. TLIs were measured 24 h after the final treatment [110]

tumor volume. Further, a 50% decrease in TLI was observed 2 h after treatment, with no change in the growth fraction estimated by PDPI [15]. In vivo treatment of first-generation transplants of C3H/HeJ spontaneous tumors with dexamethasone or methylprednisolone (10 mg/kg every 12 h for three doses) resulted in inhibition of cell proliferation followed by a maximum in TLI 18-24 h after methylprednisolone and 42-48 h after dexamethasone treatment. Administration of dexamethasone every 12 h during the recovery period following surgical removal of a primary implanted RIF-1 tumor of C3H/HeJ mice inhibited the increase in proliferative activity that was observed in the artifical lung metastases of control mice (no dexamethasone). Proliferative recovery was evident after cessation of treatment with dexamethasone [16].

Role of Recovery Kinetics in Cancer Therapy

Most cancer treatment failures are attributable not to the local primary tumor, but to the secondary sites that are usually present at the time of diagnosis [69]. Thus, effective therapy for the residual tumor cells following surgical intervention, or possibly irradiation of the primary tumor, becomes the challenge of cancer therapy [97]. The recovery kinetics of tumor and host tissue following noncurative surgery, irradiation, or chemotherapy define the time frame for depression or stimulation of proliferative activity. Reduction of the tumor mass by surgery or radiation may stimulate growth of residual tumor by increasing GF. The diverse available data suggest that the consequences of surgical excision or radiation therapy for the primary tumor may be related to the type of tumor, size or number of metastatic foci present at the time of treatment, the site of the foci, and the immune status of the host. The incidence of micrometastases apparently far exceeds the incidence of macroscopically evident metastases [70], but these small foci may be subject to control by the immune system of the host. If this is the case, then surgical excision of the primary tumor (Table 6) may yield apparent "cures" or dormancy of the metastases unless or until the host immune system is impaired [37]. Irradiation of the primary tumor may sufficiently impair host immunity to allow outgrowth of micrometastases. Metastatic foci that are macroscopic in size at the time of surgery or irradiation may be stimulated to more rapid growth.

Chemotherapy usually produces a depression of proliferative activity followed by a recovery phase – the magnitude of the depression and the interval between treatment and recovery appears to be a function of GF of the tumor, the host, the drug, and the dose. When the low-GF C3H/HeJ spontaneous mammary tumor and the high-GF 13762 transplantable murine mammary adenocarcinoma were compared, important differences in the recovery kinetics were noted [10]. Following treatment with cyclophosphamide, TLI was suppressed in both tumors, but the interval between treatment and recovery of TLI was considerably longer in the high-GF 13762 tumor than in the low-GF C3H/HeJ model. Further, there was evidence that GF of the 13762 tumors did not increase significantly above the pretreatment value, possibly indicating an absence of recruitment of nonproliferating cells. This observation suggests that kinetically directed therapeutic protocols

Table 6. Possible consequences of therapy for a local or primary tumor. (Adapted from [68])

Residual neoplastic cells	Consequences of surgery or irradiation for localized tumor
None	Cure
A few micrometastases	Cure, dormancy or outgrowth of metastases (possibly as a function of host immune status)
Micrometastases and macrometastases	Outgrowth of metastases (possibly accelerated by primary therapy)

may be useful in relatively sensitive high-GF tumors as well as the insensitive low-GF tumors.

In the experimental systems the most effective chemotherapeutic schedules were those in which drugs were administered to coincide with the kinetic recovery from single agents alone. Less effective schedules were seen when the recovery peaks were avoided in administration of therapy. Cetrain specific anticancer agents, e.g., bleomycin, may be more effective when administered to avoid this peak. In a combined modality protocol, radiation should be administered just prior to the peak of recovery for maximum effectiveness [14, 29]. The experimental data support the hypothesis that the recovery kinetics of residual tumor cells can be utilized to improve the results of therapeutic protocols for disseminated cancer. Clearly evident is the need for more rigorous data to define the recovery kinetics under clinically relevant conditions.

References

1. Abdelaal AS, Wheldon FE, Clark BM (1980) Perturbation of the growth kinetics of C3H mouse mammary carcinoma by irradiation of tumor and host and by attempted pre-immunization of host. Br J Cancer 41: 567-576
2. Agostino D, Clifton EE (1964) Anesthetic effect on pulmonary metastases in rats. Arch Surg 88: 735-739
3. Alexander P (1961) Mouse lymphoma cells with different radiosensitivities. Nature 192: 572-573
4. Alexander P, Mikulski ZB (1961) Differences in the response of leukaemia cells in tissue culture to nitrogen mustard and to dimethyl myleran. Biochem Pharmacol 5: 275-282
5. Barski G, Youn JK (1969) Evolution of cell-mediated immunity in mice bearing an antigenic tumor. Influence of tumor growth and surgical removal. JNCI 43: 111-121
6. Begg AC (1971) Kinetic and histological changes of a serially transplanted mouse tumour. Cell Tissue Kinet 4: 401-411
7. Belehradek J, Barski G, Thonier M (1972) Evolution of cell-mediated antitumor immunity in mice bearing a syngeneic chemically induced tumor. Influence of tumor growth, surgical removal and treatment with irradiated tumor cells. Int J Cancer 9: 461-469
8. Boeryd B, Rudenstam C-M (1967) Effect of heparin, plasminogen inhibitor (EACA) and trauma on tumour metastases. Acta Pathol Microbiol Scand 69: 28-34

9. Braunschweiger PG (1987) Tumor growth fraction estimation, perturbation, and prognostication. In: Gray JW, Darzynkiewicz Z (eds) Techniques in cell cycle analysis. Humana, Clifton, pp 47-71
10. Braunschweiger PG, Schiffer LM (1978) Therapeutic implications of cell kinetic changes after cyclophosphamide treatment in "spontaneous" and "transplantable" mammary tumors. Cancer Treat Rep 62: 727-736
11. Braunschweiger PG, Schiffer LM (1980a) Effect of adriamycin on the cell kinetics of 13762 rat mammary tumors and implications for therapy. Cancer Treat Rep 64: 293-300
12. Braunschweiger PG, Schiffer LM (1980b) Cell kinetic-directed sequential chemotherapy with cyclophosphamide and adriamycin in T1699 mammary tumors. Cancer Res 40: 737-743
13. Brauschweiger PG, Schiffer LM (1981) Antiproliferative effects of corticosteroids in C3H/HeJ mammary tumors and implications for sequential combination chemotherapy. Cancer Res 41: 3324-3330
14. Braunschweiger PG, Schenken LL, Schiffer LM (1979) The cytokinetic basis for the design of efficacious radiotherapy protocols. Int J Radiat Oncol Biol Phys 5: 37-47
15. Braunschweiger PG, Stragand JJ, Schiffer LM (1978) Effect of methylprednisolone on cell proliferation in C3H/HeJ spontaneous mammary tumors. Cancer Res 38: 4510-4514
16. Braunschweiger PG, Ting HL, Schiffer LM (1983) Role of corticosteroid hormones in the control of cell proliferation in residual tumor after surgical cytoreduction. Cancer Res 43: 5801-5807
17. Bresciani F (1965) A comparison of the cell generative cycle in normal, hyperplastic and neoplastic mammary gland of the C3H mouse. In: Symposium on fundamental cancer research. Cellular radiation biology. Williams and Wilkins, Baltimore, pp 547-557
18. Brown JM (1970) The effect of acute X-irradiation on the cell proliferation kinetics of induced carcinomas and their normal counterpart. Radiation Res 43: 627-653
19. Brown JM (1977) Effects of radiation and chemotherapeutic agents on the incidence and treatment of blood-borne metastases. In: Stansyl PG, Sato H (eds) Cancer metastases, approaches to the mechanism, prevention and treatment. Gann monograph on cancer research, no 20. University of Tokyo Press, Tokyo, pp 207-225
20. Burns ER (1969) On the failure of self-inhibition of growth in tumors. Growth 33: 25-45
21. Chaput B, Rella W, Vetterlein M (1974) Changes in cell mediated immune functions by growing tumor. Eur J Cancer 10: 185-188
22. Cheshire PJ (1970) The effect of multiple tumours on mammary tumour growth rates in the C3H mouse. Br J Cancer 24: 542-547
23. Combs JW, Mackey M, Bennington, JL (1971) Regulation of cell proliferation in DMBA-induced rat mammary neoplasms by the estrus cycle. Am J Pathol 62: 61(a)
24. Crile G, Deodhar SD (1971) Role of preoperative radiation in prolonging concomitant immunity and preventing metastasis in mice. Cancer 27: 629-634
25. de Lacroix WF, Lennartz KJ (1981) Changes in the proliferation characteristics of a solid transplantable tumour of the mouse with time after transplantation. Cell Tissue Kinet 14: 135-142
26. Denekamp J (1970) The cellular proliferation kinetics of animal tumors. Cancer Res 30: 393-400
27. Denekamp J, Thomlinson RH (1971) The cell proliferation kinetics of four experimental tumors after X-irradiation. Cancer Res 31: 1279-1284
28. de Ruiter J, Cramer SJ, Lelieveld P, van Putten LM (1982) Comparison of metastatic disease after local tumour treatment with radiotherapy or surgery in various tumour models. Eur J Cancer 18: 281-289

29. Dethlefsen LA (1979) Cellular recovery kinetic studies relevant to combined-modality research and therapy. Int J Radiat Oncol Biol Phys 5: 1197-1203
30. Dethlefsen LA (1980) The growth dynamics of murine mammary tumor cells in situ. In: McGrath C, Brennan MJ, Rich MA (eds) Cell biology of breast cancer. Academic, New York, pp 145-160
31. Dethlefsen LA, Prewitt JMS, Mendelsohn ML (1968) Analysis of tumor growth curves. JNCI 40: 389-405
32. Dethlefsen LA, Riley RM, Roti Roti JL (1979) Flow cytometric analysis of adriamycin-perturbed mouse mammary tumors. J Histochem Cytochem 27: 463-469
33. DeWys WD (1972) Studies correlating the growth rate of a tumor and its metastases and providing evidence for tumor-related systemic growth-retarding factors. Cancer Res 32: 374-379
34. Dickson JA, Ellis HA (1974) Stimulation of tumour cell dissemination by raised temperature (42°C) in rats with transplanted Yoshida tumours. Nature 248: 354-358
35. Dickson JA, Ellis HA (1976) The influence of tumor volume and the degree of heating on the response of the solid Yoshida sarcoma to hyperthermia (40-42°). Cancer Res 36: 1188-1195
36. Dunphy JE (1950) Some observations on the natural behavior of cancer in man. N Engl J Med 242: 167-172
37. Eccles SA, Alexander P (1975) Immunologically-mediated restraint of latent tumour metastases. Nature 257: 52-53
38. Fidler IJ, Kripke ML (1980) Tumor cell antigenicity, host immunity, and cancer metastasis. Cancer Immunol Immunother 7: 201-205
39. Fisher B (1984) The clinical scientific basis of adjuvant chemotherapy in breast cancer. In: Senn H-J (ed) Adjuvant chemotherapy of breast cancer. Springer, Berlin Heidelberg New York Tokyo, pp 8-17 (Recent results in cancer research, vol 96)
40. Fisher B, Gunduz N (1979) Further observations on the inhibition of tumor growth by *Corynebacterium parvum* with cyclophosphamide. X. Effect of treatment on tumor cell kinetics in mice. JNCI 62: 1545-1551
41. Fisher B, Gunduz N, Saffer EA (1983a) Influence of the interval between primary tumor removal and chemotherapy on kinetics and growth of metastases. Cancer Res 43: 1488-1492
42. Fisher B, Gunduz N, Saffer EA (1983b) Interrelation between tumor cell proliferation and 17-fluoresceinated estrone binding föllowing primary tumor removal, radiation, cyclophosphamide or tamoxifen. Cancer Res 43: 5244-5247
43. Fisher B, Saffer EA, Deutsch M (1986) Influence of irradiation of a primary tumor on the labeling index and estrogen receptor index in a distant tumor focus. Int J Radiat Oncol Biol Phys 12: 879-885
44. Fisher B, Saffer EA, Fisher ER (1970) Comparison of concomitant and sinecomitant tumor immunity. Proc Soc Exp Biol Med 135: 68-71
45. Frindel E, Malaise EP, Alpen E, Tubiana M (1967) Kinetics of cell proliferation of an experimental tumor. Cancer Res 27: 1122-1131
46. Gershon RK, Carter RL, Kondo K (1968) Immunologic defenses against metastases: impairment by excision of an allotransplanted lymphoma. Science 159: 646-648
47. Goldie H, Walker M, Kelley L, Gaines J (1956) Free tumor cell growth in the peritoneal cavity (ascites tumor) of mice bearing subcutaneous tumors. Cancer Res 16: 553-558
48. Goodman GJ (1957) Effects of one tumor upon the growth of another. Proc Am Assoc Cancer Res 2: 207
49. Gorelik E (1982) Antimetastatic concomitant immunity. In: Liotta LA, Hart IR (eds) Tumor invasion and metastasis. Nijhoff, Boston, pp 113-131

50. Gorelik E, Fogel M, de Baetselier P, Katzav S, Feldman M, Segal S (1982) Immunological diversity of metastatic cells. In: Liotta LA, Hart IR (eds) Tumor invasion and metastasis. Nijhoff, The Hague, pp 133-141
51. Gorelik E, Segal S, Feldman M (1978) Growth of a local tumor exerts a specific inhibitory effect on progression of lung metastases. Int J Cancer 21: 617-625
52. Gorelik E, Segal S, Feldman M (1980) Control of lung metastasis progression in mice: role of growth kinetics of 3LL Lewis lung carcinoma and immune reactivity. JNCI 65: 1257-1264
53. Gorelik E, Segal S, Feldman M (1981) On the mechanism of tumor "concomitant immunity". Int J Cancer 27: 847-856
54. Greene HSN, Harvey EK (1960) The inhibitory influence of a transplanted hamster lymphoma on metastasis. Cancer Res 20: 1094-1103
55. Gunduz N, Fisher B, Saffer EA (1979) Effect of surgical removal on the growth and kinetics of residual tumor. Cancer Res 39: 3861-3865
56. Halleraker B, Hartviet F (1971) Interaction between subcutaneous and intraperitoneal transplants of the Ehrlich carcinoma; the possible role of anti-tumor antibody. J Pathol 105: 95-103
57. Hartveit F, Halleraker B (1971) Effect of subcutaneous transplants of Ehrlich carcinoma on the survival time of mice with intraperitoneal transplants of the same tumour. J Pathol 105: 85-93
58. Hermens AF, Barendsen GW (1969) Changes of cell proliferation characteristics in a rat rhabdomyosarcoma before and after X-irradiation. Eur J Cancer 5: 173-189
59. Howes AE (1969) An estimation of changes in the proportions and absolute number of hypoxic cells after irradiation of transplanted C3H mouse mammary tumours. Br J Radiol 42: 441-447
60. Huggins C, Grand LC, Brillantes FP (1961) Mammary cancer induced by a single feeding of polynuclear hydrocarbons, and its suppression. Nature 189: 204-207
61. Janik P (1971) Cell proliferation during the course of immunological rejection of Ehrlich ascites tumour cells. Cell Tissue Kinet 4: 69-74
62. Janik P, Steel GG (1972) Cell proliferation during immunological perturbation in three transplanted tumours. Br J Cancer 26: 108-114
63. Jeejeebhoy HF (1974) Stimulation of tumor growth by the immune response. Int J Cancer 13: 665-678
64. Kaplan HS, Murphy ED (1948) The effect of local roentgen irradiation on the biological behavior of a transplantable mouse carcinoma. I. Increased frequency of pulmonary metastasis. JNCI 9: 407-413
65. Keller R (1981) Induction of macroscopic metastases via surgery. Invasion Metastasis 1: 136-148
66. Keller R (1982) Involvement of spontaneous rather than induced antitumor mechanisms in resistance to primary fibrosarcoma implantation and its secondary spread. In: Heberman RD (ed) NK cells and other natural effector cells. Academic, New York, pp 1353-1358
67. Keller R (1983) Elicitation of macroscopic metastases via surgery: various forms of surgical intervention differ in their induction of metastatic outgrowth. Invasion Metastasis 3: 183-192
68. Keller R (1985a) Repression of lymphatic metastasis by a second implant of the same tumor. Invasion Metastasis 5: 295-308
69. Keller R (1985b) Surgical intervention and metastasis. In: Metzger U, Larigiader L, Senn H-J (eds) Perioperative chemotherapy. Springer, Berlin Heidelberg New York Tokyo, pp 11-16 (Recent results in cancer research, vol 98)

70. Keller R, Hess MW (1982) Divergency between incidence of microscopic and macroscopic metastases. Virchows Arch [17] 398: 33-43
71. Ketcham AS, Kinsey DL, Wexler H, Mantel N (1961) The development of spontaneous metastases after removal of a "primary" tumor. II. Standardization protocol of 5 animal tumors. Cancer 14: 875-882
72. Ketcham AS, Wexler H, Mantel N (1959) The effect of removal of a "primary" tumor on the development of spontaneous metastases I. Development of a standardized experimental technique. Cancer Res 19: 940-944
73. Ketcham AS, Wexler H, Mantel N (1961) Studies on the effects of surgery on transplanted animal tumors and their metastases. JNCI 27: 1311-1321
74. Ketcham AS, Wexler H, Minton JP (1966) Experimental study of metastases. JAMA 198: 177-184
75. Laird AK (1964) Dynamics of tumour growth. Br J Cancer 18: 490-502
76. Laird AK (1965) Dynamics of tumour growth: comparison of growth rates and extrapolation of growth curve to one cell. Br J Cancer 19: 278-291
77. Lewis MR, Cole WH (1958) Experimental increase of lung metastases after operative trauma (amputation of limb with tumor). Arch Surg 77: 621-626
78. McCredie JA, Inch RW, Sutherland RM (1971) Differences in growth and morphology between the spontaneous C3H mammary carcinoma in the mouse and its syngeneic transplants. Cancer 27: 635-642
79. Mendelsohn ML (1965) The kinetics of tumor cell proliferation. In: Symposium on fundamental cancer research. Cellular radiation biology. Williams and Wilkins, Baltimore, pp 498-513
80. Mendelsohn ML (1962) Autoradiographic analysis of cell proliferation in spontaneous breast cancer of C3H mouse. III. The growth fraction. JNCI 28: 1015-1029
81. Mendelsohn ML (1976) Computer analyzed transit times for vertebrate cell cycle and phases. In: Altman PL, Katz DD (eds) Cell biology. Federation of American Society of Experimental Biology, Bethesda, pp 11-13
82. Mendelsohn ML, Dethlefsen LA (1973) Cell kinetics of breast cancer: the turnover of nonproliferating cells. In: Griem ML, Jensen EV, Ultman JE, Wissler RW (eds) Breast cancer: a challenging problem. Springer, Berlin Heidelberg New York Tokyo, pp 73-86 (Recent results in cancer research, vol 42)
83. Mendelsohn ML, Dohan FC, Moore HA (1960) Autoradiographic analysis of cell proliferation in spontaneous breast cancer of C3H mouse. I. Typical cell cycle and timing of DNA synthesis. JNCI 25: 477-484
84. Middle JG, Embleton MJ (1981) Naturally arising tumors of the inbred WAB/Not rat strain. II. Immunogenicity of transplanted tumors. JNCI 67: 637-643
85. Mikulska ZB, Smith C, Alexander P (1966) Evidence for an immunological reaction of the host directed against its own actively growing tumor. JNCI 36: 29-35
86. Milas L, Hunter N, Mason K, Withers HR (1974) Immunological resistance to pulmonary metastases in C3Hf/Bu mice bearing syngeneic fibrosarcoma of different sizes. Cancer Res 34: 61-71
87. Munster AM, Gale GR, Hunt HH (1977) Accelerated tumor growth following experimental burns. J Trauma 17: 373-375
88. Naito H, Ziegler MM, Tsou KC (1985) Rational selection of adjuvant chemotherapy after cytoreduction surgery for murine neuroblastoma. Cancer Res 45: 3554-3560
89. North RJ, Kirstein DP (1977) T-cell-mediated concomitant immunity to syngeneic tumors. I. Activated macrophages as the expressors of nonspecific immunity to unrelated tumors and bacterial parasites. J Exp Med 145: 275-292

90. Ogita S, Tokiwa K, Goto Y, Majima S (1985) Experimental study on the growth and proliferation kinetics of residual tumor after surgery in mouse neuroblastoma. J Pediatr Surg 20: 224-227
91. Paranjpe MS, Boon CW (1974) Kinetics of the anti-tumor delayed hypersensitivity response in mice with progressively growing tumors: stimulation followed by specific suppression. Int J Cancer 13: 179-186
92. Prehn RT, Prehn LM (1987) The autoimmune nature of cancer. Cancer Res 47: 927-932
93. Price CHG, Jeffree GM (1973) Metastatic spread of osteosarcoma. Br J Cancer 28: 515-524
94. Riley V (1975) Mouse mammary tumors: alteration of incidence as apparent function of stress. Science 189: 465-467
95. Rockwell S, Kallman RF (1972) Growth and cell population kinetics of single and multiple KHT sarcomas. Cell Tissue Kinet 5: 449-457
96. Romsdahl MM (1963) The experimental influence of operative procedures on distant metastases. Proc Am Assoc Cancer Res 4: 58
97. Schabel FM Jr, Simpson-Herren L (1984) Tumor growth kinetics and drug treatment of cancer. In: Keummerle HP (ed) Clinical chemotherapy, vol III: antineoplastic chemotherapy. Thieme-Stratton, New York, pp 16-34
98. Schatten WE (1958a) An experimental study of postoperative tumor metastases. I. Growth of pulmonary metastases following total removal of primary leg tumor. Cancer 11: 455-459
99. Schatten WE, Kramer WM (1958b) An experimental study of postoperative tumor metastases. II. Effects of anesthesia, operation, and cortisone administration on growth of pulmonary metastases. Cancer 11: 460-462
100. Schiffer LM (1978) The cell kinetics of mammary cancers. In: McGuire WL (ed) Breast cancer: advances in research and treatment, vol 2. Plenum, New York, pp 259-282
101. Schiffer LM, Braunschweiger PG, Stragand JJ (1978) Tumor cell population kinetics following noncurative treatment. In: Schabel FM Jr (ed) Antiobiotics and chemotherapy, vol 23. Karger, Basel, pp 148-156
102. Schiffer LM, Markoe AM, Nelson JSR (1973) Evaluation of the PDP index as a monitor of growth fraction during tumor therapy. In: The cell cycle in malignancy and immunotherapy. Proc of thirteenth Annual Hanford Biology Symposium, Technical Information Center, Office of Public Affairs, US Energy Research and Development Administration, pp 459-472
103. Schiffer LM, Markoe AM, Nelson JSR (1976) Estimation of tumor growth fraction in murine tumors by the primer-available DNA-dependent DNA polymerase assay. Cancer Res 36: 2415-2418
104. Shapiro J, Jersky J, Katzav S, Feldman M, Segal S (1981) Anesthetic drugs accelerate the progression of postoperative metastases of mouse tumors. J Clin Invest 68: 678-685
105. Sheldon PW, Fowler JF (1973) The effect of irradiating a transplanted murine lymphosarcoma on the subsequent development of metastases. Br J Cancer 28: 508-514
106. Sheldon PW, Fowler JF (1976) The effect of low-dose pre-operative x-irradiation of implanted mouse mammary carcinomas on local recurrence and metastasis. Br J Cancer 34: 401-407
107. Simpson-Herren L (1977) Kinetics and multiple modality therapy. First annual meeting of the Cell Kinetics Society, 11-13 March 1977, Birmingham, AL
108. Simpson-Herren L (1982) Kinetic perturbations during cancer therapy. Ann NY Acad Sci 397: 88-100
109. Simpson-Herren L, Griswold DP Jr (1970) Studies of the kinetics of growth and regression of 7,12-dimethylbenz(*a*)anthracene-induced mammary adenocarcinoma in Sprague-Dawley rats. Cancer Res 30: 813-818

110. Simpson-Herren L, Griswold DP Jr (1973) Studies of the cell population kinetics of induced and transplanted mammary adenocarcinoma in rats. Cancer Res 33: 2415-2424
111. Simpson-Herren L, Lloyd HH (1970) Kinetic parameters and growth curves for experimental tumor systems. Cancer Chemother Rep 54: 143-174
112. Simpson-Herren L, Griswold DP Jr, Corbett TH (1978) Studies of the growth, population kinetics and host lethality of $CD8F_1$ mammary adenocarcinoma. Cancer Treat Rep 62: 519-528
113. Simpson-Herren L, Sanford AH, Holmquist JP (1976) Effects of surgery on the cell kinetics of residual tumor. Cancer Treat Rep 60: 1749-1760
114. Skipper HE (1971) Kinetics of mammary tumor cell growth and implications for therapy. Cancer 28: 1479-1499
115. Sklar LS, Anisman H (1979) Stress and coping factors influence tumor growth. Science 205: 513-515
116. Steel GG (1977) Growth kinetics of tumors. Clarendon, Oxford
117. Stragand JJ, Braunschweiger PG, Pollice AA, Schiffer LM (1979) Cell kinetic alterations in murine mammary tumors following fasting and refeeding. Eur J Cancer 15: 281-286
118. Tannock IF (1970) Population kinetics of carcinoma cells, capillary endothelial cells, and fibroblasts in a transplanted mouse mammary tumor. Cancer Res 30: 2470-2476
119. Thunold S (1967) Acquired immunity after surgical removal of subcutaneous Ehrlich's ascites carcinoma. Acta Pathol Microbiol Scand 71: 564-574
120. Tyzzer EE (1913) Factors in the production and growth of tumor metastases. J Med Res 28: 309-332
121. van den Brenk HAS, Sharpington C (1971) Effect of local X-irradiation of a primary sarcoma in the rat on dissemination and growth of metastases: dose-response characteristics. Br J Cancer 25: 812-830
122. van Peperzell HA (1972) Effects of single doses of radiation on lung metastases in man and experimental animals. Eur J Cancer 8: 665-675
123. Visintainer MA, Volpicelli JR, Seligman ME (1982) Tumor rejection in rats after inescapable or escapable shock. Science 216: 437-439
124. Vollmer TL, Conley FK (1984) Effect of cyclosphosphamide on survival of mice and incidence of metastatic tumor following intravenous and intracardial inoculation of tumor cells. Cancer Res 44: 3902-3906
125. Walker A, McCallum HM, Wheldon TE, Nias AHW, Abdelaal AS (1978) Promotion of metastasis of C3H mouse mammary carcinoma by local hyperthermia. Br J Cancer 38: 561-563
126. Watson JV (1976) The perturbed cell proliferation kinetics of the EMT6/M/AC tumour in mice treated with anti-mouse lymphocyte serum. Cell Tissue Kinet 9: 565-571
127. Whitney RB, Levy JG, Smith AG (1974) Influence of tumor size and surgical resection on cell-mediated immunity in mice. JNCI 53: 111-116
128. Xu X (1987) The biological foundation of the Gompertz model. Int J Biomed Comput 20: 35-39
129. Yerushalmi A (1976) Influence on metastatic spread of whole-body or local tumor hyperthermia. Eur J Cancer 12: 455-463
130. Yuhas JM, Pazmiño NH (1974) Inhibition of subcutaneously growing line 1 carcinomas due to metastatic spread. Cancer Res 34: 2005-2010

Receptors

Hormone Receptors and Risk in Breast Cancer

D.E. Merkel, S.M. Hill, and W.L. McGuire

The Evanston Hospital, Division of Medical Oncology, 2650 Ridge Avenue, Evanston, IL 60201, USA

Introduction

It has long been appreciated that some metastatic breast cancers were susceptible to hormonal influences and would respond to hormonal manipulation. The discovery of steroid hormone receptors in some breast cancers permitted more accurate prediction of which tumors would respond to such hormonal manipulation. In recent years the prognostic importance of the estrogen receptor (ER) and progesterone receptor (PR) content of primary breast cancers has become apparent. Today, hormone receptor status can aid in predicting the risk of relapse of a primary breast cancer, the anatomic sites at risk for such relapse, and overall survival risk. Furthermore, receptor status predicts which patients will benefit from adjuvant hormonal therapy. These data are reviewed in the first section of this chapter. Given the important association between the receptor status and the natural history of breast cancer, it would seem reasonable to expect that the ligands for these receptors, circulating estrogens and progesterones, would have a similar relationship with the course of this disease. As discussed in the second section of this chapter, however, there is no clear connection between specific circulating steroid hormones and either development or progression of breast cancer. Nonetheless, direct effects of steroid hormones on breast cancer cell lines have been demonstrated in vitro.

The final section reviews recent progress in understanding the function and structure of receptor molecules. Using the techniques of molecular biology, the amino acid sequences for the various hormone receptor molecules have been determined and compared, yielding insights into their functional components. Such molecular probes may enable us to identify dysfunctional receptor molecules, a potential cause of the imperfect correlation between receptor content and clinical hormonal responsiveness. Furthermore, understanding the function of steroid hormone receptors at a molecular level may clarify the role that circulating hormones play in the pathogenesis and progression of breast cancer.

Hormone Receptors as Clinical Indicators

The first application of ER and PR determinations to the care of breast cancer patients was to aid in selection of those patients most likely to respond to hormonal

Ragaz/Ariel (Eds.), High-Risk Breast Cancer

therapy. These biochemical assays have now been available for over a decade, and with time the relationship between tumor receptor status and prognosis has become apparent. Both ER and PR status have important relationships to prognosis in primary breast cancer. Not only the duration of disease-free survival after primary therapy, but also the sites at risk for relapse, survival after relapse, and overall survival can be correlated to receptor status. In this way, steroid receptor assays can provide both valuable guides to treatment and powerful predictors of future risk in breast cancer.

Response of Metastatic Disease

By 1974 it was clear that ER-positive metastatic breast cancer was more likely to respond to a variety of hormonal manipulations than ER-negative cancers [50]. Since PR is expressed by normal breast tissue in response to estrogenic stimulation, it was felt that PR might serve as a marker for an intact estrogen response mechanism in breast cancer. In this way PR determinations might enhance the ability of ER assays to predict hormonal responsiveness. Indeed, by 1979, a number of investigators had shown that ER and PR assays, when used in combination, could better predict the response of metastatic breast cancer to endocrine therapy [55].

When these data were pooled, an overall response rate of 77% for ER-positive, PR-positive tumors was seen, in contrast to only 11% for ER-negative, PR-negative tumors. As could be predicted, ER-negative, PR-positive tumors were uncommon. Responses were also seen in 27% of patients with ER-positive, PR-negative breast cancer. Response by tumors lacking detectable PR might be due to: (a) inadequate estrogenic stimulation in postmenopausal women to cause PR expression; (b) false-negative PR determinations in premenopausal women because of receptor saturation by circulating progesterone; or (c) uncoupling of estrogen-dependent growth properties and PR expression in tumor cells. This uncoupling has recently been demonstrated in a breast cancer cell line [62].

Prognosis

ER and PR status could also be immediately correlated with other prognostically important histologic features in breast cancer. Well-differentiated tumors, and those with low nuclear grade, prominent elastosis, minimal necrosis, and absent lymphocytic infiltration are more likely to be ER-positive [26]. In some series smaller tumors are more likely to be receptor-positive [16], but this relationship has not been found by all investigators. Older patients are more likely to be ER-positive, regardless of menopausal status. The frequency of PR-positive tumors also increases with age for both premenopausal and postmenopausal groups when considered separately, as shown in Table 1 [16]. Receptor status of the primary tumor is not related to the presence or number of axillary nodal metastases.

The relationship of receptor status to prognostically important histologic characteristics suggested that ER and PR might be directly related to prognosis. In

Table 1. Age menopausal status, and proportion of receptor-positive tumors. (From San Antonio receptor data base)

Age	ER-positive (%)		PR-positive (%)	
(years)	Premenopausal	Postmenopausal	Premenopausal	Postmenopausal
25-30	26		41	
30-35	60		51	
35-40	61	36	52	33
40-45	62	45	56	33
45-50	75	60	66	32
50-55	67	70	73	39
55-60		75		49
60-65		82		53
65-70		85		59
70-75		84		63

1977 Knight et al. [43] first reported a relationship between ER status and both disease-free and overall survival in primary breast cancer. A similar worsening of prognosis in ER-negative stage I and II breast cancer patients was subsequently reported by a number of other groups [4, 77, 27, 56, 13, 47, 61, 1, 3, 35, 54, 71]. On the other hand, several studies have found either no relationship between ER and prognosis, or an initial survival advantage in the ER-positive group which was, however, lost after 4-5 years.

PR has also been strongly correlated with outcome in a limited number of studies [58, 15, 25, 48, 10, 22]. In a cohort of 189 patients with stage II breast cancer treated with adjuvant chemotherapy, the relative importance of a variety of prognostic factors was assessed by multivariate analysis. Both the number of involved axillary nodes and the PR concentration had strong independent associations with prognosis ($P<0.0001$), but the ER concentration provided no additional prognostic information [15].

Those results suggested that ER and PR might have different prognostic importance in different subsets of primary breast cancer patients. Data from the San Antonio receptor data base, shown in Table 2, support this possibility. In multivariate analyses of both disease-free survival and overall survival of 1647 stage I breast cancer patients, ER and tumor size are highly significant independent prognostic factors, but PR is not. In contrast, similar analyses of 1529 stage II breast cancer patients show the number of positive nodes, size of the primary tumors, and PR to be important prognostic factors. ER does not contribute independently to disease-free survival, but does have a significant independent relationship to overall survival [51].

One might conclude that ER and PR reflect different biologic characteristics in primary breast cancer. In stage I breast cancer, metastatic capability, perhaps associated with features such as high nuclear and histologic grades, high proliferative rate, and absent ER, may be most important. Interestingly, however,

Table 2a. Multivariate analysis of disease-free and overall survival in 1647 stage I breast cancer patients. (Modified from 51)

Prognostic factor	Disease-free survival (P)	Overall survival (P)
Estrogen receptor	<0.0001	0.0003
Size of tumor	0.0002	0.0041
Progesterone receptor	0.31	0.11
Age of patient	0.78	0.64

Table 2b. Multivariate analysis of disease-free and overall survival in 1529 stage II breast cancer patients. (Modified from 51)

Progonostic factor	Disease-free survival (P)	Overall survival (P)
Number of positive nodes	<0.0001	<0.0001
Size of tumor	<0.0001	0.0001
Progesterone receptor	0.0001	0.0001
Estrogen receptor	0.14	0.0017
Age of paitent	0.90	0.062

neither ER nor PR status is directly correlated with axillary node involvement [16]. Once metastatic capability is evident, i.e., in stage II disease, endocrine dependence as marked by PR expression becomes a more important prognostic determinant.

Response to Adjuvant Hormonal Therapy

Receptor determinations are useful not only in assessing risk in primary breast cancer, but also in predicting which patients will benefit from adjuvant hormonal therapy. Several large studies have randomized stage II breast cancer patients to adjuvant treatment with tamoxifen or no further therapy. Most studies in which receptor content of the primary tumor was measured have shown that tamoxifen-related improvement in disease-free survival occurred only in the receptor-positive subset of patients [60, 75, 47, 64]. Usually results were analyzed only in relation to ER status. In the Toronto-Edmonton Breast Cancer Study Group Trial, however, PR status was a stronger predictor of benefit from adjuvant antiestrogen therapy than was ER status [60]. In the large Nolvadex Adjuvant Trial Organisation Study [54] adjuvant therapy with tamoxifen resulted in improved disease-free and overall survival, regardless of ER status. It should be noted that ER results were available in less than half of all patients in this study, ER assays were not performed by central reference laboratories, and the PR status of these patients was not reported.

Further evidence that the receptor content of primary breast cancer can predict which patients will benefit from adjuvant hormonal therapy has come from trials which randomized patients between adjuvant chemotherapy alone and the same chemotherapy plus tamoxifen. Pearson [57] reported that improved disease-free survival was seen in the ER-positive subset of randomized stage II patients who received both chemotherapy and tamoxifen. In contrast, those ER-negative patients who received tamoxifen in addition to chemotherapy did slightly worse than those receiving chemotherapy alone. The National Surgical Adjuvant Breast Project Trial B-09 gave similar results: patients who received tamoxifen in addition to chemotherapy had a significant increase in disease-free survival if their primary tumor was ER-positive or PR-positive [25]. Younger patients with PR-negative tumors had a worsened overall survival if they were randomized to receive tamoxifen as well as chemotherapy. Here, as in the Toronto-Edmonton Trial [60], PR status was a stronger predictor of benefit from adjuvant hormonal therapy than was ER status. The Gynecological Adjuvant Breast Cancer Group also found that the addition of tamoxifen to adjuvant chemotherapy produced an increase in disease-free survival among ER-positive patients [41]. On the other hand, the Eastern Cooperative Oncology Group failed to find a difference in disease-free survival between women who received adjuvant chemotherapy or chemotherapy plus tamoxifen, regardless of receptor status [71].

Behavior of Metastatic Disease

Even after relapse, the hormone receptor status continues to provide prognostic information. The initial site of relapse is much more likely to be osseous in ER-positive primary breast cancers [61]. In contrast, the first site of recurrence for ER-negative primary tumors is more commonly in the lungs, liver, or brain. In a smaller autopsy series, de la Monte et al. [20] showed that metastases to the thyroid and parathyroid glands were more common in receptor-positive breast cancers, whereas leptomeningeal spread was more characteristic of ER-negative tumors. Patients with ER-positive primary breast cancers have also been reported to have a longer duration of survival *after* relapse than those with ER-negative primary tumors [36].

It is important to note in this respect that the receptor content of a primary tumor may not always predict that of a subsequent metastasis, and that a change in receptor status may have prognostic importance. PR status in particular is likely to be discordant between a primary tumor and a later metastasis. In one study, 44% of initially PR-positive patients, and 56% of those who then received hormonal therapy, had PR-negative breast cancer in a subsequent biopsy [30]. Those patients who were initially PR-positive, but whose later biopsies were PR-negative, had a worse prognosis than those who continued to be PR-positive.

Hormones in Breast Cancer

These correlative studies have shown that analysis of primary breast cancers for steroid receptor content can provide valuable prognostic information, but do not explain how the presence or absence of these receptors could affect the natural history of the disease. The interrelationship between receptor status, surgical stage, and prognosis suggests that perhaps ER and PR act as markers for other, as yet undescribed properties related to malignant progression; alternately, the degree of hormonal responsiveness of early breast cancer may directly influence its growth and spread, implying that the body's hormonal milieu has an important effect on cancer cells. The role of various hormones in the development and progression of breast cancer has been the subject of intensive study, but remains largely uncertain. This section will discuss circulating estrogen, progestins, and androgens, and the risk of breast cancer.

Estrogens

Estrogens have long been considered important in the development of breast cancer. Understanding of the precise role of estrogens in the cellular biology of breast cancer has lagged behind the therapeutic use of estrogens and antiestrogens, however. Current evidence of the importance of circulating estrogens in breast cancer includes epidemiologic data and studies involving human breast cancer cell lines.

Lemon and co-workers [45] originally proposed that the roles of the three main estrogens – estrone (E_1), estradiol (E_2), and estriol (E_3) – need to be considered; Cole and MacMahon [18] suggested the lifetime risk of breast cancer was reduced by an excess of E_3 relative to E_1 and E_2 occurring during the years immediately after menarche. This hypothesis is consistent with the observation that early full-term pregnancies protect against breast cancer, since during the third trimester of pregnancy concentrations of E_3 are greatly increased relative to E_1 and E_2. Cole et al. [17] observed that uniparous women have higher ratios of E_3 to E_1 and E_2 than nulliparous women of similar age. This difference is evident only in women having their first child before the age of 24 years and during the follicular phase of the cycle. Among the youngest women, the differences in the E_3 ratio between the parous and nulliparous were highly statistically significant. Despite this and other pieces of circumstantial epidemiologic evidence, the hypothesis that a high ratio of E_3 to E_1 and E_2 protects against breast cancer remains controversial.

Published epidemiologic studies have not indicated any definite relationships between breast cancer and the use of oral contraceptives. Two studies have reported a substantially increased risk for oral contraceptive users who had previous breast biopsies. Studies by Fasal and Paffenbarger [24] and Brinton et al. [8] noted an increased risk for previously biopsied postmenopausal women experiencing a natural menopause. On the other hand, a large number of both cohort and case-control studies, including the landmark Cancer and Steroid Hormone Study (1986) [81], have detected no increased relative risk of breast cancer among women exposed to oral contraceptives, regardless of the duration of exposure.

Several case-control studies have examined users of postmenopausal estrogen supplements for an increased risk of breast cancer, but have been hampered by small numbers and limited data regarding dosage and duration of use [14, 66]. A recent well-designed study found a 2.5-fold increased risk of breast cancer in women with intact ovaries who had taken a total estrogen dose in excess of 1500 mg. The increased risk could not be detected, however, in oophorectomized women. In women with surgically confirmed benign breast disease the relative risk rose to 4.8 [65]. It is clear from the lack of consistent data that more large-scale studies of women receiving postmenopausal estrogens are urgently needed.

The growth-stimulatory effects of E_2 have been studied extensively in human breast cancer cell lines. The results of different investigators are not in complete harmony, owing to the differences in culture conditions; nonetheless, growth stimulation of human breast cancer cell lines has been reported by several authors. For example, Lippman et al. [46] reported a twofold stimulation of [^{3}H] thymidine incorporation into the DNA of MCF-7 human breast cancer cells treated with estrogens. Moreover, E_2 supplementation is essential for the growth of MCF-7 cells in vivo, when these cells are inoculated into athymic nude mice [68, 79].

In addition to their mitogenic action, estrogens also modify the morphology of human breast cancer cells in vitro. A study by Vic and co-workers [73] clearly demonstrated (by scanning and transmission electron microscopy) that 10 n*M* E_2 increased surface microvilli and transformed the MCF-7 cells into a secretory phenotype. These effects were also observed in other estrogen-responsive human breast cancer cell lines (ZR-75 and T47-D), but not the BT-20 cell line, which lacks estrogen receptors.

Estromedins. Besides a direct effect on cellular growth machinery, estrogens may induce the expression of enzymes involved in DNA synthesis or cell growth [9, 2]. Furthermore, estrogens induce alterations in specific secreted proteins and growth factors. Lippman and co-workers have recently shown that secretion of insulin-like growth factor [37], and α-transforming growth activity [21, 5], is increased in response to estrogen stimulation. In addition, Rochefort et al. [74, 78] have identified a glycoprotein ($M_r = 52\,000$) that stimulates replication of MCF-7 cells in vitro. Estrogens may also affect the malignant phenotype by decreasing the production of growth factors and other proteins which would normally exert a negative effect on growth. Roberts et al. [63] have shown that β-transforming growth factor can inhibit the growth of MCF-7 breast cancer cells. Possible autocrine and paracrine effect of these estrogen-regulated proteins are the subject of ongoing research.

Progesterone

The role of progesterone in the etiology of breast cancer has received relatively less attention than that of estrogens. Several animal studies have found progesterone to be a carcinogen in rodents [53, 59]. However, Horwitz and McGuire [33] found that progesterone can stimulate tumor growth in rats only in cooperation with estrogen. Ovariectomized-adrenalectomized rats bearing 7,12-dimethylbenz(*a*)anthracene-induced mammary tumors were treated, either with estradiol alone, or with estradiol plus progesterone, or were not treated. In animals withdrawn from all hormonal supplementation, 22 of 24 tumors regressed. When estradiol was discontinued in rats receiving estradiol and progesterone, 11 of 13 tumors regressed rapidly. Conversely, when tumors growing on both estradiol and progesterone were switched to estradiol alone, 5 of 7 tumors continued to grow. Although progesterone may possibly enhance the induction of these tumors, it is not believed to play a major role in the growth of established tumors.

In humans, however, most attention has been focused on progesterone's possible protective effect against estrogens. Because ER levels in the endometrium drop during the luteal phase, at a time of increased progesterone secretion, it has been proposed [31] that increased progesterone secretion has a protective effect against estrogenic stimulation. In fact, it has been hypothesized that estrogenic stimulation in the absence of sufficient progesterone secretion may provide a favorable environment for the development of breast cancer [70].

At the present time, there is very little epidemiologic evidence that inadequate corpus luteum function, with its associated low progesterone levels, increases the risk of breast cancer [44]. In fact, studies of women at high risk for breast cancer have generally not found these women to have abnormally low luteal progesterone levels. Thus, the role of progesterone in the etiology of breast cancer and the way it interacts with estrogens and other hormones is unclear, but remains an area of continued research interest.

Androgens

Interest in the involvement of androgenic hormones in breast cancer increased after the early work of Bulbrook and colleagues [11]. In a prospective study of normal women on the island of Guernsey, Bulbrook found that women who later developed breast cancer had been excreting low levels of androgen metabolites (11-deoxy-17-oxosteroids and androsterone), particularly etiocholanolone, into the urine. It was observed that etiocholanolone excretion was lower in precancer cases than in controls. Similar data, demonstrating lower urinary excretion of androgen metabolites, have also been reported by others [52, 72].

From these data it is tempting to speculate that women with decreased production of adrenal androgens are at high risk for breast cancer. However, this cannot be the only explanation because Japanese women, who are at low risk for breast cancer, excrete lower levels for androgen metabolites than do British women, who are at high risk for breast cancer [12]. From these conflicting, but not necessarily contradictory results, it is obvious that the role of adrenal androgens in the etiology of breast cancer remains unclear.

Molecular Aspects of Steroid Hormone Receptors

As the preceding sections reveal, there remain many poorly understood aspects of the interrelationships between circulating hormones, tumor hormone receptors, and the pathogenesis and natural history of breast cancer. Tumor receptor content is not a perfect predictor of hormonal responsiveness, and many receptor-positive tumors will not respond clinically to hormonal manipulation. Tumors which lack detectable receptors have a more aggressive natural history, but the *normal* growth of breast tissue is clearly dependent on both hormones and hormone receptors. Finally, the events that occur subsequent to the binding of ligand to ER and PR are incompletely described, even in tumor cells with intact hormone response mechanisms.

Proposed Function of Steroid Receptors

The ER (M_r=65-70000) exists in low abundance in tissue-specific target cells, comprising 0.01% of the total cellular proteins. The cellular localization of the human ER has been studied by immunocytochemical techniques with a variety of monoclonal antibodies produced against the human ER [29]. Data from several laboratories [69, 42] suggest that steroids may exert their effects by binding directly to an intranuclear receptor molecule that is weakly associated with nuclear components in the absence of ligand. Binding of hormone to its receptor results in a conversion of the receptor-steroid complex to a form that associates with high affinity to one or more nuclear components. The molecular nature of this association is not known, but it is suspected that, like other steroid receptors, the ligand-occupied ER recognizes specific DNA sequences upstream of the transcriptional start sites of responsive genes.

Steroid hormone receptors can thus be thought of as target-cell-specific gene-regulatory elements. The high affinity ligand binding measured by biochemical receptor assays may not always imply accurate and efficient function of the activated receptor molecules as regulators of gene expression. Defects in this regulatory function might explain the failure of some receptor-positive tumors to respond to hormonal therapy. To explore this possibility, the structure and function of steroid receptors must first be understood on a molecular level.

Comparative Structure of Steroid Receptor Molecules

Recent cloning of the human glucocorticoid receptor [32], human ER [76], chicken PR [38], and chicken ER [49] have allowed the comparison of both nucleic acid and amino acid sequences of these steroid receptors. Since many cell types contain receptors for more than one steroid hormone [34], differences in the structure of the receptor proteins are likely to explain the functional specificity of steroids in controlling responsive cellular machinery. Comparison of amino acid sequences between receptors in this way makes it possible to suggest regions of functional significance within the receptor proteins.

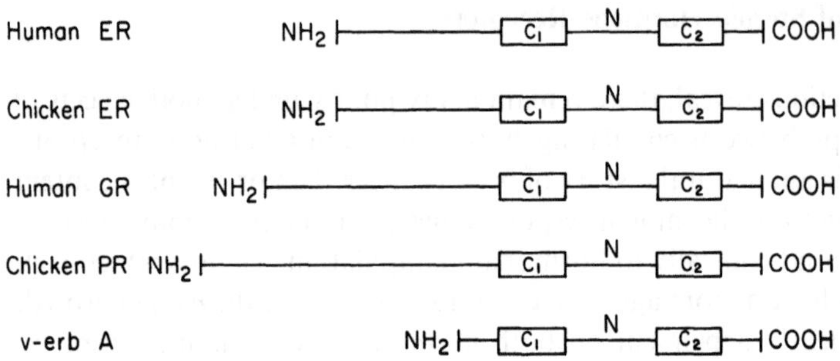

Fig. 1. Comparative amino acid sequences of chicken and human estrogen receptor (*ER*), glucocorticoid receptor (*GR*), and progesterone receptor (*PR*) proteins, and the protein coded for by the oncogene v-*erb*-A. Regions of homology are labeled C_1 and C_2. The nonhomologous, putative "hinge" region is labeled N. (Modified from Maxwell et al. 1987 [49])

The human and chicken ERs share on overall amino acid homology of approximately 75%. Another comparison [49] between chicken ER, human ER, human glucocorticoid, chicken PR, and the v-*erb*-A oncogene sequences shows an overall low homology (<20%), but significant regions of similarity. The best alignment of all the receptor sequences is illustrated in Fig. 1. This figure indicates that relative to the regions of significant homology, the carboxyl ends of the molecules are very well aligned while the proteins have heterogeneous amino termini. It was observed early on that both the human ER [28] and human glucocorticoid receptors [32] as well as chicken ER and PR [38] share a large degree of homology with the P75 *gag-erb*-A fusion product of the avian erythroblastosis virus. (This fusion protein is incapable of erythroblast transformation, but blocks their maturation and potentiates the transforming action of v-*erb* B, an epidermal growth factor receptor-like oncogene.) Two regions of what is believed to be significant homology have been identified (Fig. 1), the first consensus region (C_1) located in the central portion of the protein and the second region (C_2) located more toward the carboxyl end of the protein. The C_1 region is a 72 amino acid sequence and has a high content of cysteine and basic amino acids. The positional conservation of these nine cysteine residues among all of the steroid receptors, including v-*erb*-A, suggests a possible functional importance.

Several eukaryotic transcriptional regulatory factors contain histidine- and/or cysteine-rich motifs (similar to those seen in steroid receptors) which are believed to represent DNA-binding structures. For example, the *Xenopus* 5 S RNA transcription factor TFIIIA [49] contains a series of nine cysteine and histidine-containing motifs. These motifs are believed to fold into DNA-binding loops or "fingers," as a Zn^{2+} ion is bound between two pairs of cysteine (or histidine) residues. The amino acids between the two pairs of cysteines are thought to form a "finger" that contacts DNA by fitting into the major groove of the DNA helix. Recent evidence further supports the premise that these cysteine motifs do have DNA-binding activity when coordinating Zn^{2+} ions [40, 6].

The second region of high homology (C_2) between the receptors is a stretch of 62 amino acids located on the carboxyl side of the C_1 region. This region is 98% conserved between the human and chicken ERs. The large number of conserved amino acids in this region may provide the structure for a hormone-binding pocket, with differences at some amino acid positions resulting in hormone specificity.

Another interesting feature of the amino acid composition of the C_2 region observed by O'Malley and co-workers [49] is the number of hydrophobic residues. Even though the amino acid homologies between the steroid receptors are lower in this region than C_1, the hydropathicity plots are almost identical.

In contrast, v-*erb*-A has a different hydropathicity plot, suggesting that the C_2 domain is related to the function of these proteins as steroid receptors. It is this characteristic of the C_2 domain which distinguishes the steroid receptors from the v-*erb*-A gene product.

Regions of nonhomology such as region N between C_1 and C_2 may also have functional significance. This corresponds to the region of lowest homology between the human and chicken ER. In addition, there is no homology between the receptors and v-*erb*-A in this region. Even though the boundaries of this non-homologous region may be both structurally and functionally important, its composition may be less critical. The distance between C_1 and C_2 in the ERs is 108 amino acids. Only a single amino acid deletion is necessary to allow for the exact alignment of the C_1 and C_2 regions of v-*erb*-A with the corresponding regions in the ER proteins. In the human glucocorticoid receptor [32] and chicken PR [19], 17 and 13 amino acid insertions, respectively, are required for alignment with ER. This seems to imply that the two conserved regions (C_1 and C_2) function independently, rather than as a continuous unit.

It is known that, on binding their cognate steroid hormones, the receptors become more tightly bound to the nucleus, presumably because their affinity for specific DNA sequences is increased [80]. The underlying mechanism is unknown, but may involve communication between the hormone-binding domain and the DNA-binding domains. The nonconserved (N) region between domains C_1 and C_2 is predicted to have a highly coiled secondary structure, which could provide flexibility. Therefore, it is possible that the N region, acting as a hinge between C_1 and C_2, facilitates direct contact and communication between the latter two domains. This structural arrangement of two important functional domains separated by a hinge region has recently been described in prokaryotic and eukaryotic DNA-binding transcriptional regulatory proteins [7].

The availability of the cloned full-length ER will allow the function of ER in breast cancer to be established more precisely. Elucidation of those factors which control ER expression may help to explain why only a portion of breast cancers express ERs and how this expression can be modulated. The mechanism of steroid receptor action may be further elucidated by correlation of steroid receptor mutations with their effects on gene transcription, by the construction of chimeric receptors between the ER and glucocorticoid receptor or PR sequences, and by X-ray crystallographic analysis of the purified receptor.

Conclusion

The expression of ER and PR are intimately related to the course of clinical breast cancer. In addition to providing useful predictive information on the likelihood that hormonal treatment will be successful, receptors can be used to estimate future risk of progression. The presence of hormone receptors does not, however, assure hormonal responsiveness in all cases. In fact, the reason why hormonal receptors should be so strongly predictive of the natural history of breast cancer is uncertain. Studies of the natural ligands for these receptors, circulating estrogens and progesterones, have not shed light on this question, though it is clear that some breast cancer cells are dependent on estrogens for growth in vitro. Recent investigations have begun to elucidate the molecular structure and define the functional components of these receptors, and may lead to a better understanding of the way in which estrogen, progesterone, and their receptors influence risk in breast cancer.

References

1. Adami HO, Graffman S, Lindgren A, Sallstrom J (1985) Prognostic implications of estrogen receptor content in breast cancer. Breast Cancer Res Treat 5:293-300
2. Aitken SC, Lippman ME (1985) Effect of estrogen and antiestrogens on growth regulatory enzymes in human breast cancer in tissue culture. Cancer Res 45: 1611-1620
3. Alanko A, Heinonen E, Scheinin T, Tolppanen E-M, Vihko R (1985) Significance of estrogen and progesterone receptors, disease-free interval, and site of first metastasis on survival of breast cancer patients. Cancer 56: 1696-1700
4. Allegra JC, Lippman ME, Simon R, Thompson EB, Barlock A, Green L, Huff KK, Do HMT, Aitken SC, Warren R (1979) Association between steroid hormone receptor status and disease-free interval in breast cancer. Cancer Treat Rep 63: 1271-1277
5. Bates SE, Lippman ME, McManaway ME, Dickson RB (1976) Characterization of estrogen responsive transforming activity in human breast cancer cell lines. Cancer Res 46: 1703-1707
6. Blumberg H, Eisen A, Sledziewski A, Bader D, Young ET (1987) Two zinc fingers of a yeast regulatory protein shown by genetic evidence to be essential for its function. Nature 328: 443-445
7. Brent R, Ptashne M (1985) An eukaryotic transcriptional activator bearing the DNA specificity of a prokaryotic repressor. Cell 43: 729-736
8. Brinton LA, Williams RR, Hoover RN, Stegens NL, Feinleib M, Fraumeni JF (1979) Breast cancer risk factors among screening program participants. J N C I 62: 37-44
9. Bronzert DA, Monaco ME, Pinkus L, Aitkens S, Lippman ME (1981) Purification and properties of estrogen responsive cytoplasmic thymidine kinase from human breast cancer. Cancer Res 41: 604-610
10. Bryan RM, Mercer RJ, Bennett RC, Rennie GC, Lie TH (1984) Progesterone receptors in breast cancer. Aust NZ J Surg 54: 209-213
11. Bulbrook RD, Hayward JL, Spicer CC (1971) Relation between urinary androgen and corticoid excretion and subsequent breast cancer. Lancet ii: 395-398
12. Bulbrook RD, Thomas BS, Utsunomiya J, Yamaguchi E (1967) The urinary excretion of 11-deoxy-17-oxosteroids and 17-hydroxycorticosteroids by normal Japanese and British women. J Endocrinol 38: 401-407

13. Caldarola L, Calderini P, Voltrrani P, Di Carlo F, Gaglia P (1983) The correlation between estrogen receptor status, axillary-node metastases and disease-free interval after surgery in primary breast cancer. Ital J Surg Sci 13: 179-185
14. Casagrande J, Gerkins V, Henderson BE (1976) Exogenous estrogens and breast cancer in women with natural menopause. J N C I 56: 839-841
15. Clark GM, McGuire WL, Hybay CA, Pearson OH, Marshall JS (1983) Progesterone receptors as a prognostic factor in stage II breast cancer. N Engl J Med 309: 1343-1347
16. Clark GM, Osborne CK, McGuire WL (1984) Correlations between estrogen receptor, progesterone receptor, and patient characteristics in human breast cancer. J Clin Oncol 2: 1102-1109
17. Cole P, Brown JB, MacMahon B (1976) Oestrogen profiles of parous and nulliparous women. Lancet ii: 596-598
18. Cole P, MacMahon B (1969) Oestrogen functions during early reproductive life in the etiology of breast cancer. Lancet i: 604-606
19. Conneely OM, Sullivan WP, Toft DD, Birnbaumer M, Cook RG, Maxwell BL, Zarucki-Shultz T, Greene GL, Schrader WT, O'Malley BW (1986) Molecular cloning of the chicken progesterone receptor. Science 233: 767-770
20. de la Monte SM, Hutchins GM, Moore GW (1984) Estrogen and progesterone receptors in prediction of metastatic behavior of breast carcinoma. Am J Med 76: 11-17
21. Dickson RB, Huff KK, Spencer EM, Lippman ME (1986) Induction of epidermal growth factor-related polypeptides by 17-β estradiol in MCF-7 human breast cancer cells. Endocrinology 118: 138-142
22. Di Fronzo G, Cappelletti V, Coradine D, Ronchi E, Scavone G (1984) Prognostic significance of progesterone receptors alone or in association with estrogen receptors in human breast cancer. Tumori 70: 159-164
23. Edwards DP, Chamness GC, McGuire WL (1979) Estrogen and progesterone receptor proteins in breast cancer. Biochim Biophys Acta 560: 457-486
24. Fasal E, Paffenbarger RS (1975) Oral contraceptives as related to cancer and benign lesions of the breast. J N C I 55: 767-773
25. Fisher B, Redmond C, Brown A, Wickerham DL, Wolmark N, Allegra J, Escher G, Lippman M, Savlov E, Wittliff J, Fisher ER (1983) Influence of tumor estrogen and progesterone receptor levels on the response to tamoxifen and chemotherapy in primary breast cancer. J Clin Oncol 1: 227-241
26. Fisher ER, Osborne CK, McGuire WL, Redmond C, Knight WA III, Fisher B, Bannayan G, Walder A, Gregory EJ, Jacobsen A, Queen DM, Bennett DE, Ford HC (1981) Correlation of primary breast cancer histopathology and estrogen receptor content. Breast Cancer Res Treat 1: 37-41
27. Godolphin W, Elwood JM, Spinelli JJ (1981) Estrogen receptor quantitation and staging as complementary prognostic indicators in breast cancer: a study of 583 patients. Int J Cancer 28: 677-683
28. Green S, Walter P, Kumor V, Krust A, Bornert JM, Argos P, Chambon P (1986) Human estrogen receptor cDNA: sequence, expression and homology to v-*erb* A. Nature 320: 134-139
29. Greene GL, Sobel NB, King WJ, Jensen EV (1984) Immunochemical studies of estrogen receptors. J Steroid Biochem 20: 51-56
30. Gross GE, Clark GM, Chamness GC (1984) Multiple progesterone receptor assays in human breast cancer. Cancer Res 44: 836-840
31. Gurpide E (1976) Hormones and gynecologic cancer. Cancer 38: 503-508
32. Hollenberg SM, Weinberger C, Ong ES, Cerelli G, Oro A, Lebo R, Thompson EB, Rosenfeld MG (1984) Primary structure and expression of a functional glucocorticoid receptor cDNA. Nature 318: 635-641

33. Horwitz KB, McGuire WL (1977) Progesterone and progesterone receptor in experimental breast cancer. Cancer Res 37:1733-1738
34. Horwitz KB, McGuire WL (1978) Estrogen control of progesterone receptor in human breast cancer. J. Biol Chem 253: 2223-2228
35. Howatt JMT, Harris M, Swindell R, Barnes EM (1985) The effect of oestrogen and progesterone receptors on recurrence and survival in patients with carcinoma of the breast. Br J Cancer 51: 263-270
36. Howell A, Harland RNL, Bramwell VHC, Swindell R, Barnes DM, Redford J, Wilkinson MJS, Crowther D, Sellwood RA (1984) Steroid hormone receptors and survival after first relapse in breast cancer. Lanceti: 588-591
37. Huff KK, Knabbe C, Kaufman D, Gabby KH, Dickson RB (1986) Hormonal regulation of insulin-like growth factor I (IGF-1) secretion from MCF-7 human breast cancer cells. Endocrine Soc Ann Meeting (abstr 310)
38. Jeltsch JM, Krozowski Z, Quirin-Stricker C, Gronemeyer H, Simpson RJ, Garnier JM, Krust A, Jacob F, Chambon PC (1986) Cloning of the chicken progesterone receptor. Proc Natl Acad Sci USA 83: 5424-5428
39. Jensen EV, Suzuki T, Kawashima T, Stumpf WE, Jungblut PW, DeSombre ER (1968) A two-step mechanism for the interaction of estradiol with rat uterus. Proc Natl Acad Sci USA 59: 632-638
40. Johnston M (1987) Genetic evidence that zink is an essential co-factor in the DNA binding domain of GALA protein. Nature 328: 353-355
41. Kaufmann M, Maass H, Kubli F, Jonat W, Caffier H, Melchert F, Hilfrich J, Mahlke M, Stosiek U, Brunnert KW, Kleine W, Schorscher H, Howlweg-Majert P, Stiglmayer R, Wander HF (for the Gynecologic Adjuvant Breast Cancer Group) (1984) Risk adapted adjuvant chemo-hormonotherapy in operable nodal positive breast cancer. In: Jones SE, Salmon SE (eds) Adjuvant therapy of cancer VI. Grune and Stratton, Orlando, pp 369-378
42. King WJ, Greene GL (1984) Monoclonal antibodies localize oestrogen receptor in the nuclei of target cells. Nature 307: 745-749
43. Knight WA III, Livingston RB, Gregory EJ, McGuire WL (1977) Estrogen receptor as an independent prognostic factor for early recurrence in breast cancer. Cancer Res 37: 4669-4671
44. Korenman SG (1981) Reproductive endocrinology and breast cancer in women. In: Pike MC, Siiteri PK, Welsch CW (eds) Hormones and breast cancer. (Banbury Report 8). Cold Spring Harbor, New York, pp 71-85
45. Lemon HM, Wotiz HH, Parsons L, Mozden PJ (1966) Reduced estradiol excretion in patients with breast cancer prior to endocrine therapy. JAMA 196: 1128-1136
46. Lippman ME, Bolan G, Monaco M, Pinkus L, Engel L (1976) Model systems for the study of estrogen action in tissue culture. J Steroid Biochem 7: 1045-1051
47. Ludwig Breast Cancer Study Group (1984) Randomized trial of chemoendocrine therapy, endocrine therapy, and mastectomy alone in postmenopausal patients with operable breast cancer and axillary node metastasis. Lancet i: 1256-1260
48. Mason BH, Holdaway IM, Mullins PR, Yee LH, Kay RG (1983) Progesterone and estrogen receptors as prognostic variables in breast cancer. Cancer Res 43:2985-2990.
49. Maxwell BL, McDonnell DP, Conneely OM, Shultz T, Greene GL, O'Malley BW (1987) Structural organization and regulation of the chicken estrogen receptor. Mol Endocrinol 1: 25-35
50. McGuire WL, Carbone PP, Sears ME, Eschert GC (1975) Estrogen receptors in human breast cancer: an overview. In: MCguire WL, Carbone PP, Vollmer EP (eds) Estrogen receptors in human breast cancer. Raven, New York, pp 1-7

51. McGuire WL (1986) Prognostic factors in primary breast cancer. In: Bulbrook RD (ed) Cancer surveys – advances and prospects in clinical, epidemiological and laboratory oncology, vol 5(3). Oxford University Press, Oxford, pp 527-536
52. Miller H, Durant JA (1968) The values of urine steroid hormone assays in breast cancer. Clin Biochem 1: 287-298
53. Muhlbock O, Boot LM (1967) The mode of action of ovarian hormones in the induction of mammary cancer in mice. Biochem Pharmacol 16: 627-630
54. Nolvadex Adjuvant Trial Organisation (1985) Controlled trial of tamoxifen as single adjuvant agent in management of early breast cancer. Lancet i: 836-840
55. Osborne CK, Yochmowitz MG, Knight WL (1980) The value of estrogen and progesterone receptors in the treatment of breast cancer. Cancer 46: 2884-2888
56. Paterson AGH, Zuck VP, Szafran O, Lees AW, Hanson J (1982) Influence and significance of certain prognostic factors on survival in breast cancer. Eur J Cancer Clin Oncol 18: 937-943
57. Pearson OH, Hubay CA, Marshall JS, Gordon NH, McGuire WL, Mansoour EG, Hermann RE, Jones JC, Flynn WJ, Eckert C, and 24 participating investigators (1983) Adjuvant endocrine therapy, cytotoxic chemotherapy, and immunotherapy in stage II breast cancer: five-year results. Breast Cancer Res Treat 3: 61-68
58. Pichon M-F, Pallud C, Brunet M, Milgrom E (1980) Relationship of presence of progesterone receptors to prognosis in early breast cancer. Cancer Res 40: 3357-3360
59. Poel WE (1968) Progesterone enhancement of mammary development as a causal model of co-carcinogenesis. Br J Cancer 22: 867-873
60. Pritchard KI, Meakin JW, Boyd NF, Ambus U, DeBoer G, Dembo AJ, Paterson AHG, Suterland DJA, Wilkinson RH, Bassett AA, Evans WK, Beale FA, Clark RM, Keane TJ (1984) A randomized trial of adjuvant tamoxifen in postmenopausal women with axillary node positive breast cancer. In: Jones SE, Salmon SE (des) Adjuvant therapy of cancer IV. Grune and Stratton, Orlando, pp 339-347
61. Qazi R, Chuang J-LC, Drobyski W (1984) Estrogen receptors and the pattern of relapse in breast cancer. Arch Intern Med 1344: 2365-2376
62. Reiner GC, Katzenellenbogen BS (1986) Characterization of estrogen and progesterone receptor and the dissociated regulation of growth and progesterone receptor stimulation by estrogen in MDA-MB-134 human breast cancer cells. Cancer Res 46: 1124-1131
63. Roberts AB, Anzano MA, Wakefield LM, Roche NS, Stern DF, Sporn MB (1985) Type B transforming growth factor a bifunctional regulator of cellular growth. Proc Natl Acad Sci USA 82: 119-123
64. Rose C, Thorpe SM, Andersen KW, Pedersen BV, Mouridsen HT, Blichert-Toft M, Rasmussen BB (1985) Beneficial effect of adjuvant tamoxifen therapy in primary breast cancer patients with high oestrogen receptor values. Lancet i: 16-19
65. Ross R, Paganini-Hill A, Mack TM, Pfeffer R, Arthur M, Henderson BE (1980) A case-control study of menopausal estrogen therapy and breast cancer. JAMA 243: 1635
66. Sartwell PE, Arthes FG, Tonascia JA (1977) Exogenous hormones, reproductive history and breast cancer. J N C I 59: 1589-1592
67. Schrader WT, Birnbaumer ME, Hughes MR, Weigel NL, Grody WW, O'Malley BW (1981) Studies on the structure and function of the chicken progesterone receptor. Recent Prog Horm Res 37: 583-633
68. Shafie SM (1980) Estrogen and the growth of breast cancer: new evidence suggests indirect action. Science 209: 701-702
69. Sherridan PJ, Buchanan JM, Anselmo VC, Martin PM (1979) Equilibrium: the intracellular distribution of steroid receptors. Nature 282: 579-582

70. Sherman BM, Korenman SG (1974) Inadequate corpus luteum function: a pathophysiological interpretation of human breast cancer epidemiology. Cancer 33: 1306-1312
71. Taylor SG IV, Kalish LA, Olsen JE, Cummings F, Bennett JM, Falkson G, Tormey DC, Carbone PP (1985) Adjuvant CMFP versus CMFP plus tamoxifen versus observation alone in postmenopausal node-positive breast cancer patients: three-year results of an Eastern Cooperative Oncology Group Study. J Clin Oncol 3: 144-154
72. Thijssen JHH, Poortman J, Schwarz F (1975) Androgens in postmenopausal breast cancer: excretion, production and interaction with estrogen. J Steroid Biochem 6: 729-734.
73. Vic P, Vignon F, Derocq D, Rochefort H (1982) Effects of estradiol on the ultrastructure of the MCF-7 human breast cancer cells in culture. Cancer Res 42: 667-673
74. Vignon F, Capony F, Chambon M, Friess G, Garcia M, Rochefort H (1986) Autocrine growth stimulation of the MCF-7 breast cancer cells by the estrogen-regulated 52K protein. Endocrinology 118: 1537-1545
75. Wallgren A, Baral E, Carstensen J, Friberg S, Glas U, Hjalmar ML, Kaigas M, Nordenskjld B, Skoog L, Theve N-O, Wilking N (1984) Should adjuvant tamoxifen be given for several years in breast cancer? In: Jones SE, Salmon SE (eds) Adjuvant therapy of cancer IV. Grune and Stratton, Orlando, pp 331-337
76. Walter P, Green S, Greene G, Krust A, Bonert JM, Jettsch JM, Staub A, Jensen E, Scrace G, Waterfield M, Chambon P (1985) Cloning of the human estrogen receptor DNA. Proc Natl Acad Sci USA 82: 7889-7893
77. Westerberg H, Gustafson SA, Nordenskjold B, Silfversward C, Wallgren A (1980) Estrogen receptor level and other factors in early recurrence of breast cancer. Int J Cancer 26: 429-433
78. Westley B, Rochefort H (1980) A secreted glycoprotein induced by estrogen in human breast cancer cell lines. Cell 20: 353-362
79. White AC, Levy JA, McGrath CM (1982) Site-selective growth of hormone-responsive human breast carcinoma in athymic nude mice. Cancer Res 42: 906-912
80. Zaret KS, Yamamoto KR (1984) Reversible and persistent changes in chromatin structure accompany activation of a glucocorticoid-dependent enhancer element. Cell 38: 29-38
81. Centers for Disease Control (1983) Long-term Oral contraceptive use and the risk of breast cancer. JAMA 249: 1591-1595

Overview of the Prognostic and Clinical Correlates of Steroid Hormone Receptors in Human Breast Cancer

L.L. Shek and W. Godolphin

Department of Pathology, The University of British Columbia and Vancouver General Hospital, Vancouver, V5Z 1M9, Canada

Introduction

Analysis of (estrogen receptors) ER in human breast cancer has shown two main clinical applications: patient selection for endocrine therapy and prediction of the clinical course of the disease. Jensen and his colleagues [52] showed that breast cancer tissue possessed the same specific receptor mechanism for estrogen as did other estrogen target tissues. This work presented a working model of steroid action at the molecular level, applicable to female reproductive tissue including the breast. It was an extension of Folca's observation that breast cancer patients with a favorable response to adrenalectomy incorporated more radioactive hexestrol into their tumors in vivo than those who did not respond [30]. Such research contributed a mechanistic explanation for Beatson's observation [5] that oophorectomy caused tumor regression in two premenopausal patients with advanced breast cancer.

Jensen's model states that response of target tissues to steroid hormones depends on the presence of specific, high affinity protein receptors in the cytoplasm, to which the activating hormone binds to exert an inductive effect on protein synthesis, including the ER themselves. They found that most, but not all women whose breast tumors contained receptors responded to endocrine ablation or hormone administration, whereas neither manipulation brought significant remission in patients with negligible amounts of receptors [49]. Others soon confirmed the results [69, 72, 93]. The ER status, then, met the need for a method of predicting which patients had a reasonable chance of hormonal treatment success [51].

Current thinking on this model of steroid hormone action, based on receptor-steroid complex translocation differs with respect to the nature and location of the receptor protein. There is evidence that unoccupied steroid receptors are nuclear proteins bound to some yet undefined nuclear components with low affinity which are extractable in low ionic strength homogenization media. This affinity to nuclear components is greatly increased after receptor conformational change due to interaction with the steroid hormone [35]. More recent immunocytochemical studies with monoclonal ER-specific antibodies support this concept [58].

The most common technique for receptor quantitation is based on steroid binding to radiolabeled ligands. Tumor tissue is homogenized and the supernatant

Ragaz/Ariel (Eds.), High-Risk Breast Cancer

prepared is incubated with increasing concentrations of [^{3}H] estradiol, with and without an estrogen analog which competitively inhibits high affinity specific binding of the [^{3}H] estradiol. Serum furnishes components which have variable affinities and specificities for the ligand and thus interfere with receptor binding. This nonspecific binding is corrected for mathematically in the calculations of the number of binding sites. Dextran-coated charcoal is used to remove absorbed unbound or loosely bound estradiol. Results from scintillation counting of the charcoal supernatants, now containing bound estradiol in the presence and absence of the competitor, are expressed as specific estradiol binding per milligram protein. The EORTC Breast Cancer Cooperative Group [26] suggested this specific estradiol binding to be quantitatively more accurate when expressed on a per milligram cytosol protein basis, which corrects for serum protein contamination. The clinical classification by ER status is often unaltered, but if uncorrected, specific estradiol binding per tumor cell is underestimated. Furthermore, this quantitative base has been empirically found to have a strong correlation with results expressed on a per milligram DNA basis, the latter being a reflection of tumor epithelial cellularity [47]. Finally, a constant (K_D) is derived which provides a measure of the affinity of the estrogen-receptor complex.

The concern that conventional steroid binding assay technically cannot detect receptors already bound with endogenous or exogenous steroids has prompted the development of new methodologies using monoclonal antibodies to the ER protein. Two major areas have been intensely investigated. One is the biochemical enzyme immunoassay (ER-EIA) based on the "sandwich" principle, utilizing two monoclonal ER-specific antibodies purified from the human breast cancer cell line MCF-7 that react with separate and nonoverlapping antigenic sties on the receptor protein [36]. One of those specific antibodies (Ab 1) is attached to a polystyrene bead incubated with the tumor cytosol. Ab 1 associates with the free or estrogen-bound receptor. The tumor cytosol is further incubated with the second monoclonal antibody (Ab 2) tagged with either radioactive iodine or sulfur or an enzyme such as peroxidase, and associates with the receptor Ab 1-bead at a different antigenic site on the receptor. The amount of bead-bound receptor is quantitated by scintillation counting (if the tag is radioactive iodine or sulfur) or by spectrophotometric assay (if the tag is peroxidase) [53]. Some apparent advantages of this assay include its simplicity relative to biochemical methods, less influence by receptor lability, and possibly better quality control [20]. Results from the ER-EIA have been shown to correlate well with the steroid binding assay [22, 55, 64].

The second use of monoclonal ER-specific antibodies is immunohistochemical determination of ER in fixed, frozen tissue sections. Localization of ER is visualized by the intensity and distribution of specific staining. The staining results from the presence of a bridging antibody (anti-rat IgG), which provides an attachment site for a peroxidase-antiperoxidase complex. The latter interacts with a substrate such as diaminobenzidine and hydrogen peroxide to produce a staining level that varies with the number of receptors present. This immunoperoxidase staining is frequently noted to be localized in the nucleus [59, 75]. Although evaluation of the staining is semiquantitative in nature, this method has demonstrated strong qualitative and quantitative correlations with the steroid binding assay, as well as with patient prognosis for recurrence and survival [21].

In 1974 a gathering of twelve independent research groups produced a consensus that ER is a more reliable predictor of hormonal response than other diagnostic factors [70]. Despite different assay methods and different thresholds for a "significant" receptor level, patients classified ER+ responded to endocrine therapy at a rate of 52%-58%, whereas ER− tumors responded at about 5% [77]. The independence of ER from other prognostic factors like nodal status, clinical stage, relapse-free survival, and location of primary, at least in stage II patients [19], was confirmed.

Initial optimism about the clinical value of receptor status was tempered by a large proportion (up to 50%) of patients with ER+ tumors who did not respond objectively. Contributing factors to this discrepancy may be methodological, including variation in results by different assay techniques [40], interlaboratory differences in cutoff points defining ER status [33], and in the reference parameters used to report quantity of receptors [37], as well as differences in judgment of objective responses [70].

Factors that Influence Receptor Measurement

Tumor heterogeneity within an ER+ tumor also influences potential response to hormonal treatment. The idea of heterogeneous cell populations in breast tumors is not new. McGuire and Chamness [76] reported that individual epithelial cells may or may not retain the functional characteristic of receptor production during malignant transformation. A particular tumor specimen may have enough receptor-containing cells to yield a positive assay, but cells whose growth is not under hormonal control (i.e., ER− cells) may dominate and influence the clinical course while the ER+ cells are selectively eliminated by hormonal therapy [62]. A microsample technique was recently used to examine intratumoral regional variability in ER levels, and results showed that the average coefficient of variation for intratumoral ER level was a striking 86%, and that 35% of overall ER+ tumors lacked receptors in some regions of the sample [103]. Measuring this type of heterogeneity of intratumor distribution of ERs is beyond the capacity of the conventional biochemical ER assay.

Temporal ER stability in vivo also relates to tumor heterogeneity. An 85% concordance has generally been found in sequential determinations, independent of the length of elapsed time between assays. This indicates that ER status of the primary tumor can predict hormonal response of a recurrent lesion which may be inaccessible to biopsy [38]. In the absence of adjuvant therapy, the receptor phenotype rather than receptor quantity remains generally the same as before a recurrence, even though primary breast tumors are comprised of both ER+ and ER− cells. A recent study by Jakesz et al. [48] examined the effect of intervening therapy on receptor levels in subsequent biopsies. They reported reductions in both ER and progesterone receptor (PR) levels sufficient to change from positive to negative in patients who received endocrine intervention; this resulted in a discordance rate of 45%. The effect of intervening cytotoxic chemotherapy is less clear [101], since ER status changed at a rate of 32%, but PR status of the second biopsy did not. This and other studies reporting the trend of ER+ conversion to ER− [46, 66, 85, 101] support the hypothesis that selective pressure is exerted against ER+ cells by hormonal therapy, resulting in receptor loss as the disease progresses and becomes more autonomous [62]. It must be emphasized that only nodal and soft tissue metastases were studied owing to their accessibility for biopsy. Those ER+ tumors that tend to first metastasize to osseous sites [10] may not necessarily display similar receptor status conversion.

Prospective studies are needed to clarify the clinical significance of receptor changes over time. The reliability of the receptor status of the primary tumor for therapeutic and prognostic purposes could then be ascertained. In addition to an adequate sample size, assay methodology for the sequential biopsies must be nearly identical for proper interpretation of results. An assessment of whether the receptor change is accompanied by increasing histologic differentiation would be informative. It is unclear whether prognosis is different in patients whose tumors have undergone either a spontaneous or treatment-induced change from ER+ to ER− status, as compared with patients with ER− tumors which remain ER− at the second biopsy.

Several other factors influence the level of steroid hormone receptors. Both the incidence and quantity of ER in breast tumors are higher in postmenopausal than in premenopausal women [70, 107]. This relationship is confounded by age [14]. In fact, age but not menopausal status was significantly associated with ER concentration in a multiple regression analysis. Elwood and Godolphin [25] demonstrated that ER level becomes significantly higher with increasing age within both pre- and postmenopausal categories; patients of similar age (45-54 years old) had similar ER levels, regardless of menopausal status. After age is controlled for, ER status is found not to correlate with variables such as use of exogenous hormones, parity, age at first birth, ethnic origin, body weight, and family history of breast cancer. At variance with these results is a study by Lesser et al. [68], who reported a statistically significant correlation between age and receptor level only in the postmenopausal group. Their failure to control for age as a confounding factor when correlating ER with other epidemiologic variables seriously biased the analyses. Well-known associations between ER status and contraceptive hormone usage and menopausal estrogen usage illustrate this point. Oral contraceptives are used by premenopausal and hence younger women, thus the age factor rather than the use of such hormones per se may be the primary contribution to the lower ER concentration. Similarly, lower ER levels seen in postmenopausal women who were estrogen users at diagnosis, compared with those who had used estrogens, but not at the time of diagnosis, may be due to relative age differences, with the latter being the older group. The significant association between race and ER status may also be an artifact of age.

The mechanism that underlies the age-receptor relationships is not yet fully elucidated, although it is often said that masking of receptor sites by high endogenous estrogen level in the premenopausal state is partially responsible for the phenomenon [107]. This is not supported by Edery et al. [23], who concluded that estrogen regulates its own receptor synthesis since estradiol concentration is higher in ER+ than ER− tumors. Receptor "masking" is also not supported by Saez et al. [89], who suggested that lower ER in premenopausal women may be due to counteracting effects of cyclic progesterone on the stimulatory action of estrogens. It is possible that in the postmenopausal state where these cyclical variations of progesterone and estrogen are absent, syntheses of both ER and PR may be prompted by extraglandular origins of estrogens. In support of this concept, it was found that ER+/PR+ postmenopausal women demonstrated a positive correlation between ER levels and circulating estrogens. Mason et al. [73] reported that plasma estrone, and to a lesser extent plasma estradiol, exhibit quantitative relationships with ER levels in postmenopausal women. All these results appear to conflict with the observation that patients with higher plasma estradiol have fewer numbers of binding sites [84]. Some concern had been raised regarding possible discrepancy between ER results on biopsy and mastectomy specimens. Receptors are thermolabile and may be more prone to degradation due to devascularization and warm ischemia during the mastectomy [39]. A recent examination of this problem, albeit with rather small numbers, has found that proper handling of mastectomy specimens resulted in ER determinations in good agreement with their biopsied counterparts [67].

A critical factor that inherently affects ER determination is the malignant epithelial cell content of the specimen. This epithelial cellularity is important since ER is found in tumor cells as opposed to stromal elements or nontumorous tissue [102]. The conventional biochemical assay homogenizes all cells in the tumor. Results are commonly expressed on a per milligram cytosol protein basis which at best approximates the amount of ER measured minus any nontumor cell protein that has varying affinity for the radiolabeled estradiol, without an accurate assessment of cellularity of the specimen. The consequence may be clinically significant if a false-negative assay is generated by a tumor specimen containing sparse numbers of ER+ carcinoma cells [103]. This problem has been studied by a field-by-field graticule cell counting method [83], and by semiquantitative estimation of the proportion of tumor cells in order to correct for measured ER [6, 43]. These studies do not entirely reinforce each other. Howat et al. [43] found cellularity to be unrelated to the mere presence or absence of ER, but the highest ER values were found in the most cellular tumors, statistically significant in the postmenopausal and overall patient groups. Mumford et al. [83] reported a correlation between cellularity and ER concentration in postmenopausal, but not in premenopausal or in overall groups.

Estrogen Receptors: Correlation with Pathology

From a pathologist's point of view, histologic characteristics of a tumor are a measure of the cancer's anatomic extent and its biologic aggressiveness. A biochemist's view is that the presence of ER and/ or PR is evidence that the breast cancer cell, like its normal counterpart, has retained its dependence on estrogenic stimulation for growth, in contrast with one that might not produce the receptor because it has escaped hormone dependency [50]. The common belief is that the greater the mimicry of normal breast epithelium, the less the anticipated biologic aggressiveness. A causal relationship cannot yet be ascribed to the presence of certain histologic features and ER in the primary tumor, but the question of whether there are correlations between the pathologist's findings and the biochemist's findings was posed as soon as the predictive importance of ER was realized. The earliest correlations tested were between ER and the two features: histologic type and histologic grade. There is no strong association between major histologic types and ER status, perhaps with the exception of variants such as lobular, tubular and papillary carcinomas that have a tendency to be ER+ [28, 43], and medullary carcinoma that associates with low or negative ER [94]. Significant correlations between ER status and cellular differentiation are usually found [28, 80], even when this differentiation is expressed as an ultrastructural index that is different from histologic grading [65].

Three other morphological factors, elastosis, necrosis, and fibrosis have received attention. A positive correlation between the presence of elastosis and clinically significant amounts of ER is usually found [32]. A recent study found a direct quantitative relationship between the two, but refuted any prognostic significance of elastosis [87]. Tumors having marked necrosis tend to be ER−, as only viable cells harbor the receptors. Extensive necrosis may be indicative of aggressive growth and is one manifestation of vascular invasion. A marked degree of tumor necrosis in ductal carcinoma (not otherwise specified) is directly correlated with higher rates of locoregional recurrence, metastases, or death [27]. Carter et al. [11] found that tumors with both necrosis and an infiltrating border associate with higher 10-year mortality rate than circumscribed tumors without necrosis. The influence of tumor fibrosis on prognosis is uncertain, but a positive correlation between degree of fibrosis and ER content has been found [43]. In contrast to these histologic parameters, the anatomic extent of the primary disease, as indicated by clinical staging, primary tumor size, and nodal status is not correlated with ER.

Correlation studies between tumor ER and the kinetics of cell proliferation, as measured by thymidine labeling index, have consistently shown an inverse relationship [95, 100]. Thymidine labeling index also positively correlates with tumor size, nuclear anaplasia, tumor necrosis, and inflammatory cellular infiltration [78]. Theoretically, inability to retain ER and high rates of cellular replication are the results of tumor cell dedifferentiation [79]. The mean proportion of cells engaged in DNA synthesis (S-phase fraction) increases in ductal carcinoma as the tumor becomes more poorly differentiated, and this fraction is still higher in the predominantly ER− medullary carcinoma [81]. The prognostic role of cell kinetics was also confirmed, but it appears that while recurrence-free survival is better in all patients with low labeling index than in those with high labeling index, low labeling index confers overall survival advantage only in premenopausal and perimenopausal patients [96]. However, the number of postmenopausal patients examined was relatively small in this subset analysis (node-negative patients only).

In contrast to the generally accepted relation between ER and response to hormonal therapy, no such agreement exists with regard to chemotherapy. Cytotoxic antineoplastic drugs are theoretically most effective against rapidly proliferating cells, and correlational studies demonstrate an inverse relationship between ER status and in vitro thymidine labeling index. Hence, it was easy to assume that ER− tumors would be most likely to respond to cytotoxic chemotherapy. Lippman et al. [71] reported a significantly higher response rate to chemotherapy among ER− than ER+ patients, and were supported by others [54]. However, patients with ER+ tumors have also been found to have superior response to chemotherapy [57, 82, 92]. Still others have found no significant differences [7, 41, 88].

Clarification of this unresolved controversy is needed since usual clinical practice is institution of chemotherapy to ER− patients since they are unlikely to respond to hormonal therapy. There are, however, contrary data which indicate that a subgroup of ER+ patients would derive comparable benefit from chemotherapy. Kiang [56] attributed the apparent contradiction in such responses to differences in patient population, and suggested prospective randomized studies of a large homogeneous population of patients with a standardized regimen of chemotherapy. Kiang had criticized Lippman for selectively including "life-threatening types of visceral involvement in patients with receptor-rich tumors" compared with less aggressive types of visceral involvement in those with receptor-poor tumors [57]. Although no such selection was obvious in Kiang's groups, half of their receptor-rich group was composed of patients whose receptor status was determined after hormonal therapy followed by chemotherapy [57]. Both Kiang and Lippman based their observations on metastatic tumors, which are not directly comparable to Hilf's or Bonadonna's results derived from primary tumors [7, 41].

A major contributing factor to the controversy over the relationship between ER and the response to chemotherapy is the nonuniformity of end events examined. Some studies used objective response criteria and others in recurrence rates [41]. A comparison of the responsiveness of ER+ tumors versus ER− tumors lacks validity unless a control group with similar non-chemotherapy-treated patients exists [29]. There is also a need to distinguish between chemotherapy given in an adjuvant setting and that given for distant disease recurrence [16].

Considering the treatment of high risk breast cancer, one must be conscious of a distinction between the response and prolongation of survival. Response to cytotoxic chemotherapy does not lead to longer survival. If the question is "does ER predict for response to chemotherapy?" then a prospective study is needed with relatively long follow-up to assess the extent and duration of response. On the other hand, if the question is "does ER predict longer survival?" then a careful interpretation of survival plots will be needed as ER+ patients may have better survival owing to the biologic nature of the tumor and not to the response to chemotherapy.

The concept of "proportional gain" [16] is useful in casting new light on the problem that ER status may not predict for chemotherapeutic response until longer follow-up. Thus, ER+ patients, representing a group with good prognosis, may have at any time a lesser treatment gain than the ER− group (poor prognosis), even though the proportional gain is the same. The absolute gain, which may be as great in the ER+ as in the ER− group may not be evident until much later. Therefore, it is vital to make a clear distinction between a response and a survival improvement as a direct result of chemotherapy, as opposed to other factors, like biology of disease, etc. For instance, premenopausal ER+ patients may, in addition to a response to chemotherapy, also benefit from obliteration of ovarian function which may contribute to a longer recurrence-free survival, while in the ER− counterparts the response reflects the effects of chemotherapy itself.

Another aspect that has been overlooked by past studies is the impact of dichotomized ER information. Quantitative ER may better predict chemotherapeutic results. If the relative proportion of ER+ to ER− cells in a tumor is important in determining response, then simple ER status (positive or negative) would not adequately indicate the likelihood of response to chemotherapy. Therefore, if ER+ tumors are stratified into concentration ranges, it is possible that patients in the low positive range may have different response to adjuvant chemotherapy from those in the high to very high level range. Such a hypothesis is suggested by the greater prognostic accuracy when ER is used quantitatively. Not only is the survival better in patients with increasing ER concentration, but a significant difference in survival exists also within the ER− tumors stratified into low negative (i.e., $ER \leqslant 1$) and high negative (i.e., $2 \leqslant ER \leqslant 9$) categories [34].

Estrogen Receptor and Prognosis

Present data indicate that ER status allows for discrimination of those patients at higher risk for disease recurrence, independent of certain clinical characteristics (menopausal status, size of primary, nodal status). A very high risk group of ER− patients with positive axillary nodes who might benefit from adjuvant therapy was defined [61, 74]. Subsequent studies also found ER+ patients to have significantly longer recurrence-free survival, regardless of lymph node involvement [4, 15, 63, 31].

More dissension arose among studies which examined subset behavior. The observation that a difference in the recurrence-free survival between ER+ and ER− subgroups was seen only in the premenopausal group, regardless of nodal status [91], was contradicted by Crowe et al. [17] who found that, in ER+ patients, recurrence-free survival was significantly longer only in the postmenopausal, node-negative group. Howat and Barnes [42] found, in the node-negative subgroup, no difference in recurrence rates between ER+ and ER− patients. They also found that ER+ patients with 1-3 nodes have a recurrence rate similar to patients with no nodes, while on the other hand, ER− patients with 1-3 nodes recurred at a higher rate. The recurrence rate, however, between ER+ and ER− subgroups was no longer different when patients with $\geqslant 4$ nodes were examined.

Other data suggest the futility of using ER to predict the risk of relapse. No difference was found in recurrence-free survival between ER+ and ER− patients when analyzed by menopausal status [9], or by stage [97]. To confuse the issue, further differences which existed during early months of follow-up did not persist with later follow-up [2, 43, 90].

There is much greater agreement that ER positivity confers advantage to overall survival after initial surgery. ER+ patients are found to have considerably longer survival than ER− patients [45, 98, 104]. Some studies had implied that

ER + patients experience longer survival because they respond favorably to hormonal therapy given at disease recurrence [3, 44]. Accordingly, ER + patients who did not demonstrate objective response to hormonal therapy have postrecurrence survival comparable to ER − patients [44, 106]. It is, however, arguable whether response is a direct and sole explanation for prolonged survival after recurrence, or whether patients defined to be ER + at primary diagnosis are prognostically better than ER − patients, even when hormonal therapy was not given. One explanation for the lack of response to hormonal therapy in ER + patients may be the changes of receptor quantity over the course of the disease in some breast tumors. Another possibility is that an objective response to treatment is difficult to ascertain accurately in patients with nonmeasurable disease, i.e., bone metastases [99], that are more often disseminated from ER + primary tumors [10]. Therefore, the initial response to treatment may not necessarily reflect the long-term prognosis.

Clark et al. have shown, in their multivariate analyses of stage II patients, that the positive nodes and PR concentration were the only two important predictors for recurrence-free survival, even though ER status and ER concentration were also significant when assessed in univariate analysis [12]. An additional set of patients ($N = 229$) with a different demographic profile who were not treated in a randomized clinical trial was subsequently analyzed with the previous patient group (N = 189). Not only did ER status attain statistical significance as a predictor for recurrence-free survival, but it was actually more important than PR in predicting overall survival [13]. The significance of PR as a prognosticator has not always been confirmed [44, 45], perhaps because cutoff points for defining PR-positivity have ranged from 5 to 15 fmol per milligram cytosol protein or greater. Studies have shown that improved recurrence-free survival was seen only in patients with PR + tumors who had received adjuvant CMF chemotherapy (cyclophosphamide, methotrexate, and 5-fluorouracil) [86], or adjuvant tamoxifen therapy when axillary nodes were positive [18].

Comments on Methodology of Studies Analyzing Data on Estrogen Receptors

Despite the great volume of studies analyzing ER and the outcome, the issue is not entirely clear as most studies have some identifiable problem preventing clear conclusion. These shortcomings include small sample size, short follow up [60, 61], insufficient information on exclusion criteria, or testing from an old population with a high proportion of disease-nonspecific mortality [1].

Although most studies describe objective criteria for identifying recurrences and death, several are less accurate on the date of first recurrence – a time point in the clinical course often subject to observer variation [24]. In contrast, the date of death is usually confirmable from death certificates or autopsy reports. To achieve interstudy comparability, a cohort should be identified at a sufficiently early and uniform point in the natural history of the disease. A concern relates to the use of the date of primary surgery as opposed to the date of diagnosis to assemble such a cohort. Most studies are retrospective and the time from mastectomy is often chosen as a date of diagnosis, as in most instances it can be more conveniently traced in the retrospective analysis. The trend in western Canada during the last decade is toward longer delay time between diagnosis and primary surgical treatment. With such a practice one must be aware that waiting time from diagnosis to mastectomy may vary widely such that interstudy comparisons of recurrence-free survival cannot be done reliably. Further complications arise if ER results from primary tumors and metastases are combined, such as in a study by Alanko et al. [3] who correlated recurrence-free survival with ER results from 84% of patients who had the assay on a primary tumor, and 16% on metastases. Criteria for defining ER positivity also vary greatly, from >3.1 and 4.1 fmol per milligram cytosol protein for premenopausal and postmenopausal patients, respectively [105], to >18 [8] and 20 [104].

Summary

The presence as well as the quantity of ER in the primary breast tumor is informative of the potential biologic behavior of the tumor. The tendency of ER+ tumors to be histologically better differentiated and to have a relatively lower growth rate, as compared with ER− tumors, is the basis for biologic differences which may influence the response to therapy and survival of breast cancer patients. Continued research on the elucidation of the subcellular localization of ER and their interaction with genomic entities will yield greater understanding of the relation between biology and clinical behavior.

Since some of these factors are highly associated and the expression of one may depend on another, a multivariate analysis of 859 patients with complete data on prognostic variables was conducted. Nodal status was the important independent factor, but also TNM stage, ER concentration, and tumor necrosis were critical for survival predictions (Table 1), while the remaining factors have not provided further prognostic information. The combined effects of the four variables determines the wide range of outcome. The predicted 5-year survival for patients with TNM I ranged from 36% (N4+, $\log_e$ [ER]=0, marked necrosis) to 96% (N0, $\log_e$ [ER]

Table 1. Cox model on overall survival ($N=859$) by multivariate stepwise regression analysis

Order of entry	Variable	Coefficient	P1
1	Nodal status: 1-3 nodes	0.47	0.009
	⩾4 nodes	1.17	<0.0001
2	TNM stage: II	0.41	0.02
	III	1.14	<0.0001
	IV	2.06	<0.0001
3	$\log_e$ [ER]	−0.22	<0.0001
4	Marked necrosis	0.65	0.0003

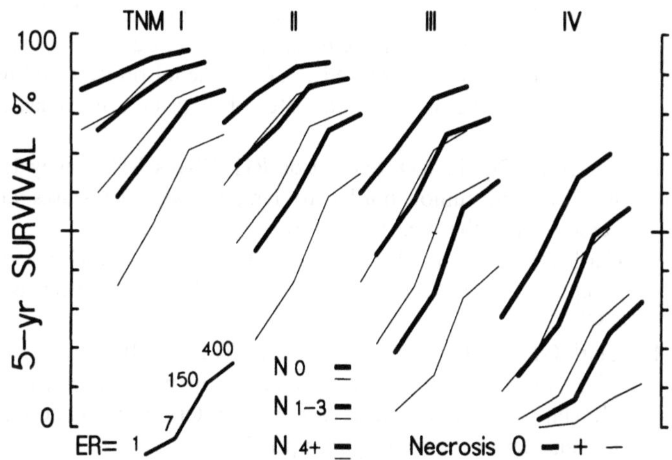

Fig. 1. Predicted 5-year survival based on the Cox model shown in Table 1. Predicted *curves* are displayed on TNM stage, subdivided by nodal status, ER concentration, and marked/absent necrosis. Four ER concentrations are arbitrarily chosen to illustrate the effect of increasing ER quantity. [Shekk LM, Godolphin W (1988) Cancer Res 48: 5565-5569]

= 6, no necrosis) and from 0% to 70% for the same cateogories in TNM IV (Fig. 1). The systematic application of such clinical, histopathologic, and tumor receptor information greatly aids in identifying the risk in patients who are otherwise considered to have comparably staged breast cancer.

References

1. Aamdal S, Bormer O, Jorgensen O, Host H, Eliassen G, Kaalhus O, Pihl A (1984) Estrogen receptors and long term prognosis in breast cancer. Cancer 53: 2525-2529
2. Adami HO, Graggman S, Lindgren A, Sallstrom J (1985) Prognostic implication of estrogen receptor content in breast cancer. Breast Cancer Res Treat 5: 293-300
3. Alanko A, Heinonen E, Scheinin T, Tolppanen EM, Vihko R (1985) Significance of estrogen and progesterone receptors, disease-free interval, and site of first metastases on survival of breast cancer patients. Cancer 56: 1696-1700
4. Allegra JC, Lippman ME, Simon R, Thompson EB, Barlock A, Green L, Huff KK, Do HM, Aitken SC, Warren R (1979) Association between steroid hormone receptor status and disease-free interval in breast cancer. Cancer Treat Rep 63: 1271-1277
5. Beatson GT (1896) On the treatment of inoperable cases of carcinoma of the mamma: suggestions for a new method of treatment, with illustrative cases. Lancet ii: 104-107
6. Black R, Prescott R, Bers K, Hawkins A, Stewart H, Forrest P (1983) Tumor cellularity, estrogen receptors and prognosis in breast cancer. Clin Oncol 9: 311-318
7. Bonadonna G, Valagussa P, Tancini G, Di Fronzo G (1980) Estrogen receptor status and response to chemotherapy in early and advanced breast cancer. Cancer Chemother Pharmacol 4: 37-41
8. Brooks JL, Ryan JA Jr, Bauermeister DE (1983) Prognostic significance of hormone receptors in early recurrence of breast cancer. Am J Surg 145: 599-603

9. Butler JA, Bretsky S, Menendez-Botet C, Kinne DW (1985) Estrogen receptor protein of breast cancer as a predictor of recurrence. Cancer 55: 1178-1181
10. Campbell FC, Blamey RW, Elston CW, Nicholson RI, Griffiths K, Haybittle JL (1981) Oestrogen-receptor status and sites of metastasis in breast cancer. Br J Cancer 44: 456-459
11. Carter D, Pipkin RD, Shephards RH, Elkins RC, Abbey H (1978) Relationship of necrosis and tumor border to lymph node metastases and 10-year survival in carcinoma of the breast. Am J Surg Pathol 2: 39-46
12. Clark GM, McGuire WL, Hubay CA, Pearson OH, Marshall JS (1983) Progesterone receptors as a prognostic factor in stage II breast cancer. N Engl J Med 309: 1343-1347
13. Clark GM, McGuire WL, Hubay CA, Pearson OH, Carter AC (1983) The importance of estrogen and progesterone receptor in primary breast cancer. In: Mirand EA, Hutchinson WB, Mihich E (eds) 13 th International cancer congress, part E. Cancer management Liss, New York, pp 183-190
14. Clark GM, Osborne CK, McGuire WL (1984) Correlations between estrogen receptor, progesterone receptor, and patient characteristics in human breast cancer. J Clin Oncol 2: 1102-1109
15. Cooke T, George D, Shield R, Maynard P, Griffiths K (1979) Oestrogen receptors and prognosis in early breast cancer. Lancet i: 995-997
16. Coppin CML, Swenerton KD (1983) Selective treatment in breast cancer. In: Stoll BS (ed) Cancer treatment: end point evaluation. Wiley, Chichester
17. Crowe JA, Hubay CA, Pearson OH, Marshall JS, Rosenblatt J, Mansour EG, Hermann RE, Jones JC, Flynn WJ, McGuire WL: (1982) Estrogen receptor status as a prognostic indicator for stage I breast cancer patients. Breast Cancer Res Treat 2: 171-176
18. Dembo AJ, Pritchard KI, De Boer G, Meakin JW, Boyd NF, Ambus U, Evans WK, Wilkinson RH, Bassett AA, Sutherland DJ, Mobbs BG (1985) Prognostic factors in postmenopausal women with axillary node positive breast cancer. Proc Annu Meet Am Soc Clin Oncol 4: 70 (abstr)
19. DeSombre ER, Carbone PP, Jensen EV, McGuire WL, Wells SA, Witliff JL, Lipsett MB (1979) Steroid receptors in breast cancer. N Engl J Med 301: 1011-1012
20. DeSombre ER, Greene GL, King WJ, Jensen EV (1984) Estrogen receptors, antibodies and hormone dependent cancer. In: Gurpide E, Calandra R, Levy C, Soto RJ (eds) Hormones and cancer. Liss, New York, pp 1-21
21. DeSombre ER, Thorpe SM, Rose C, Blough RR, Andersen KW, Rasmussen BB, King WJ (1986) Prognostic usefulness of estrogen receptor immunocytochemical assays for human breast cancer. Cancer Res [Suppl] 46: 4256s-4264s
22. Di Fronzo G, Miodini P, Brivio M, Cappelletti V, Coradini D, Granata G, Ronchi E (1986) Comparison of immunochemical and radioligand binding assays for estrogen receptors in human breast tumors. Cancer Res [Suppl] 46: 4278s-4281s
23. Edery M, Goussard J, Dehennin L, Scholler R, Reiffsteck J, Drosdowsky MA (1981) Endogenous oestrogen-17β concentration in breast tumours determined by mass fragmentography and by radioimmunoassay: relationship to receptor content. Eur J Cancer 17: 115-120
24. Editorial (1984) Steroid receptors and prognosis of breast cancer. Lancet i: 887-888
25. Elwood JM, Godolphin W (1980) Oestrogen receptors in breast tumors: associations with age, menopausal status and epidemiological and clinical features in 735 patients. Br J Cancer 42: 635-644
26. EORTC Breast Cancer Cooperative Group (1973) Standards for the assessment of estrogen receptors in human breast cancer. Eur J Cancer 9: 379-381

27. Fisher ER, Palekar AS, Gregorio RM, Redmond C, Fisher B (1978) Pathological findings from the National Surgical Adjuvant Breast Project (protocol no 4) IV. Significance of tumor necrosis. Hum Pathol 9: 523-530
28. Fisher ER, Redmond CK, Liu H, Rockette H, Fisher B (1980) Correlation of estrogen receptor and pathologic characteristics of invasive breast cancer. Cancer 45: 349-353
29. Fisher B, Redmond CK, Wickerham DL, Rockette HE, Brown A (1983) Relations of estrogen and/or progesterone receptor content of breast cancer to patient outcome following adjuvant chemotherapy. Breast Cancer Res Treat 3: 355-364
30. Folca PJ, Glascock RF, Irvine WT (1961) Studies with tritium-labelled hexoestrol in advanced breast cancer: comparison of tissue accumulation of hexoestrol with response to bilateral adrenalectomy and oophorectomy. Lancet ii: 796-798
31. Forrest APM, Black RB, Humeniuk V, Cant ELM, Hawkins RA, Prescott RJ, Roberts MM, Shivas AA, Stewart JH, Smith AF, Summerling M (1980) Preoperative assessment and staging of breast cancer: preliminary communications. J R Soc Med 73: 561-566
32. Glaubitz LC, Bowen JH, Cox EB, McCarty KS Jr (1984) Elastosis in human breast cancer. Correlation with sex steroid receptors and comparison with clinical outcome. Arch Pathol Lab Med 108: 27-30
33. Godolphin W (1982) The clinical utility of estrogen receptor analyses. In: Burchiel SW, Rhodes BA, Friedman BE (eds) Tumor imaging. The radioimmunochemical detection of cancer. Masson, New York, pp 231-239
34. Godolphin W, Elwood JM, Spinelli JJ (1981) Estrogen receptor quantitation and staging as complementary prognostic indicators in breast cancer: a study of 583 patients. Int J Cancer 28: 677-683
35. Gorski J, Welshons WV, Sakai D, Hansen J, Walent J, Kassis J, Schull H, Stack G, Campen C (1986) Evolution of a model of estrogen action. Recent Prog Horm Res 2: 297-329
36. Greene GL, Nolan C, Engler JP, Jensen EV (1980) Monoclonal antibodies to human estrogen receptors. Proc Natl Acad Sci USA 77: 5115-5119
37. Hahnel R, Twaddle E (1978) Estradiol binding by human breast carcinoma cytosols: the influence of commonly used reference parameters on the results. Eur J Cancer 14: 125-131
38. Hahnel R, Twaddle E (1985) The relationship between estrogen receptors in primary and secondary breast carcinomas and in sequential primary breast carcinomas. Breast Cancer Res Treat 5: 155–163
39. Hasson J, Luhan PA, Kohl MW (1981) Comparison of estrogen receptor levels in breast cancer samples from mastectomy and frozen section specimens. Cancer 47: 138-139
40. Heuson JC, Paridaens R, Sylvester R, Leclerq G (1981) Discrepancies between institutions in clinical correlations. In: Sarfaty GA, Nash AR, Keightley DD (eds) Estrogen receptor assays in breast cancer: laboratory discrepancies and quality assurance. Masson, New York, pp 1-19
41. Hilf R, Feldstein ML, Gibson SL, Savlov ED (1980) The relative importance of estrogen receptor analysis as a prognostic factor for recurrence or response to chemotherapy in women with breast cancer. Cancer 45: 1993-2000
42. Howat JMT, Barnes DM (1981) Oestrogen receptor status and management of breast cancer. Lancet i: 1317
43. Howat JMT, Barnes DM, Harris M, Swindell R (1983) The association of cytosol oestrogen and progesterone receptors with histological features of breast cancer and early recurrence of disease. Br J Cancer 47: 629-640

44. Howat JMT, Harris M, Swindell R, Barnes DM (1985) The effect of oestrogen and progesterone receptors on recurrence and survival in patients with carcinoma of the breast. Br J Cancer 51: 263-270
45. Howell A, Harland RNL, Bramwell VHC, Swindell R, Barnes DM, Redford J, Wilkinson MJS, Crowther D, Selwood RA (1984) Steroid hormone receptors and survival after first relapse in breast cancer. Lancet i: 588-591
46. Hull DF, Clark GM, Osborne CK, Chamness GC, Knight WA III, McGuire WL (1983) Multiple estrogen receptor assays in human breast cancer. Cancer Res 43: 413-416
47. Jacobson BE (1981) Investigation of estrogen receptor protein in human mammary carcinoma for the establishment of a routine clinical assay. Can J Med Technol 43: 17-33
48. Jakesz R, Dittrich C, Hanusch J, Kolb R, Lenzhofer R, Moser K, Rainer H, Reiner G, Schemper M, Spona J (1985) Simultaneous and sequential determinations of steroid hormone receptors in human breast cancer. Ann Surg 201: 305-310
49. Jensen EV (1974) Some newer endocrine aspects of breast cancer. N Engl J Med 291: 1252-1254
50. Jensen EV (1981) Hormone dependency of breast cancer. Cancer 47: 2319-2326
51. Jensen EV, DeSombre ER (1977) The diagnostic implications of steroid binding in malignant tissues. Adv Clin Chem 19: 57-81
52. Jensen EV, DeSombre ER, Jungblut PW (1967) Estrogen receptors in hormone responsive tissues and tumors. In: Wissler RW, Dao TL, Wood S Jr (eds) Endogenous factors influencing host-tumor balance. University of Chicago Press, Chicago
53. Jensen EV, Greene GL, Closs LE, DeSombre ER, Nadji M (1982) Receptors reconsidered: a 20-year perspective. Rec Prog Horm Res 38: 1-40
54. Jonat W, Maass H (1978) Some Comments on the necessity of receptor determination in human breast cancer. Cancer Res 38: 4305-4306
55. Jordan VC, Jacobson HI, Keenan EJ (1986) Determination of estrogen receptor in breast cancer using monoclonal antibody technology: results of multicenter study in the United States. Cancer Res [Suppl] 46: 4237s-4240s
56. Kiang DT (1984) Correlation between estrogen receptor proteins and response to chemotherapy in patients with breast cancer. Cancer Treat Rep 68: 577-579
57. Kiang DT, Frenning DH, Goldman AI, Ascensao VF, Kennedy BJ (1978) Estrogen receptors and responses to chemotherapy and hormonal therapy in advanced breast cancer. N Engl J Med 299: 1330-1334
58. King WJ, Greene GL (1984) Monoclonal antibodies localize estrogen receptor in the nuclei of target cells. Nature 307: 745-747
59. King WJ, DeSombre ER, Jensen EV, Greene GL (1985) Comparison of immunocytochemical and steroid-binding assays for estrogen receptors in human breast tumors. Cancer Res 45: 293-304
60. Kinne DW, Ashikari R, Butler A, Menendez-Botet C, Rosen PP, Schwartz M (1981) Estrogen receptor protein in breast cancer as a predictor of recurrence. Cancer 10: 2364-2367
61. Knight WA III, Livingston RB, Gregory EJ, McGuire WL (1977) Estrogen receptor as an independent prognostic factor for early recurrence in breast cancer. Cancer Res 37: 4669-4671
62. Leake RE (1984) Clinical aspects of steroid receptor assays. Med Lab Sci 41: 257-261
63. Leake RE, Laing L, McArdle C, Smith D (1981) Soluble and nuclear oestrogen receptor status in human breast cancer in relation to prognosis. Br J Cancer 43: 67-71
64. Leclercq G, Bojar H, Goussard J, Nicholson RI, Pichon MF, Piffanelli A, Pousette A, Thorpe S, Lonsdorfer M (1986) Abbott monoclonal enzyme immunoassay measure-

ment of estrogen receptors in human breast cancer: a European multicenter study. Cancer Res [Suppl] 46: 4235s-4236s

65. Le Doussal V, Pinchon MF, Pallud C, Hacene K, Gest J, Milgrom E (1984) Relationship between ultrastructure and receptor content of primary breast cancer. Histopathology 8: 89-103
66. Lee YN (1982) Variability of steroid receptors in multiple biopsies of breast cancer: effect of systemic therapy. Breast Cancer Res Treat 2: 185-193
67. Leight GS Jr, Wells SA Jr, McCarty KS Jr (1984) Sex steroid receptor concentration in breast carcinoma tissue: effect of devascularization during mastectomy. Surgery 95: 256-260
68. Lesser ML, Rosen PP, Senie RT, Duthie K, Menendez-Botet C, Schwartz MK (1981) Estrogen and progesterone receptors in breast carcinoma: correlations with epidemiology and pathology. Cancer 48: 299-309
69. Leung BS, Fletcher WS, Lindell TD, Wood DC, Krippaehne WW (1973) Predictability of response to endocrine ablation in advanced breast carcinoma. A correlation to estrogen receptor and steroid sulfurylation. Arch Surg 106: 515-519
70. Lippman ME (1976) Steroid hormone receptors in human malignancy. Life Sci 18: 143-152
71. Lippman ME, Allegra JC, Simon R, Barlock A, Green L, Huff KK, Do HM, Aitken SC, Warren R (1978) The relationship between estrogen receptor and response rate to cytotoxic chemotherapy in metastatic breast cancer. N Engl J Med 298: 1223-1228
72. Maass H, Engel B, Hohmeister H, Lehmann F, Trams G (1972) Estrogen receptors in human breast cancer tissue. Am J Obstet Gynecol 113: 377-382
73. Mason RC, Miller WR, Hawkins RA (1985) Plasma oestrogens and oestrogen receptors in breast cancer patients. Br J Cancer 52: 793-796
74. Maynard PV, Blamey RW, Elston CW, Haybittle JL, Griffiths K (1978) Estrogen receptor assay in primary breast cancer and early recurrence of the disease. Cancer Res 38: 4292-4295
75. McCarty KS Jr, Szabo E, Flowers JL, Cox EB, Leight GS, Miller L, Konrath J, Soper JT, Budwit DA, Creasman WT, Seigler HF, McCarty KS Sr (1986) Use of a monoclonal anti-estrogen receptor antibody in the immunohistochemical evaluation of human tumors. Cancer Res [Suppl] 46: 4244s-4248s
76. McGuire WL, Chamness GC (1973) Role of estrogen receptor in breast cancer. Adv Exp Med Biol 36: 113-136
77. McGuire WL, Carbone PP, Vollmer EP (eds) (1975) Estrogen receptors in human breast cancer. Raven, New York, pp 1-9
78. Meyer JS (1986) Cell kinetics in selection and stratification of patients for adjuvant therapy of breast carcinoma. NCI Monogr 1: 25-28
79. Meyer JS, Rao BR, Stevens SC, White WL (1977) Low incidence of estrogen receptors in breast carcinomas with rapid rates of cellular replication. Cancer 40: 2290-2298
80. Millis RR (1980) Correlation of hormone receptors with pathological features in human breast cancer. Cancer 46: 2869-2871
81. Moran R, Black M, Alpert L (1984) Correlation of cell-cycle kinetics, hormone receptors, histopathology and nodal status in human breast cancer. Cancer 54: 1586-1590
82. Mortimer J, Reimer R, Greenstreet R, Groppe C, Bukowski R (1981) Influence of estrogen receptor status on response to combination chemotherapy for recurrent breast cancer. Cancer Treat Rep 65: 763-766

83. Mumford CH, Elston CW, Campbell FC, Blamey RW, Johnson J, Nicholson RI, Griffiths K (1983) Tumor epithelial cellularity and quantitative oestrogen receptor values in primary breast cancer. Br J Cancer 47: 549-552
84. Nagai R, Kataoka M, Kobayashi S, Ishihara K, Tobioka N, Nakashima K, Naruse M, Saito K, Sakuma S (1979) Estrogen and progesterone receptors in human breast cancer with concomitant assay of plasma 17β-estradiol, progesterone, and prolactin levels. Cancer Res 39: 1834-1840
85. Raemaekers JM, Beex LV, Koenders AJ, Pieters GF, Smals AG, Benraad TH, Kloppenborg PW (1984) Concordance and discordance of estrogen and progestereone receptor content in sequential biopsies of patients with advanced breast cancer: relation to survival. Eur J Cancer Clin Oncol 20: 1011-1018
86. Raemaekers JM, Beex LV, Pieters GF, Smals AG, Benraad TH, Klopenborg PW (1987) Progesterone receptor activity and relapse-free survival in patients with primary breast cancer: the role of adjuvant chemotherapy. Breast Cancer Res Treat 9: 191-199
87. Rasmussen BB, Pedersen BV, Thorpe SM, Rose C (1985) Elastosis in relation to prognosis in primary breast carcinoma. Cancer Res 45: 1428-1430
88. Rubens RD, King RJ, Sexton S, Minton MJ, Hayward JL (1980) Oestrogen receptor and response to cytotoxic chemotherapy in advanced breast cancer. Cancer Chemother Pharmacol 4: 43-45
89. Saez S, Martin PM, Chouvet CD (1978) Estradiol and progesterone receptor levels in human breast adenocarcinoma in relation to plasma estrogen and progesterone levels. Cancer Res 38: 3468-3473
90. Saez S, Cheix F, Asselain B (1983) Prognostic value of estrogen and progesterone receptors in primary breast cancer. Breast Cancer Res Treat 3: 345-354
91. Samaan NA, Buzdar AU, Aldinger KA, Schultz PN, Yang KP, Romsdahl MM, Martin R (1981) Estrogen receptor: a prognostic factor in breast cancer. Cancer 47: 554-560
92. Samal BA, Brooks SC, Cummings G, Franco L, Hire EA, Martino S, Singhakowinta A, Vaitkevicius VK (1980) Estrogen receptors and responsiveness of advanced breast cancer to chemotherapy. Cancer 46: 2925-2927
93. Savlov ED, Wittliff JL, Hilf R, Hall TC (1974) Correlations between certain biochemical properties of breast cancer and response to therapy: a preliminary report. Cancer 33: 303-309
94. Silfversward C, Gustafsson JA, Gustafsson SA, Humla S, Nordenskjold B, Wallgren A, Wrange O (1980) Estrogen receptor concentrations in 269 cases of histologically classified human breast cancer. Cancer 45: 2001-2005
95. Silvestrini R, Daidone MG, DiFronzo G (1979) Relationship between proliferative activity and estrogen receptor in breast cancer. Cancer 44: 665-670
96. Silvestrini R, Daidone MG, Gasparaini G (1985) Cell kinetics as a prognostic marker in node-negative breast cancer. Cancer 56: 1982-1987
97. Skinner JR, Wanebo HJ, Betsill WL, Wilhelm MC, Drake CR, Macleod RM (1982) Evaluation of the pathologic and prognostic correlates of estrogen receptors in primary breast cancer. Ann Surg 196: 636-641
98. Stewart JF, Rubens RD, Millis RR, King RJ, Hayward JL (1983) Steroid receptors and prognosis in operable (stage I and II) breast cancer. Eur J Cancer Clin Oncol 19: 1381-1387
99. Stoll BA (1985) Mechanisms in endocrine therapy of bone metastases. J R Soc Med [Suppl] 78: 11-14
100. Straus MJ, Moran R, Muller RE, Wotiz HH (1982) Estrogen receptor heterogeneity and the relationship between estrogen receptor and the tritiated thymidine labeling index in human breast cancer. Oncology 39: 197-200

101. Toma S, Leonessa F, Paridaens R (1985) The effects of therapy on estrogen receptors in breast cancer. J Steroid Biochem 23: 1105-1109
102. Underwood JCE (1985) Oestrogen receptor status and cellular composition of breast cancer. Lancet i: 1274-1275
103. van Netten JP, Algard FT, Coy P, Carlyle SJ, Brigden ML, Thornton KR, Peter S, Fraser T, To MP (1985) Heterogeneous estrogen receptor levels detected via multiple microsamples from individual breast cancers. Cancer 56: 2019-2024
104. Vollenweider-Zerargui L, Barrelet L, Wong Y, Lermarchand-Beraud T, Gomez F (1986) The predictive value of estrogen and progesterone receptors' concentrations on the clinical behaviour of breast cancer in women: clinical correlation on 547 patients. Cancer 57: 1171-1180
105. Walt AJ, Singhakowinta A, Brooks SC, Cortez A (1976) The surgical implications of estrophile protein estimations in carcinoma of the breast. Surgery 80: 506-512
106. Williams MR, Todd JH, Nicholson RI, Elston CW, Blamey RW, Griffiths K (1986) Survival patterns in hormone treated advanced breast cancer. Br J Surg 73: 752-755
107. Wittliff JL (1984) Steroid hormone receptors in breast cancer. Cancer [Suppl] 53: 630-643

Pathology

Identification of Risk Factors by Conventional Pathologic and Some Ancillary Techniques in Women with Breast Cancer

E.R. Fisher

Institute of Pathology, Shadyside Hospital, Pittsburgh University, Pittsburgh, PA, USA

Conventional Pathologic Discriminants of Risk

In 1971 the National Surgical Adjuvant Breast Project (NSABP) initiated a protocol to evaluate whether total mastectomy with and without postoperative irradiation was as efficacious as radical mastectomy in the primary treatment of patients with stage I and II breast cancer. Patients were randomized so that those with clinically negative axillae were treated by either radical mastectomy, total (simple) mastectomy and irradiation including the axilla, or total mastectomy without axillary intervention. Those with clinically positive axillary nodes were also randomized into groups receiving either radical mastectomy or total mastectomy and irradiation. Accrual of 1665 evaluable patients was completed in 1974. No significant difference in survival has been noted 10 years after mastectomy in the various treatment arms of each of the two strata [21]. This collection represents one of the best available sources for exploring the natural history and pathologic discriminants or markers for the prognosis of breast cancer.

Pathologic examination of all specimens was initially performed by pathologists of participating institutions according to guidelines established by a predesigned protocol [24]. Stained sections and blocks of the tumor, nipple, skin overlying the tumor, lymph nodes when present, and one randomly selected block from each of the four quadrants of breast were forwarded to the pathology headquarters for a detailed review, including special histologic and tinctorial features. A total of 38 pathologic and 6 clinical characteristics were examined [24]. Preliminary analyses revealed at least 20 pathologic features which might influence survival. Attempts to rank these prognostic discriminants revealed the nodal status, as determined pathologically, to be the dominant factor in this regard. Further, it was observed that women with only 1-3 regional lymph nodes positive for metastases fared better than those with involvement of 4 or more. This latter group was subdivided into those with 4-6, 7-12, and 13 or more positive nodes since different 5-year treatment failure rates and survival were demonstrated in these various subgroups of the 4 or more nodal patients [18]. Because of the prognostic importance of nodal status and the recognition of an approximately 40% false-positive and false-negative error in clinical estimates, it was considered imperative to perform the analyses only on the 614 patients subjected to radical mastectomy in whom the lymph nodes and other appropriate material were available for pathologic study.

Ragaz/Ariel (Eds.), High-Risk Breast Cancer

Disease-free survival for 10 years following mastectomy is strongly related to nodal status, and when positive, to the numbers of nodes containing metastases (Fig. 1) [31]. Inspection of the figure reveals that the curves of the various categories reach a relative plateau after 4-5 years. Indeed the differences in survival at 5 and 10 years in the node-negative group was only 5%, in the 1-3 positive category it was 8%, and in those with 4 or more nodal metastases only 2%. With the 5-year postoperative period as the "zero" point it becomes apparent that survival for 5 years assures less risk for subsequent treatment failure, regardless of nodal status. This information gives credence to the value of 5-year estimates of survival in women with breast cancer.

Although nodal status is clearly the dominant influence on survival it should be emphasized that some pathologic characteristics such as perineural tumor extension, sinus histiocytosis, nipple involvement, and type of tumor border, which are found to be related to nodal status, are not found to be associated with treatment failure. It is therefore imprudent, as has been occasionally practiced, to conclude that because a marker is related to nodal status it is pari passu associated with survival. On the other hand, cancers which have been designated as types 1, 2, and 4 scar cancers (see later in this chapter) and the presence of tumor mucin reactive to the periodic acid-Schiff stain are related to treatment failure, but not nodal status. Similarly, in analyses in which nodal status is controlled, disease-free survival was found to be statistically greater for women whose tumors measured less than 2 cm than in those in whom the cancers exceeded this size. However, the magnitude of this difference was only 15% and no stepwise relationship to survival was noted for tumors larger than 2 cm. It has been estimated that approximately 10% of patients with large tumors would have been disease free if their tumors had been removed when less than 2 cm [22]. This information indicates that other biologic character-

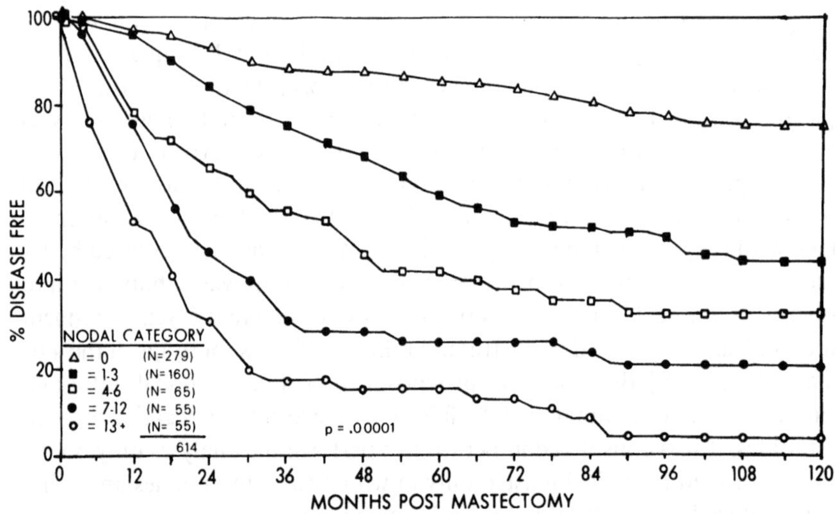

Fig. 1. Probability of disease-free survival according to number of regional nodal metastases

istics of the tumor as well as perhaps host factors may play a greater role in prognosis than size per se.

When life tables of probability of disease-free survival were prepared according to nodal status, several significant characteristics were observed which allowed for further discrimination in these categories. As noted in Table 1 the presence of a germinal center predominance pattern (Fig. 2) in the regional nodes of women

Table 1. Pathologic markers related to 10-year treatment failure according to nodal category

Absent	*P*
Nodal germinal center predominance	0.004
Histologic grade III	0.02
1-3 Nodes	
None with significance	
⩾4 Nodes	
Tumor size (> 2 cm)	0.01
Histologic grade III	0.02

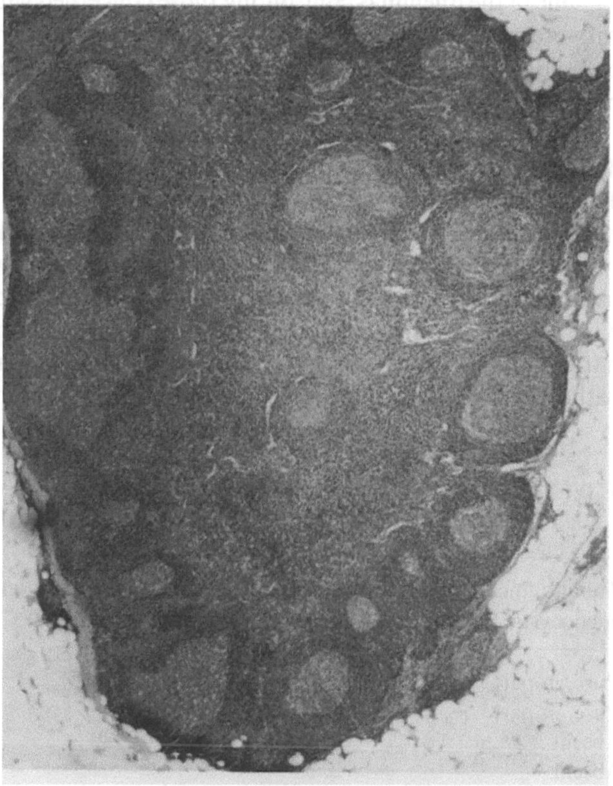

Fig. 2. Regional lymph node exhibiting germinal center predominance, an adverse finding in the node-negative patient. ×25

designated as stage I (absent nodal metastases) was an adverse finding at both 5 and 10 years after mastectomy. Such a nodal appearance connotes humoral antibody formation. Whether this indeed occurs and represents evidence of blocking antibodies to cell-mediated immunity in this situation is speculative. Cancers estimated to be of high histologic grade (poorly differentiated) were also associated with treatment failure in the node-negative patient. A similar experience has been noted by others [3]. Several methods of grading breast cancers have been utilized. Our algorithm represents a simplified modification of these, emphasizing nuclear characteristics expressed as nuclear grade which is based on the most dedifferentiated forms present and the presence or absence of tubular differentiation (Table 2) [24, 27]. We have found this scheme to be highly reproducible. Since well-differentiated or grade I tumors of the breast are uncommon we have chosen to incorporate these with cancers of intermediate grade into one group regarded as being well differentiated. This simplification has proven to be practical and importantly minimizes observer error in distinguishing between grades 1 and 2, and between grades 2 and 3 (Fig. 3). Although estimation of nuclear grade alone or presence or absence of tubule formation may be utilized for assessments of differentiation, better discrimination is offered when the two are combined as histologic grade, particularly at the 10th postoperative year. In our opinion most difficulty in grading tumors results from suboptimal technical preparation of slides for such evaluation.

One of the dilemmas confronting those concerned with the treatment of patients with breast cancer is whether to administer adjuvant chemotherapy to patients with pathologic stage I disease. Reports have suggested that high risk stage I patients can be identified by the presence of lymphatic invasion [7, 61, 62, 70]. However, only two of the groups [7, 70] mention whether lymphatics in the vicinity of the dominant mass or in quadrants remote from the dominant mass were involved. This distinction is important since lymphatic extension into remote breast quadrants represents a histologic manifestation of so-called inflammatory or rapidly progressive breast cancer, a form of the disease associated with an extremely high treatment failure rate and other ominous features. Also the sample sizes studied have been relatively small. A more disquieting concern relative to the role of intralymphatic extension as a discriminant is the lack of unanimity among pathologists concerning the recognition of this phenomenon [38]. It is true that

Table 2. NSABP scheme for histologic grading of breast cancer

Tubules (including adenocystic forms)	Nuclear grade	Histologic grade
Pure, in part	1	1
Pure, in part	2, 3	2
Absent	1	2
Absent	2, 3	3

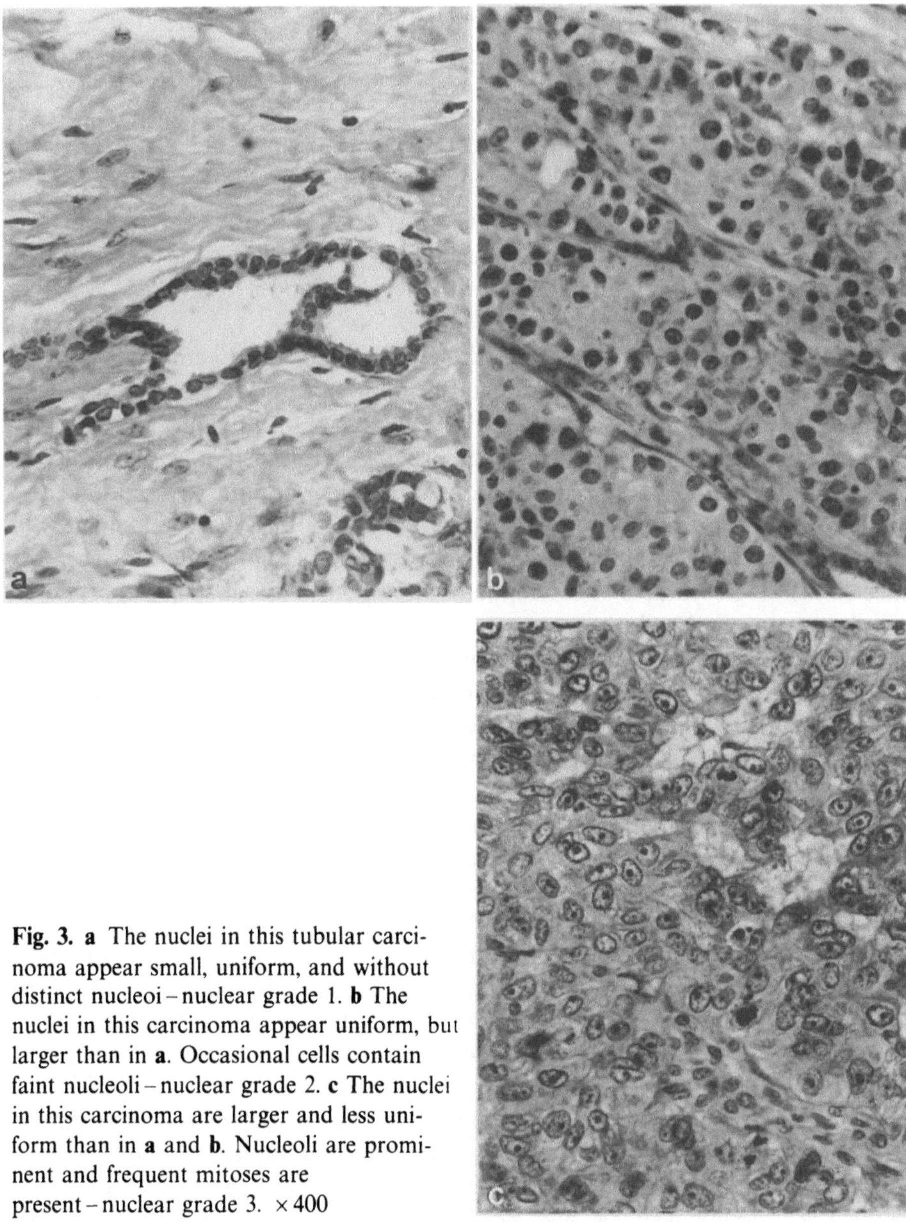

Fig. 3. **a** The nuclei in this tubular carcinoma appear small, uniform, and without distinct nucleoi – nuclear grade 1. **b** The nuclei in this carcinoma appear uniform, but larger than in **a**. Occasional cells contain faint nucleoli – nuclear grade 2. **c** The nuclei in this carcinoma are larger and less uniform than in **a** and **b**. Nucleoli are prominent and frequent mitoses are present – nuclear grade 3. ×400

many breast cancers contain aggregates of tumor cells in tissue spaces which may simulate intralymphatic extension. However, this effect appears to be related to fixation, appearing more commonly in tissues preserved in formalin or alcohol than in Bouin's fluid or those fixatives containing heavy metals. Careful observation of these artifactual spaces reveals an absence of lining endothelia. Our experience has taught us to regard such questionable examples of this phenomenon as being negative. True lymphatic extension is more clearly perceived at the periphery of the cancer. Our data reveals lymphatic extension to be more closely related to nodal metastases than treatment failure. Indeed, 33% of the tumors from patients surviving for 10 years possessed such extension, and others [15] have observed lymphatic extension in 63% of 25-year survivors. Lastly, it is not surprising to us that lymphatic extension does not appear as a significant discriminant for treatment failure when it is appreciated that nodal metastases measuring < 1.3 mm may be found in approxxmately one-quarter of cases by extended pathologic examination of lymph nodes regarded by conventional study as being negative [33]. Yet, survival is similar to that noted in patients with negative nodes examined by either conventional or extended methods.

It is germane to inquire why the pathologic features noted here have not been utilized as a guide to the administration of chemotherapeutic agents in women with stage I disease. Their use was considered in the design of the node-negative NSABP protocols 13 and 14 which are now in progress. However, it was decided to randomize the patients of this relatively low risk group according to receptor status. It was recognized that many if not most practicing pathologists are unfamiliar with technique of histologic grading. Since values of estrogen and progesterone receptors reflected histologic features of differentiation (see later in this chapter), appraisal of these latter appeared to be more practical and objective.

As observed at 5 years [28], no pathologic discriminants or markers could be identified in patients in the 1-3 positive node category 10 years after mastectomy, although trends of a relationship of survival to tumor size, histologic grade, and scar types were noted. The failure to detect any statistically significant discriminant for treatment failure in patients with 1-3 positive nodes is perplexing and enigmatic. Indeed, other analyses performed by us more often than not reveal associations in patients with absent or 4 or more nodal metastases, but not the 1-3 group. It is relevant in this regard, however, to recognize that the size of the nodal metastases in almost 25% of these patients is less than 1.3-2 mm. Such sizes have been noted to be associated with survival indistinguishable from that of patients without nodal metastases. This dilution of the 1-3 group contributes to this failure to detect any statistically significant prognostic discriminants in this group of patients.

A tumor size > 2.0 cm as well as one that exhibits a high or most malignant histologic grade have been found to represent adverse discriminants of breast cancers accompanied by 4 or more nodal metastases. Unfortunately, the sample sizes were too small to explore these possible discriminants in the various subdivisions of the 4 or more nodal category. On the other hand, unlike the 5-year results [28], tumor necrosis was no longer found to represent a prognostic characteristic in any nodal category in the 10th year. Except for the presence of 13 or more nodal metastases and the presence of types 1, 2, and 4 scar cancers, no other characteristics were observed which might provide insight into which patients at 5 years may or may not exhibit treatment failure by the 10th postoperative year. There is evidence [26, 48] that some cancers of breast may evolve from an otherwise banal lesion designated as nonencapsulated lesion or radial scar (Fig. 4). The frequency of such an event has been estimated to be about 35%-50%. Although five types of scar-related cancer can be identified, the more classical form which we

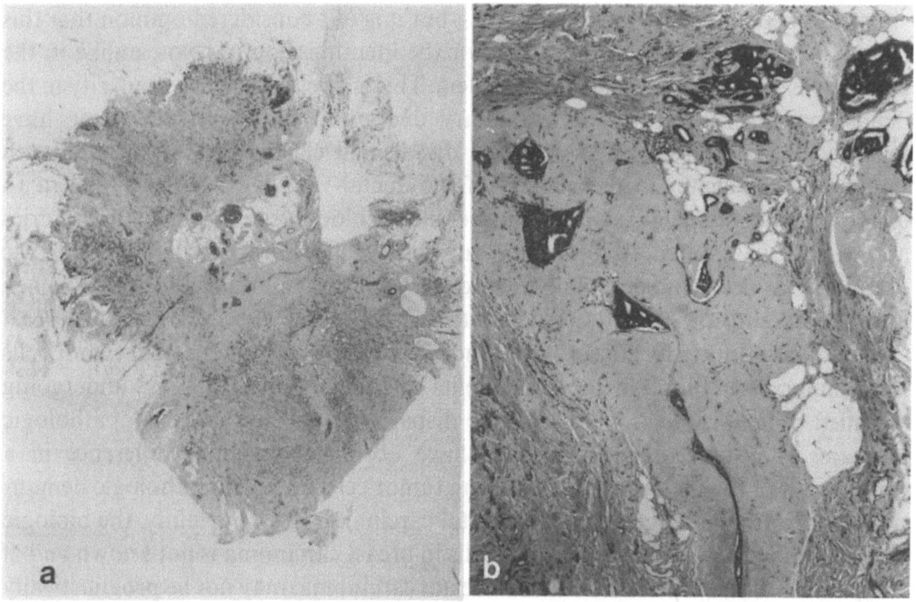

Fig. 4. a Low power appearance of so-called scar cancer 1. The relatively acellular central core and peripheral spiculated infiltration of breast and fatty tissue is apparent. × 10. **b** Higher magnification of central core, demonstrating its acellular hyaloelastic nature which is also characteristic of the banal nonencapsulated sclerosing lesion or radial scar of breast. × 100

designate as type 1, and its variants, types 2 and 4, are associated with better treatment failure rates than other scar forms or those cancers lacking evidence of origin from the banal radial scar. Further, this survival appears independent of nodal status. The majority of the cancers comprising these scar types exhibit a prominent or marked tubular component. It is therefore not surprising that types 1 and 4 scar cancers have better survival rates since they are very well differentiated. Other histologic types of breast cancer, notably the mucinous and papillary forms in addition to tubular carcinoma, have been observed to exhibit more favorable treatment failure rates. The medullary, lobular invasive, infiltrating ductal carcinoma, not otherwise specified (NOS), and tubular combinations, as well as other combination tumor types, are intermediate in this regard, with the NOS having the worst prognosis. Multivariate analysis reveals that the influence of these various types of breast cancer on survival is more closely related to histologic grade than histologic type per se.

The prognostic significance of recognizing blood vessel invasion in breast cancers is controversial. Reports reveal an incidence of such an extension in 21%-46%, although our own estimate of this event is only 4%. This dichotomy appears to be related to the criteria employed for its identification. It is important to note that in our studies we have relied on the more classical features of tumor thrombus, tumor covered by endothelial cells in a vascular space, or presence of neoplastic cells in an unequivocal vein or capillary [24]. Recourse to elastic tissue stains has been made by all investigators, but it is our considered opinion that this technique, when applied to the breast for the identification of veins, unlike in the colon, does not greatly resolve this problem. This is due to the close similarity in the deposition of elastic fibers in mammary ducts and blood vessels. Some have regarded the presence of distorted and disoriented elastic fibers associated with tumor cell aggregates in the vicinity of the ductal-vascular bundles sufficient to connote blood vessel invasion. In another study, blood vessel invasion in "arteries and veins" was stated to be scored as positive [78]. Intra-arterial neoplastic extension has been conventionally regarded as a curiosity, and in our opinion when found represents an artifact. Our low estimates of blood vessel extension in breast carcinoma is admittedly conservative. Indeed, we have identified actual tumor cells in mammary vein blood in 26% of patients with stage I and II disease undergoing modified radical mastectomy [39]. The disparity in this and the histopathologic estimates is not surprising, since we have observed a similar difference in a comparison of the incidence of circulating tumor cells and histopathologic demonstration of vascular extension in colorectal carcinoma [34]. Certainly, the biologic significance of such circulating tumor cells in breast carcinoma is not known and, if comparable to the experience with colorectal carcinoma, may not be prognostically significant [16]. Of course it should also be recalled that only about 50% of patients with angioinvasive thyroidal carcinoma will die of their disease, although diagnosis is based on the presence of blood vessel invasion. Indeed, not all tumor emboli represent metastases!

Despite the range in purported incidence of blood vessel invasion in breast cancer, as well as the inability to relate tumor emboli to metastases, all studies suggest that blood vessel invasion represents an adverse pathologic discriminant for breast cancer. In our own data, such a phenomenon was observed in 13 or 3.6% of the cases without recurrence and only 28 (7.8%) of those with treatment failure. Again, although this characteristic appears in exploratory contingency tables to be related to nodal status and 10-year treatment failure, it loses its statistical significance in regard to the latter in node-adjusted life tables or when patients are stratified according to nodal category. This, of course, may be related to the relatively few examples of blood vessel invasion in the various subsets. Results of a study utilizing less stringent criteria for blood vessel invasion, which generated a higher incidence of this event, have failed to alter our conclusions concerning its prognostic significance.

Conventional Pathologic Discriminants of Chemotherapeutic Responsiveness

During the search for pathologic markers for survival in patients with breast cancer, information was being accumulated concerning the effectiveness of adjuvant chemotherapy in patients with stage II disease (regional nodal metastases). Noteworthy was the apparent responsiveness of premenopausal, but not postmenopausal, women to such treatment. Although a variety of reasons are advanced as possible explanations for this dichotomy, none appeared to be satisfactory. On the other hand, our own pathologic studies had revealed that, generally, breast cancers in postmenopausal women were better differentiated than those in their younger counterparts [24]. The pathologic observation was consonant with the more frequent high estrogen receptor (ER) content of cancers in postmenopausal women. We demonstrated that this marker appeared to represent a biochemical reflection of tumor differentiation [25, 30]. Lastly, it has long been recognized that poorly differentiated neoplasms respond more favorably to radiation than well-differentiated forms, and many of the chemotherapeutic agents used were considered to possess at least some radiomimetic properties. These considerations prompted us to attempt to correlate the pathologic characteristics of the cancers in women receiving adjuvant chemotherapy with their response [29]. Patients with poorly differentiated tumors who were treated with L-phenylalanine mustard (P) with methotrexate (PM), and 5-fluorouracil (PMF) exhibited satistically greater survival as compared with control subjects (Figs. 5 and 6). Increase in survival was evident in women < 49 years as well as those > 50 years of age, and was particularly pronounced in those with 4 or more nodal metastases and whose tumors were poorly differentiated. No other independent discriminants were constantly found which allowed for such a discrimination of chemotherapeutic responsiveness. Thus, there are certain groups of postmenopausal women who do exhibit a response to chemotherapeutic agents, and general conclusions concerning the efficacy of such therapy may be misleading. Our results suggest that chemotherapy should be reserved for patients with poorly differentiated tumors, regardless of age. Conversely, evidence is accumulating that well-differentiated tumors may be more responsive to endocrine manipulation [19].

Identification of the pathologic discriminants for disease-free survival and responsiveness to adjuvant therapy underscores the importance of the "routine"

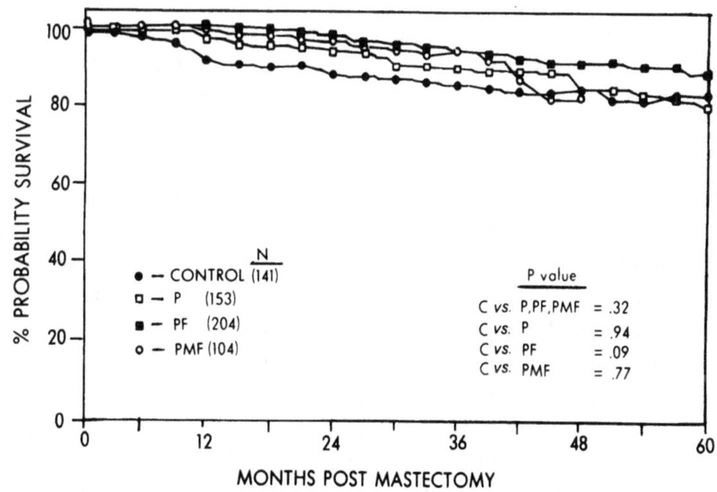

Fig. 5. Probability of survival after chemotherapy in all patients with well-differentiated tumors

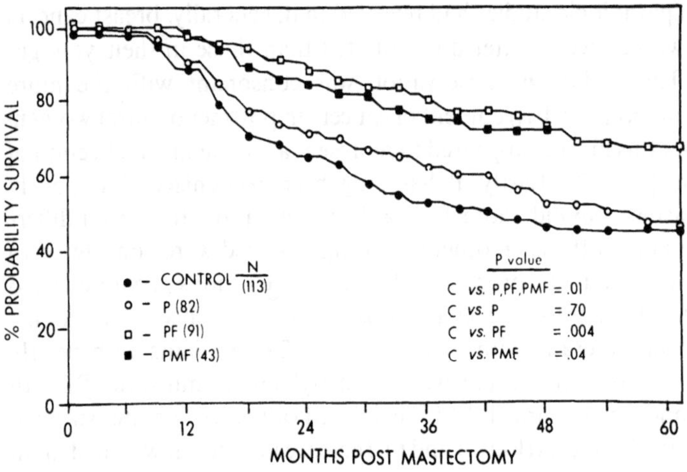

Fig. 6. Probability of survival after chemotherapy in women aged > 50 years with poorly differentiated tumors and ⩾ 4 nodal status

pathologist's role in contributing to the care of patients with breast cancer, as well as the design of protocols for evaluating treatment schemes. Finally, it should be noted that the prognostic characteristics enumerated neither require any special or sophisticated techniques for their identification nor is the practice unduly time-consuming.

Estrogen and Progesterone Receptors as Markers of Risk and their Relationship to Pathologic Discriminants

The role of receptor status in the treatment and prognosis of patients with breast cancer is well recognized. Yet, the "power" of this marker may not be as strong as is commonly believed. Indeed, it has been estimated that approximately 65% of women whose cancers possess ER will exhibit a response to ablative or additive antiestrogen treatment, whereas 10% lacking this marker will do so [54]. It has been suggested that this relative inconsistency may be due to the importance of other receptors and markers, the heterogeneity of tumor cell populations, defective cytoplasmic receptor proteins, or their exclusively nuclear disposition [54]. It has also been suggested [73] that perhaps our definition of responsiveness may be unrealistic; and we have noted responsiveness to be more closely related to quantitative rather than qualitative assessments [20]. The relationship between receptors and responsiveness is improved to approximately 80% when both ER and progesterone receptors (PR) are positive [20, 53, 66]. Although ER and PR are generally complementary, patient age has been consistently found to be more related to the former. Responsiveness to a chemotherapeutic regimen containing the antiestrogen tamoxifen appears to be more closely related to PR than ER in premenopausal women [20].

Combined assays for both ER and PR have revealed a relatively high incidence of discordant values [23, 32]. In our experience 30% of assays appear discordant with 17% being ER+/PR− and 13% the converse [32]. It is uncertain whether these findings represent a methodological [71] error or actually an incomplete synthetic process in which PR is viewed as an end product of estrogen-dependent ER activity [46, 54]. However, cancers with discordant receptors lack pathologic features noted in those cancers containing concordant ER and PR [32]. Further, life table analyses (Fig. 7) have revealed disease-free survival of women whose cancers had discordant values to be intermediate between that of women in whom these markers were ER+/PR+ and ER−/PR− [32]. This information suggests that a discordant receptor status is more indicative of an aberration of ER metabolism or a biologic phenomenon rather than a methodological error.

Attempts to assess the consistency of ER determinations in a primary breast cancer have disclosed similar values in 76-84% of such cancers that have been sequentially studied [67, 69]. Agreement of ER status has also been noted between the primary growth and nodal metastases in 62%-86% [67, 69, 77]. Assays performed on other metastases have revealed ER values comparable to the primary cancer in 74% of instances, despite variable time intervals between such assessments [69]. It has been estimated that approximately one-third of all positive ER assays will become negative after chemotherapy or endocrine therapy [2, 67, 77].

The question arises whether receptors represent independent discriminants or biochemical reflections of identifiable pathologic characteristics of breast cancers. The more frequent incidence of such markers in cancers in women > 50 years, a group in which breast cancers are generally better differentiated than those in younger women (< 49) [24], might be cited as being suggestive in this regard. Further, as noted previously in this chapter, responsiveness to chemotherapy has been found to be more frequent in younger than older women, whereas endocrine therapy appears more effective in women > 50 years [20]. These variations in

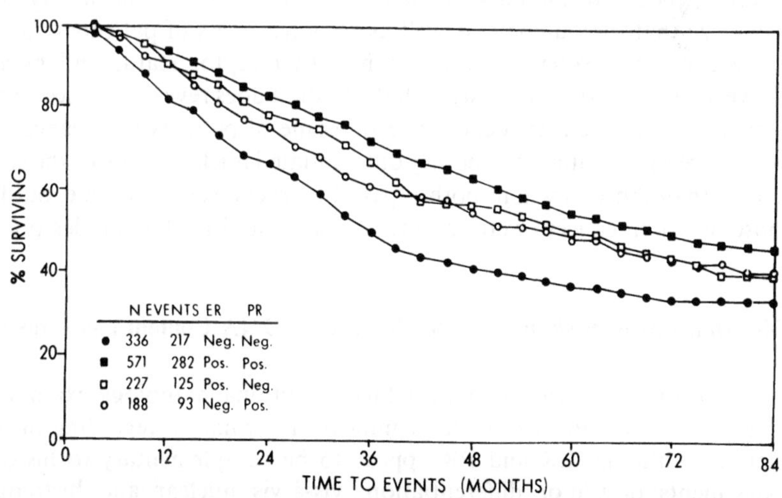

Fig. 7. Probability of disease-free survival related to concordant or discordant ER/PR status

response have also been found to be related to pathologic features reflecting tumor differentiation [20, 29].

Correlation of ER status and the pathologic characteristics of breast cancers have almost universally revealed significant associations between the former and features of tumor differentiation [1, 25, 30, 50, 63] as well as other techniques reflecting this phenomenon, viz., tumor labeling index [59], ultrastructural characteristics [76], and DNA content [37]. Similar pathologic associations have now been observed with PR as well as ER. ER+/PR+ cancers, when compared with those in which both receptors are negative, have been noted to possess low (best differentiated) nuclear and histologic grades, mild or absent lymphoid infiltration, absent necrosis, and moderate or marked elastosis in descending order of significance when ranked by logistic regression analyses [32]. Between 70% and 80% of positive ER or PR values can be predicted when four or five conforming pathologic features are found. Nuclear grade alone is predictive in approximately 70% of instances. Most studies have revealed the lobular invasive and tubular types of breast cancer to be related to a positive receptor status, whereas the medullary variant is often negative. In our experience these relationships appear to be more closely related to the degree of differentiation of these tumor types rather than their identifying structural or topographic appearances.

Studies of the interrelationship of nodal and receptor status have been inconsistent [9, 14, 19, 41, 49, 66]. Our own investigation in this regard has disclosed little or no association between negative ER/PR and increasing numbers of nodal metastases [23, 32]. Whether ER/PR status will allow for the recognition of stage I patients who will benefit from adjuvant therapy has not been conclusively demonstrated. Randomized clinical trials addressing this issue are now in progress.

Interestingly, histograms depicting the frequency of well- and poorly differentiated nuclear grades and quantitative measurements of ER and PR have confirmed the reliability of clinically regarding cancers with > 10 fmol/mg as being positive [32]. Further, the frequency of well-differentiated nuclei was found to be directly related to amounts of these receptors. It is not surprising therefore to recognize that the outcome as well as responsiveness of patients treated with the antiestrogen tamoxifen correlate with both receptor status and nuclear grade. However, multivariate analysis in that situation does reveal that these markers may exert an independent influence. The outcome of patients with cancer containing positive receptor values, but poorly differentiated nuclear grade or the converse was poorer than those in whom both types of markers were favorable, but better than those in whom cancers were receptor-negative and nuclear grades poor [19].

Discriminants of Risk as Revealed by Tumor DNA Content and Growth Rates

It would appear inarguable that careful conventional pathologic examination of the breast cancer specimen provides significant information regarding prognosis and therapy. Although ER and PR appear to be complementary to histopathologic assessments of tumor differentiation, vis-à-vis nuclear and histologic grades, as noted previously, in some situations they appear to represent independent variables. This experience reflects the utility of multiple markers in assessing prognosis and therapy of patients with breast cancer.

That alterations in nuclear DNA characterize many cancer cells has long been recognized. Further, some early studies utilizing Feulgen cytomicrospectrophotometry have suggested a relationship between DNA abnormalities and survival in patients with breast cancer [4]. Techniques for exploring cell cycle kinetics have also been utilized by a number of investigators to obtain more precise information concerning the growth rate of breast cancers. That variation in this characteristic occurs among breast cancers and may have prognostic value has been appreciated by physicians caring for patients with this disease, and indeed several schemes have evolved for making such a clinical appraisal [11, 12]. One of the most commonly employed methods for assessing the growth rate of cancers utilizes the in vitro incubation of tritiated thymidine with tumor tissue and subsequent microradioautography, the result being expressed as thymidine labeling index (TLI). Studies by Meyer and co-workers [56, 57, 58] have revealed that TLI correlates well with the histopathologic characteristics reflecting differentiation and receptor status as well as survival. However, this group more recently [58] regarded TLI as a weak predictor of metastases. Some have suggested that TLI may be similar to, if not a more significant prognostic discriminant than nodal status or pathologic features of tumor differentiation [72, 75]. These apparent inconsistencies as well as the need to identify predictive markers warrant further investigation of the kinetics as well as DNA abnormalities of breast cancer cells.

One of the more recent and obviously popular techniques for identifying DNA composition and growth rates of breast cancer is flow cytometry. The reader is referred to several overviews concerning the basic methodology and general application of this technique [8, 10, 45, 52]. Its principal attractions are that it represents a departure from the subjectivity of conventional pathologic assessments; it has the capability of quantitatively assessing these parameters; and at least in some hands is easily performed. With apparently only one exception [40] thus far, ploidy and growth rate expressed as S-phase or proliferative index have been found to be closely correlated. A similar concordance might be noted in regards to TLI and flow cytometric determinations [51]. This information suggests that the degree of aggressiveness of a cancer, if indeed ploidy relates to such a phenomenon, and growth rate, reflected by S-phase, or proliferative index, are not independent. Such a conclusion would represent a "violation" of Foulds' [36] "rules" 2 and 3 which offer that characteristics of a tumor such as biologic activity and size may progress independently [51]. It does not, however, in the author's opinion, totally vitiate the significance of Foulds' averments concerning tumor progression.

The extant literature relating to the use of flow cytometry in studying breast cancer reveals notable inconsistencies in results, surprisingly small sample sizes studied, and a certain vagueness of terminology. For instance, some investigators designate "abnormal" DNA as representing aneuploidy. Yet from a classical standpoint, aneuploidy refers to a chromosome number that is not an exact multiple of the haploid 23. It is difficult to determine from some reports whether the "aneuploidy" observed represents polyploidy (an exact multiple of the haploid number) or true aneuploidy. So-called aneuploidy has been found to occur in

50%-90% of breast cancer studies [6, 8, 13, 17, 35, 40, 44, 55, 60, 74]. Individual cancers may exhibit a variety of chromosomal aberrations. Thus, the technique may quantitatively, as well as qualitatively express the heterogeneous composition of breast cancers [68]. Interestingly, ploidy has not been observed to change in time when primary tumors have been studied by multiple biopsies [5, 6]. Similarly, tumor ploidy as well as S-phase or growth rates appear to be concordant in primary and metastatic sites [47, 64]. Ploidy has been noted to be correlated with morphological assessment of differentiation in all but one study [6] in which this parameter has been assessed. It is therefore not surprising that poorly differentiated types of breast cancers such as the medullary form are frequently aneuploid, whereas the well-differentiated tubular and mucinous varieties are often diploid. On the other hand, no consistent relationships between ploidy and nodal status, tumor size, patient age, or menopausal or receptor status have been noted. The few studies relating ploidy to disease-free survival have disclosed fewer recurrences of disease with diploid tumors in menopausal women [44] or those with cancers measuring less than 2 cm [17]. In the former study Cox's regression analysis failed to disclose the DNA index to be independent of lymph node status as a prognostic discriminant. Kinetic information expressed as S-phase or proliferative index has also been found to correlate with morphological expression of tumor differentiation; faster growing tumors more frequently being poorly differentiated [6, 47, 51, 65]. A negative ER, but not PR [51], has also been observed to be associated with faster growing cancers. No correlation of S-phase tumor size, nodal status, or number of positive nodes has been found.

It should be evident that the data thus far derived from flow cytometic studies are quite inconsistent as well as incomplete. There is no scrutable evidence as yet concerning the direct relationship of chromosomal abnormalities and growth rates of tumors to survival. Investigations in this regard have been limited by relatively small numbers of cases, and the follow-up periods of observation have been relatively short (4 years or less). It is expected, however, that the application of techniques [42, 43] allowing for determinations on archival material, vis-à-vis paraffin-embedded tumor tissue, will alleviate this shortcoming. Whether determinations of ploidy or DNA content and growth rates by flow cytometry represent singular, independent markers or a more arcane manner of measuring those found by conventional pathologic examination and/or ER and PR assessment and tumor labeling in vitro remains to be demonstrated.

Our own introduction to the use of flow cytometry for the study of breast cancers raises some doubt that the technique is as "easy" as some maintain. This may limit its widespread use. Despite these caveats, there is little doubt that flow cytometry in a research setting should provide additional insight into the biologic characteristics of tumor growth and behavior, and hopefully therapy.

References

1. Alanko A, Makinen J, Scheinen TM, Tolppanen E, Vihko R (1984) Correlation of estrogen and progesterone receptors and histological grade in human primary breast cancer. Acta Pathol Microbiol Immunol Scand 91: 311-315
2. Allegra J C, Barlock A, Huff K H, Lippman ME (1980) Changes in multiple or sequential estrogen receptor determinations in breast cancer. Cancer 45: 792-794
3. Andersen JA, Fischermann K, Hou-Jensen K et al. (1981) Selection of high-risk groups among prognostically favorable patients with breast cancer: an analysis of the value of prospective grading of tumor anaplasia in 1048 patients. Ann Surg. 194: 1-3
4. Auer G, Caspersson T, Wallgren A (1980) DNA content and survival in mammary carcinoma. Anal Quant Cytol 2: 161-165
5. Barlogie B, Drewinke B, Schumann J, Gohde W, Dosik G, Johnson DA, Freirech EJ (1980) Cellular DNA content as a marker of neoplasia in man. Am J Med 69: 195-203
6. Bedrossian CWM, Raber M, Barlogie B (1981) Flow cytometry and cyto morphology in primary resectable breast cancer. Anal Quant Cytol 3: 112-116
7. Bettelheim R, Neville AM (1981) Lymphatic and vascular channel involvement within infiltrative breast carcinomas as a guide to prognosis at the primary surgical treatment. Lancet ii: 631
8. Blijam GH, Schuette B (1983) Flow cytology in oncology: a review with emphasis on DNA flow cytometry in human solid tumors. Neth J Med 26: 314-320
9. Bishop HM, Blamey RW, Elston CW, Haybittle JL (1979) Relationship of estrogen receptor status to survival in breast cancer. Lancet ii: 283-284
10. Braglan RC (1983) Flow cytometry. Arch Pathol Lab Med 107: 1-6
11. Boyd NF, Meakin JW, Hayward JL, Brown TC (1981) Clinical estimation of the growth rate of breast cancer. Cancer 48: 1037-1042
12. Charlson ME, Feinstein AR (1974) The auxometric dimension: a new method for using rate of growth in prognostic staging of breast cancer. JAMA 228: 180-185
13. Cornelisse CJ, deKoning HR, Moolenaar AJ, van de Velde CJ, Ploem JS (1984) Image and flow cytometric analysis of DNA content in breast cancer. Int Acad Cytol 6: 9-18
14. Crowe JP, Hubay CA, Pearson OH, Marshall JS, Rosenblatt J, Mansour EG, Hermann RE, Jones JC, Flynn WJ, McGuire WL (1982) Estrogen receptor status as a prognostic indicator for stage I breast cancer patients. Breast Cancer Res Treat 2: 171-176
15. Dawson PJ, Ferguson DJ, Karrison T (1982) The pathologic findings of breast cancer in patients surviving 25 years after radical mastectomy. Cancer 50: 2131-2138
16. Engell HD (1955) Cancer cells in the circulating blood. Acta Chir Scand [suppl] 201: 1-70
17. Ewers S, Langstrom E, Baldetorp B, Killander D (1984) Flow-cytometric DNA analysis in primary breast carcinomas and clinicopathological correlations. Cytometry 5: 408-419
18. Fisher B, Bauer M, Wickerham DL, Redmond CK, Fisher ER (1983) Relation of number of positive axillary nodes to the prognosis of patients with primary cancer: an NSABP update. Cancer 52: 1551-1557
19. Fisher B, Fisher ER, Redmond CK, Brown (1986) Tumor nuclear grade, estrogen or progesterone receptor alone or in combination; their value as indicators of outcome following adjuvant therapy for breast cancer. Breast Cancer Res Treat 7: 147-160
20. Fisher B, Redmond C, Brown A, Wickerham DL, Wolmark N, Allegra J, Escher G, Lippman M, Savlov E, Witliff J, Fisher ER (1983) Influence of tumor estrogen and progesterone receptor levels on the response to tamoxifen and chemotherapy in primary breast cancer. J Clin Oncol 1: 227-241

21. Fisher B, Redmond C, Fisher ER, Bauer M, Wolmark N, Wickerham L, Deutsch M, Montague E, Margolese R, Foster R (1985) Ten-year results of a randomized clinical trial comparing radical mastectomy and total mastectomy with or without radiation. N Engl J Med 312: 674-681
22. Fisher B, Slack NH, Bross IDJ (1969) Cancer of the breast – size of neoplasm and prognosis. Cancer 24: 1071-1080
23. Fisher B, Wickerham DL, Brown A, Redmond CK (1983) Breast and progesterone receptor values. Their distribution, degree of concordance, and relation to number of positive axillary nodes. J Clin Oncol 1: 349-358
24. Fisher ER, Gregorio RM, Fisher B (1975) The pathology of invasive breast cancer: a syllabus derived from findings of the National Surgical Adjuvant Breast Project (protocol no 4). Cancer 36: 1-85
25. Fisher ER, Osborne CK, McGuire WL, Redmond CK, Knight WA III, Fisher B, Bannayan G, Wlafer A, Gregory EJ, Jacobsen A, Quees DM, Bennett DE, Ford HC (1981) Correlation of primary breast cancer histopathology and estrogen receptor content. Breast Cancer Res Treat 1: 37-41
26. Fisher ER, Palekar AS, Sass R, Fisher B (1983) Pathologic findings from the National Surgical Adjuvant Breast Project (protocol no 4): IX. Scar cancers. Breast Cancer Res Treat 3: 39-59
27. Fisher ER, Redmond C, Fisher B (1980) Histologic grading of breast cancer. Pathol Annu 15: 239-251
28. Fisher ER, Redmond C, Fisher B (1980) Pathologic findings from the National Surgical Adjuvant Breast Project (protocol no 4): VI. Discriminants for five year treatment failure. Cancer 46: 908-918
29. Fisher ER, Redmond C, Fisher B (1983) Pathologic findings from the National Surgical Adjuvant Breast Project. VIII. Relationship of chemotherapeutic responsiveness to tumor differentiation. Cancer 51: 181-191
30. Fisher ER, Redmond C, Liu H, Rockette H, Fisher B (1980) Correlation of estrogen receptor and pathologic characteristics of invasive breast cancer. Cancer 45: 349-353
31. Fisher ER, Sass R, Fisher B (1984) Pathologic findings from the National Surgical Adjuvant Breast Project (protocol 4). X. Discriminants for tenth year treatment failure. Cancer 53: 712-723
32. Fisher ER, Sass R, Fisher B (1987) Pathologic findings from the National Surgical Adjuvant Breast Project (NSABP): correlations with concordant and discordant estrogen and progesterone receptors. Cancer 59: 1554-1559
33. Fisher ER, Swamidoss S, Lee CH, Rockette H, Redmond C, Fisher B (1978) Detection and significance of occult axillary node metastases in patients with invasive breast cancer. Cancer 42: 2025-2031
34. Fisher ER, Turnbull RB (1955) The cytologic demonstration and significance of tumor cells in the mesenteric venous blood in patients with colorectal carcinoma. Surg Gynecol Obstet 100: 102-108
35. Foss SD, Thorud E, Shoaib MC, Petersen E, Hoie J, Knudsen OS (1984) DNA flow cytometry in primary breast carcinoma. Acta Pathol Microbiol Immunol Scand 92: 475-480
36. Foulds L (1957) Tumor progression (1957) Cancer Res 17: 355-356
37. Fraschini G, Johnson T, Williamson K, Gallagher H, Raber H, Blumenschein G, Barlogie B (1984) Proliferative activity and ploidy of primary breast cancer in relationship to estrogen receptor (ER) and nuclear grade. Proc Am Assoc Cancer Res 25: 35
38. Gilchrist KW, Gould VE, Hirschl S, Imbriglia JE, Patchefsky AS, Penner DW, Pickren J, Schwartz IS, Wheeler JE, Barnes JM, Mansour EG (1982) Interobserver variation in the

identification of breast carcinoma in intramammary lymphatics. Hum Pathol 13: 170-172
39. Golinger RC, Gregorio RM, Fisher ER (1977) Tumor cells in venous blood draining mammary carcinomas. Arch Surg 112: 707-798
40. Haag D, Goerttler K, Tschahargane (1984) The proliferative index (PI) of human breast cancer as obtained by flow cytometry. Pathol Res Pract 178: 315-322
41. Hahnel R, Woodings T, Vivian AB (1979) Prognostic value of estrogen receptors in primary breast cancer. Cancer 44: 671-675
42. Hedley DW, Friedlander ML, Taylor IW, Rugg CA, Musgrove EA (1983) Method for analysis of cellular DNA content of paraffin-embedded pathological material using flow cytometry. J Histochem Cytochem 31: 1333-1335
43. Hedley DW, Friedlander ML, Taylor IW (1985) Application of DNA flow cytometry to paraffin-embedded archival material for the study of aneuploidy and its clinical significance. Cytometry 6: 327-333
44. Hedley DW, Rugg CA, Ng AB, Taylor IW (1984) Influence of cellular DNA content on disease-free survival of stage II breast cancer patients. Cancer Res 44: 5395-5398
45. Herman C, Vooijs GP, Baak JPA, Boon ME (1984) Quantitative cytologic and histologic techniques to assist in cancer evaluation. Methods Achiev Exp Pathol 11: 73-95
46. Horwitz KB, McGuire WL (1975) Predicting response to endocrine therapy in human breast cancer: hypothesis. Science 189: 726-727
47. Kute TE, Muss HB, Hopkins M, Marshall R, Case D, Kammire L (1985) Relationship of flow cytometry results to clinical and steroid receptor status in human breast cancer. Breast Cancer Res Treat 6: 113-121
48. Linell F, Ljunberg O, Andersson I (1980) Breast cancer: aspects of early stages, progression and related problems. Acta Pathol Microbiol Scand [Suppl 272]: 1-233
49. Maillot K, Horke W, Prestele H (1982) Prognostic significance of the steroid receptor content in primary breast cancer. Arch Gynecol 231: 185-190
50. McCarty KS Jr, Barton TK, Fetter BF, Woodard BH, Mossler HA, Reeves W, Daly J, Wilkinson WE, McCarthy KS Sr (1980) Correlation of estrogen progesterone receptors with histologic differentiation in mammary carcinoma. Cancer 46: 2851-2858
51. McDivitt RW, Stone KR, Craig RB et al. (1985) A comparison of human breast cancer cell kinetics measured by flow cytometry and thymidine labeling. Lab Invest 3: 287-291
52. McGuire WL, Dressler LG (1985) Emerging impact of flow cytometry in predicting recurrence and survival in breast cancer patients. JNCI 75: 405-410
53. McGuire WL, Horwitz KB (1978) Progesterone receptors in breast cancer. In: McGuire WL (ed) Hormones, receptors and breast cancer. Raven, New York, pp 31-42
54. McGuire WL, Horwitz KB, Pearson OH, Segaloff A (1977) Current status of estrogen and progesterone receptors in breast cancer. Cancer 39: 2934-2947
55. Mellin W, Vollmer E, Nienhaus H, Grundmann E (1985) Flow cytometic DNA analysis and immunohistological detection of proliferation patterns in breast carcinoma and in proliferating mastopathy. Verh Dtsch Ges Pathol 69: 540-543
56. Meyer JS, Friedman E, McCrate MM, Bauer WC (1983) Prediction of early course of breast carcinoma by thymidine labeling. Cancer 51: 1879-1886
57. Meyer JS, Lee J (1980) Relationship of S-phase fraction of breast carcinoma in relapse to duration of remission, estrogen receptor content, therapeutic responsiveness, and duration of survival. Cancer Res 40: 1890-1896
58. Meyer JS, Prey MU, Babcock DS, McDivitt RW (1986) Breast carcinoma cell kinetics, morphology, stage and host characteristics. Lab Invest 54: 41-51
59. Meyer JS, Rao BR, Stevens SC, White WL (1977) Low incidence of estrogen receptor in breast carcinoma with rapid rates of cellular replication. Cancer 40: 2290-2298

60. Moran RE, Black MM, Alpert L, Straus MJ (1984) Correlation of cell-cycle kinetics, hormone receptors, histopathology, and nodal status in human breast cancer. Cancer 54: 1586-1590
61. Nealon TF, Nkongho A, Grossi CE, Ward R, Nealon C, Gillooley JF (1981) Treatment of early cancer of the breast (TINOMO) on the basis of histopathologic characteristics. Surgery 89: 279-289
62. Nime FA, Rosen PP, Thaler HT, Ashikar R, Urban JA (1977) Prognostic significance of tumor emboli in intramammary lymphatics in patients with mammary carcinoma. Am J Surg Pathol 1: 25-30
63. Noshimura R, Misuni A, Kimura A, Tokunaga T, Akagi M (1982) Relationship between the content of estrogen and progesterone receptors and the pathological characteristics in human breast cancer. Jpn J Surg 12: 191-197
64. Olszewski W, Darzynkiewicz, Rosen PP, Claps ML, Melamed MR (1982) Flow cytometry of breast carcinoma. III. Possible altered kinetics in axillary lymph node metastases. Anal Quant Cytol 4: 275-278
65. Olszewski W, Drykniewicz Z, Rosen PP, Schwartz MK, Melamed MR (1981) Flow cytometry of breast carcinoma: II. Relation of tumor cell cycle distribution to histology and estrogen receptor. Cancer 48: 985-988
66. Osborne CK, Fisher ER, Redmond C, Knight WA, Yochmowitz MG, McGuire WL (1981) Estrogen receptor, a marker for human breast cancer differentiation and patient prognosis. In: Leavitt WW (ed) Hormones and cancer. Adv Exp Med Biol 138: 377-385
67. Peetz ME, Nunley DL, Moseley HS, Keenan EJ, Davenport CE, Fletcher WS (1982) Multiple simultaneous and sequential estrogen receptor values in patients with breast cancer. Am J Surg 143: 591-594
68. Prey MU, Meyer JS, Stone KR, McDivitt RW (1985) Heterogeneity of breast carcinomas determined by flow cytometric analysis. J Surg Oncol 29: 35-39
69. Rosen PP, Menendez-Botet CJ, Urban JA, Fracchia A, Schwartz MK (1977) Estrogen receptor protein (ERP) in multiple tumor specimens from individual patients with breast cancers. Cancer 39: 2194-2200
70. Roses DF, Bell DA, Flotte TJ, Taylor R, Ratech H, Dubin H (1982) Pathologic predictors of recurrence in stage I (TINOMO) breast cancer. Am J Clin Pathol 78: 817-820
71. Sarrif AM, Durant JR (1981) Evidence that estrogen-receptor negative, progesterone-receptor positive breast and ovarian carcinomas contain estrogen receptor. Cancer 48: 1215-1220
72. Silvestrini R (1984) The cell kinetics of breast cancer. In: Bonadonna G (ed) Breast cancer: diagnosis and management. Wiley, London, pp 5-13
73. Stoll BA (1977) "False-positive" oestrogen receptor assay in breast cancer Lancet 977-978
74. Thorud E, Fossa DS, Vaage S, Kaalhus O, Knudsen OS, Bormer O, Shoaid MC (1986) Primary breast cancer. Flow cytometric DNA pattern in relation to clinical and histopathological characteristics. Cancer 57: 808-811
75. Tubiana M, Pejovic MH, Chavaudra N, Contesso G, Malaise EP (1984) The long-term significance of the thymidine labeling index in breast cancer. Int J Cancer 33: 441-445
76. Tulasan AH, Hamann M, Prestele H, Ramming I, Maillot K, Egger H (1982) Correlations of the receptor content and ultrastructure of breast cancer cells. Arch Gynecol 231: 177-184
77. Webster DJ, Bronn DG, Minton JP (1978) Estrogen receptor levels in multiple biopsies from patients with breast cancer. Am J Surg 136: 337-338
78. Weigand RA, Isenberg WM, Russo J, Brenna MJ, Rich MA (1982) Blood vessel invasion and axillary lymph node involvement as prognostic indicators for breast cancer. Cancer 50: 962-969

Mammography

The Role of Mammographic Screening in the Control of Breast Cancer: An Overview

L. Tabár

Mammography Department, Central Hospital, 79 182 Falun, Sweden

Introduction

Breast cancer is not only the common malignancy of women, accounting for 24%–25% of all female malignancies, but its incidence is rising. As we have no clear understanding of the aetiology of breast cancer, *primary prevention* is not possible. To date, there is no method that effectively defines those women who will develop breast cancer. Roberts et al. reported "When all risk factors were combined, 48% of all women fell into a 'high risk' category, but only 55% of the cancers were in this group. We conclude, that selective screening of high risk groups is not a viable alternative to population screening" [9].

Efforts to control breast cancer have been primarily directed at improving *therapy*. Recent review articles have emphasized the importance of prevention rather than treatment, stating "... some 35 years of intense effort focused largely on improving treatment must be judged as a qualified failure. Results have not been what they were intended and expected to be" [2]. "A shift in research emphasis, from research on treatment to research on prevention, seems necessary if substantial progress against cancer is to be forthcoming," and "there are many grounds for believing that when any major disease is tackled on a national scale, the chief effort should be to prevent its occurrence. To put most of the effort into treatment is to deny all precedent" [3].

Since we cannot prevent the occurrence of breast cancer, the only hope that mortality from breast cancer can be reduced is to diagnose and treat this disease at a stage when the balance between the tumor and the host is more favourable; removal of the cancer while it is still in its early stages is the most promising way to achieve a significant change in the current breast cancer situation (secondary prevention).

The only diagnostic method which has the ability to detect breast cancer at an early stage with high sensitivity is superb quality mammography interpreted by a well-trained radiologist. The cases presented in Figs. 1 and 2 demonstrate the mammographic appearance of an invasive ductal carcinoma of less than 1.0 cm (Fig. 1) and a ductal carcinoma in situ with minimal invasion (Fig. 2).

The evidence that regular mammographic examination of asymptomatic women can bring about a significant decrease in breast cancer mortality can be considered as one of the important achievements in modern medicine, since there are only a few forms of established breast cancer which can be effectively controlled.

Ragaz/Ariel (Eds.), High-Risk Breast Cancer

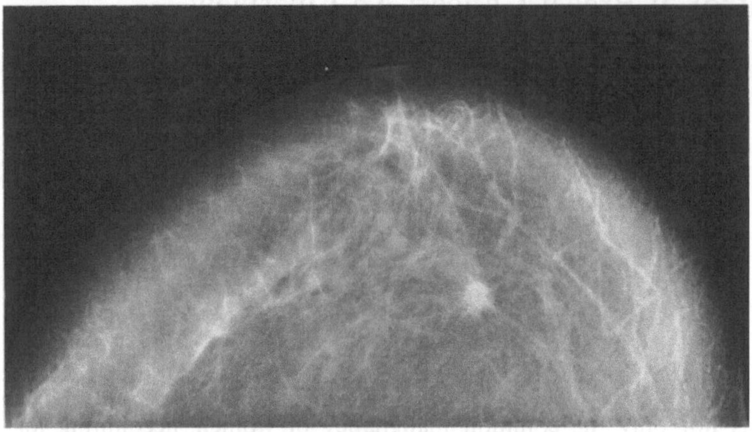

Fig. 1. Mammography of the right breast, craniocaudal projection, 4 cm from the nipple, in the medial half of the breast, there is a 9 × 9 mm solitary, stellate lesion, mammographically characteristic of a malignant tumor. Histology: invasive ductal carcinoma, 10 mm diameter

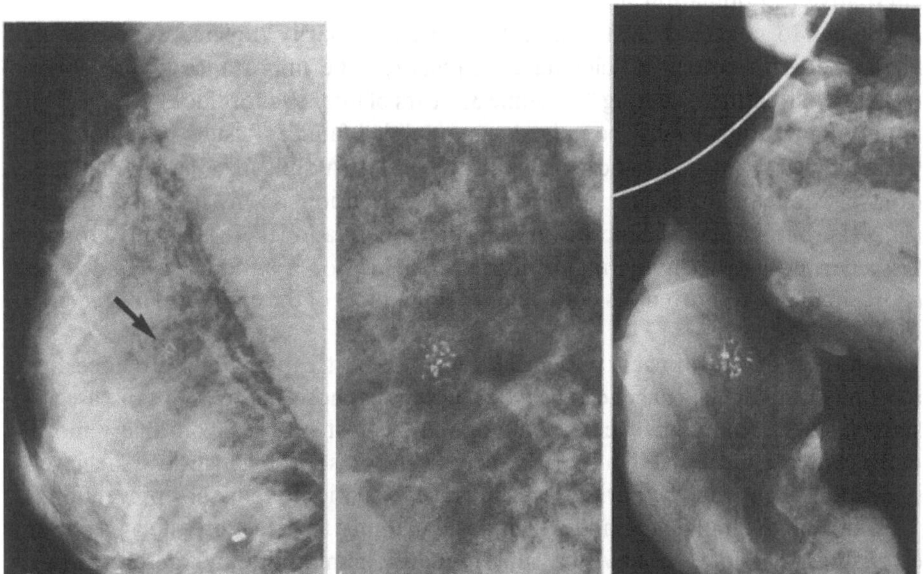

Fig. 2. a Right breast, detail of the mediolateral oblique projection; 4 cm from the nipple, in the upper half of the breast, there is a small cluster of calcifications. **b** Microfocus magnification of the calcification group seen in **2a**. Mammographically malignant-type calcifications. **c** Operative specimen radiograph. Histology: comedocarcinoma with minimal invasion

The large-scale, randomized, controlled trials carried out in the United States [10] and Sweden [12], and also the nonrandomized studies in Holland [4, 13] and Italy [8] provided evidence that the course of breast cancer could be altered by diagnosing and treating it at an earlier stage.

The Health Insurance Plan of Greater New York (HIP) Study

This prospective, randomized, controlled trial was an outstanding contribution to the efforts to control cancer. The study was scientifically designed to determine the impact of combined physical examination and mammography on mortality from breast cancer and was carried out during the years 1963-69. The study group consisted of 31 000 women aged 40-64 at randomization. Participating women were invited to attend screening with mammography and physical examination of the breast. A total of 20 166 (66.7%) participated in the first round of screening; the women were asked to attend three additional annual follow-ups. In all, 11 971 (39.6%) attended all four screenings. The control group of 31 000 individually randomized, age-matched women was not offered the screening examination. The possible biases of early detection (lead-time bias, length-biased sampling, selection bias, etc.) could not render the screening results invalid since the study was randomized and controlled and the end point was mortality from breast cancer. The significantly reduced mortality from breast cancer in the study group as compared with the control group, reported by S. Shapiro, P. Strax and L. Venet, [12] in 1971 has been maintained through 18 years of follow-up [11]. The recent update also confirmed mortality reduction for screened women aged 40-49. The HIP study has clearly answered the question it set out to investigate. It demonstrated that the natural history of breast cancer could be altered through early detection and therefore interest in breast cancer screening has been greatly stimulated.

The Swedish Kopparberg (W)-Östergötland (E) Trial (W-E Study)

The results of the HIP study awoke considerable interest in Sweden and this was soon followed by a request for mass screening with mammography. Additionally, a successful pilot study in Sandviken, Sweden showed the advantages of a simple and effective screening procedure [7]. The National Board of Health and Welfare of Sweden considered the initiation of an additional trial to be important, since there remained many unanswered questions. In fact, new studies were needed to determine the reproducibility of the results in different settings, the relative contributions of physical examination and mammography, the cost:benefit and risk:benefit ratios with modern, screen-film mammography. Additionally, the potential effect of screening on mortality from breast cancer varies considerably in different countries since there are great differences in the annual age-adjusted breast cancer mortality rates among different countries.

For these reasons a population-based, randomized, controlled trial was started in two Swedish counties; in Kopparberg (W), 1977, and in Östergötland (E), 1978, to investigate the impact of single-view mammographic screening upon mortality from breast cancer. A total of 134 867 women, 40-74 years old at randomization were enrolled into the study and were divided at random into two groups. The design and methodology of the trial have been described elsewhere [13]. The similarities and differences between the HIP study and the Swedish W-E trial are summarized in Table 1.

By the end of 1984 there was a highly significant reduction (25%) in the absolute rate of stage II or more advanced cancers ($P<0.001$). By the end of 1984 there was a 31% reduction in breast cancer mortality in the study group (invited to screening) as opposed to the control group ($P<0.013$, two-sided test). This was accompanied by a highly significant reduction ($P<0.001$) in the rate of stage II and more advanced breast cancers (25%). Both these differences began to emerge some 4 years after the randomization and have subsequently increased in magnitude. To date, the W-E study is the only randomized controlled trial using mammography as the sole screening modality that has demonstrated a significant decrease in mortality from breast cancer [13].

Detailed examination of the study revealed the following interesting observations: one-third of the breast cancer deaths in the study group occurred among those women who did not attend screening; the risk of dying from breast cancer was 2.4- to 2.9-fold higher among the nonattenders than in the control group. The decrease in breast cancer mortality was more than 60% among women who were screened as compared with those never screened. Evaluation of the data from Kopparberg county showed that the interval cancer group had the same case fatality rate as the control group. These data confirmed and extended the findings from the HIP study and the data contradict the hypothesis that the prognosis is worse in interval cancer than in breast cancer diagnosed in clinically referred patient material. Therefore, our observations do not support the suggestion of aggressive management of interval cancer [5]. The mortality from all causes other than breast cancer is the same (relative risk = 1.00) in both the study and the control group, for both counties combined.

Nonrandomized Studies with Published Data

To date, three such studies have been reported. Two from the Netherlands and one from Italy. All of them used the matched case-control method to determine the relative risk of dying from breast cancer among women who were screened compared with women who were never screened. The relative risk was calculated to be 0.30 (95% confidence interval 0.13, 0.70) in the Utrecht study and 0.48 (95% confidence interval 0.23, 1.00) in the Nijmegen study, both from the Netherlands. The relative risk of dying from breast cancer in the study period for "screened versus never screened women" was 0.53 (95% confidence interval 0.29, 0.95) in Florence, Italy [4, 14, 8].

Table 1. Similarities and differences between the HIP study and the Swedish W-E trial

	HIP study	Swedish W-E study
Study size	Study group: 31 000 Control group: 31 000	Study group: 78 085 Control group: 56 782
Basis for randomization	Individual basis	Small administrative units
Age limits (years)	40-64	40-74
Length of interval between two consecutive examinations	1 year	Age 40-49 at randomization: 24 months Age 50-74 at randomization: 33 months
Examination method	Physical examination and complete mammography	No physical examination Single-view (mediolateral oblique) mammography
Attendance rate at 1st screening	66.7%	89.2%
Attendance rate at 2nd, 3rd, etc. screenings	Attendance at all 4 screenings: 39.6%	2nd screening: 83.3% 3rd screening: 84.0%

Ongoing Trials

There are randomized, controlled breast cancer screening studies under way in Sweden, the United Kingdom and Canada, that have not yet reported mortality data. Their results will contribute to the reproducibility question; the design is somewhat different in all these studies and there are substantial differences among health care systems and cultures which combine to influence the mortality from breast cancer.

Evaluation of the Available Data

The results of the two randomized, controlled trials, the HIP study and the W-E trial, provided evidence that early detection of breast cancer alters the natural history of the disease. The W-E study in Sweden also demonstrated that breast cancer mortality could be reduced by using mammography as the only screening method. The results of the three nonrandomized, controlled trials provide further evidence that the course of breast cancer could be altered by early detection and treatment.

After the results of these studies were published, great interest in mammographic screening was generated in several countries. The immediate practical questions were the age limits (who should be screened) and the length of interval between two consecutive screening examinations (how often should women be screened). The HIP and the W-E studies have demonstrated that screening is effective in women aged 40-64 (HIP) and 40-74 (W-E). Neither of these studies was designed to evaluate any particular age subgroups. The HIP study was designed to determine the efficacy of screening women aged 40-64 years at entry and the decision on sample size was based on this objective. Accordingly, age-specific comparisons are subject to large sampling error and the study samples have little power to detect even sizable differences [11].

Consequently, any conclusions about the effect of screening on age subgroups are unjustified. If there is a need to find out whether screening is effective in a particular age subgroup, then a study has to be designed and carried out specifically to answer this question.

It has only recently become clear how the patient's age at the time of diagnosis influences mortality from breast cancer [1, 6]. Prognosis of breast cancer is best when the diagnosis is made on women in their 40s; it is significantly worse when the diagnosis is made in the 50-59 age group and progressively deteriorates with advancing age. These results may help to explain the age-specific effect of screening on mortality observed in both the HIP and the W-E studies. Because it takes breast cancer a longer time to kill women in the 40-49 age group, the difference in mortality will not be discernible at 5 or 6 years of follow-up. On the contrary, the poor survival rates in women over 50 accelerate the emergence of the mortality difference between the study and control groups.

A thorough review of the available data and a better understanding of the disease indicate that the long-term benefit of screening is evident in all age subgroups. Therefore, there is no justification for eliminating any age subgroup from screening.

The long interscreening interval in the W-E study made it possible to examine how long it would take for the breast cancer incidence in the screened population to return to the expected incidence, seen in the population of women without screening. When analysing the proportional interval cancer rate and the rate of advanced cancers at the time of second, third and subsequent screenings, we can estimate the "optimum interval time" between two consecutive screenings. As the interval cancer rate returns to the rate in the control group more rapidly in women under 50 than in women over 50, the recommended length of interval for screening women aged 40-50 should be shorter (12-18 months) than for women over 50 (should not exceed 2 years).

Principal Requirements in Screen-Film Mammography

When mammography is properly performed and interpreted screening has a high sensitivity and specificity. Poor mammographic technique and/or inadequate interpretation will result in low sensitivity and specificity. This will cause the greatest harm to screening results, lowering the cost effectiveness and raising the risk: benefit ratio. Not only will many cancers be missed, but there will also be a large number of false-positive cases, with the resulting unnecessary recalls and biopsies. In the first round of screening of the W-E study the cancer per biopsy ratio was one to two and from the second round of screening the ratio has increased to three cancers in every four biopsies.

Screen-film mammography involves a chain of events. The final product, the mammogram, cannot be better than the weakest link in the chain. These links are the following:

1. The dedicated mammography unit, specially designed and constructed for mammography. There are a number of dedicated mammography machines, which provide the potential of producing a state-of-the-art mammogram.
2. The use of mammographic screen-film combinations leads to a dramatic reduction in radiation dose and a considerable improvement in diagnostic image quality.
3. The dedicated film processor. Being a soft tissue examination method, mammography is most sensitive to variations in exposure and processing. In order to differentiate the subtle soft tissue density differences on the mammogram, a high contrast image is needed. Mammographic films need more aggressive processing than most other radiologic films. Film processing is generally the weakest and most troublesome link in the chain of the mammographic system.
4. The specially trained X-ray technician. Positioning of the patient so that as much of the breast as possible appears on the film, and so that the breast is compressed to as thin a layer as possible without pain, is no easy task to perform.
5. The chain is forged and maintained by the radiologist who has a special interest and training in mammography. It is the responsibility of the radiologist: (a) to select the proper equipment and screen-film combination; (b) to ensure that the correctly exposed film is also properly processed; (c) to arrange special training in mammography for the technician; and (d) to obtain the necessary education and training and to keep it up to date.

Conclusion

Mammography is a noninvasive examination which is relatively easy to perform. It is simple, acceptable to the patient, has a high sensitivity and specificity, is reproducible, cost effective and has a very low risk : benefit ratio. The radiation risk is only hypothetical, while the benefit is well established. There are few, if any, diagnostic methods which have been evaluated by the strict criteria that mammography as a screening method has already undergone.

We are now faced with the challenge of applying this method on a wide scale, as one of the most successful interventions in controlling breast cancer. But the personnel responsible for undertaking the examination have to be adequately trained. Women should understand the benefits they can gain from regular mammographic screening and examination, so that they will be sufficiently motivated to attend. Women should be informed about these considerable achievements of modern medicine; they should also be aware that the smaller cancers detected at mammographic examination can often be removed by breast-conserving surgery or treated by less radical methods.

References

1. Adami HO, Malker B, Holmberg L, Persson I, Stone B (1986) The relation between survival and age at diagnosis in breast cancer. N Engl J Med 315: 559-563
2. Bailar JC III, Smith EM (1986) Progress against cancer? N Engl J Med 314: 1226-1232
3. Cairns J (1985) The treatment of diseases and the war against cancer. Sci Am 253: 31-39
4. Colette HJA, Day NE, Rombach JJ, De Waard F (1984) Evaluation of screening for breast cancer in a non-randomized study (The DOM-project) by means of a case control study. Lancet i: 1224-1226
5. Holmberg LH, Tabár L, Adami HO, Bergström R (1986) Survival in breast cancer diagnosed between mammographic screening examinations. Lancet ii: 27-30
6. Host H, Lund E (1986) Age as a prognostic factor in breast cancer. Cancer 57: 2217-2221
7. Lundgren B, Jacobsson S (1976) Single view mammography. A simple and efficient approach to breast cancer screening. Cancer 38: 1124-1129
8. Palli D, Del Turco MR, Bulatti E, Carli S, Ciatto S, Toscani L, Maltoni G (1986) A case-control study of the efficacy of a non-radomized breast cancer screening program in Florence (Italy). Int J Cancer 38: 501-504
9. Roberts MM, Alexander FE, Huggins A, Muir BB (1987) Risk factors and their relevance to screening for breast cancer. 4th EORTC breast cancer working conference, London. June 30-July 3 (abstract)
10. Shapiro S, Venet W, Strax P, Venet L, Roeser R (1985) Selection, follow-up and analysis in the Health Insurance Plan-study: a randomized trial with breast cancer screening. NCI Monogr 67: 65-74
11. Shapiro S (1986) Final results of the breast cancer screening randomized trial: the Health Insurance Plan (HIP) of Greater New York study. Manuscript presented at the UICC Workshop on Screening for Breast Cancer. Helsinki April 5-7
12. Shapiro S, Strax P, Veneti L (1971) Periodic breast cancer screening in reducing mortality from breast cancer. JAMA 215: 1777-1785

13. Tabár L, Fagerberg CJG, Gad A (1985) Reduction in mortality from breast cancer after mass screening with mammography: randomized trial from the Breast Screening Group of the Swedish National Board of Health and Welfare. Lancet i: 829-832
14. Verbeek ALM, Hendriks JHCL, Holland R (1984) Reduction of breast cancer through mass screening with modern mammography: first results of the Nijmegen project, 1975-81. Lancet i: 1222-1224

The Role of Screening Mammography in Determining Risk in Breast Lesions

A.B. Miller

National Breast Screening Study, Department of Preventive Medicine and Biostatistics, University of Toronto, Toronto, Canada

Introduction

Screening is generally defined as "the presumptive identification of unrecognized disease or defect by the application of tests, examinations or other procedures that can be applied rapidly." A screening test is not intended to be diagnostic, rather a positive finding will need to be confirmed by special diagnostic procedures [26].

In the context of screening for breast cancer, mammography is usually and correctly described as the most sensitive screening test. However, in practice, the main objective of screening involves the detection of an abnormality and separating those in a population who have the abnormality from those who do not. Our approach should preferably be to apply the appropriate screening test and manage those with a detected abnormality in such a way that the probability of death from breast cancer is substantially reduced. We will not do this simply by detecting breast cancers, but by identifying the women who are destined to develop breast cancer and whose breast cancers would cause death if these cancers were not found as a result of screening. In the context of this volume, high risk breast cancer is regarded as breast cancer with a high probability of resulting in death. Most, but not all, breast cancers if untreated will result in death, but with many breast cancers, modern treatment will prevent or postpone death from the disease. The hope with screening is that an appreciable additional proportion of breast cancers will be detected at such a stage in their natural history that death which would have otherwise occurred in the absence of screening will be prevented.

In practice, therefore, screening is likely to be beneficial for only a relatively small proportion of any population. Those women who are destined never to develop breast cancer will not benefit, unless reassurance that at the time of screening they do not have detectable breast cancer is regarded as some form of benefit. Women in this group who will be disadvantaged as a result of screening are those in whom an abnormality is detected which is subsequently shown not to be due to breast cancer, but for whom a biopsy is performed.

For those women destined to develop breast cancer, only one group will benefit; those in whom breast cancer is found at an early stage in the natural history of the disease who would otherwise have died in the absence of early detection. Those who would never have died, even if not detected until the normal stage in the natural history, those whose breast cancers will inevitably result in death in spite of early

Ragaz/Ariel (Eds.), High-Risk Breast Cancer

detection, and those who are found to have breast cancer, but in whom, in practice, breast cancer would have never presented because it was growing so slowly that it would not be detected before the woman died of a competing cause, will also achieve no benefit. Indeed, there is a subsegment among these groups who may suffer a disadvantage, namely those whose cancers are initially missed by screening who are falsely reassured that they do not have cancer, but who are subsequently found to have it, possibly at a later stage in the natural history than if they had never been screened.

In this chapter I shall concentrate on the role of screening mammography in relation to those cancers destined to cause death, but where death will be prevented by earlier treatment following mammographic detection. Inevitably, it will be necessary where data are available to compare the role of mammography with other screening modalities, particularly physical examination of the breast. I shall draw on published experience where available and also the experience in the ongoing National Breast Screening Study in Canada [14]. Before directly addressing these issues, however, it is necessary to discuss some of the methodological problems which confound interpretation of some of the data available in the literature.

Biases Associated with Screening

There are four basic screening biases that I shall discuss in relation to mammography; (a) lead time; (b) length bias; (c) overdiagnosis bias; and (d) selection bias [12]. In practice, these biases operate only in relation to use of survival as a measure of effect. Survival is defined as the probability that the person will remain alive after a defined interval in relation to the total group being considered with a disease. This is the inverse of case fatality. The preferred measure to evaluate the effect of screening is mortality [17]. Mortality is defined as the proportion of a defined population who die of the disease in question in a defined time period. These two terms are often considered interchangeable, but they clearly are not. The probability of detection of a disease is influenced by screening. Hence, if you take as your denominator for assessing the proportion who remain alive or die of the disease those detected, inevitably there are going to be differences associated with the action of screening if survival or case fatality is used as the measure. If, however, you use mortality as your measure, then whether or not disease is detected in the population is irrelevant in terms of the outcome, as basically you are looking at the numbers of deaths from the disease of interest, in this case breast cancer, in relation to the total population who have the opportunity to be screened. It is, however, of importance to discuss these biases related to survival as many have become confused by the arguments surrounding them, especially in relation to mammography.

Lead time is defined as the interval between the time of detection by screening and the time at which the disease would have been diagnosed in the absence of screening. In other words, if the period by which screening advances diagnosis is pushed back 1 year, then inevitably persons diagnosed by mammography will survive 1 year longer, even if there is no long-term benefit. The amount of lead time gained as a result of the use of mammography is difficult to assess in a population in which more than one screening modality is used, but in studies in which only mammography has been used the lead time for mammography itself can be determined. In most studies such calculations suggest that on average lesions diagnosed by mammography are found between 1 and 3 years earlier than they normally would be [9]. In general, the impression is that the lesions diagnosed by mammography alone, as distinct from those that would have been diagnosed if, for example, physical examination had been used, have a longer lead time. Thus, survival is better, but this does not necessarily demonstrate that the eventual outcome will be better.

Length bias relates to the fact that screening tests tend to identify selectively the slowly developing abnormalities in the population and miss the rapidly progressive abnormalities that are more likely to present with symptoms before the initiation of the program or between screening examinations. This bias has perhaps been particularly associated with mammographic screening. It is indeed common experience that the lesions identified by mammographic screening are smaller, and are less likely to have involved nodes. Often in retrospect, if a series of films are available, lesions might have been detected one or two examinations prior to the point of actual diagnosis, or perhaps even earlier. This has raised the question in many people's minds as to whether mammography does indeed identify the high risk lesions. I shall return to this issue later in this chapter.

An extreme example of length bias is what is called overdiagnosis bias. This simply relates to the possibility that screening may bring to light lesions which would never have presented in the woman's lifetime in the absence of screening. We are basically referring here either to extremely slowly progressive lesions or to lesions which in the absence of screening might have eventually regressed. The idea that cancer might regress in an individual may be surprising, but there are indications, especially from studies which have evaluated screening for cancer of the cervix [4], and also screening for lung cancer [10] that overdiagnosis, at least within the first 8-9 years of a screening program, can be a major feature.

The fourth bias is selection bias. This is primarily related to the type of person who enters a screening program and is not directly related to mammography. People volunteer for screening and they may have characteristics that differ from the general population. One characteristic which has to be remembered, even for breast cancer, is that although women may volunteer because they have risk factors for breast cancer they tend to be more health conscious. Such women might have done very much better than the general population in the absence of screening. Selection bias may not only be influenced by the woman, but by her physician who may play a part in the decision whether a woman receives mammography.

Research on Screening

Because of the screening biases just discussed, assessment of the results of screening by mammography or any other modality cannot be made by assessment of survival.

To assess mortality usually requires a specially designed investigation. This is not the place to discuss the design of such studies in detail except to note that the best method that we have available currently for assessing the results of any approach to screening is the randomized controlled trial, similar to the use of the randomized trial as a means of assessing new therapy [17]. A randomized trial to assess screening can either be based on women who present for screening who are then randomized to be screened or not – this is basically the design used in the National Breast Screening Study in Canada [14]; or randomization is performed to invite women to attend for screening or not. The latter was the design used in the pioneering HIP study [20], and in the Swedish W-E randomized trial discussed by Tabar in this volume. Randomization may be either individually based, as in the HIP study and the National Breast Screening Study in Canada, or may be based on the randomization of clusters as in Sweden.

An alternative to the randomized trial which can be used in the evaluation of programs started without randomization as part of their design is to perform a case-control assessment. In this approach, deaths from breast cancer that occur in the community are identified, together with corresponding controls in the same community who have not died; their use of the screening procedure, for example, mammography, are compared [19]. If the cases and controls were comparable in all other respects, finding a lower frequency of screening in those who died compared with the controls would be evidence in favor of a benefit from screening. The difficulty with this approach is the complexity of separating out the various biases associated with selection, including the possibility of greater risk of the disease and greater health consciousness in those who select screening. It is, therefore, a less satisfactory approach than the randomized trial approach which is simply uninfluenced by most of these biases.

An even less satisfactory approach is to evaluate trends in mortality from breast cancer in areas where screening has been performed compared with nonscreened areas. This is the approach, for example, being used in the trial in the United Kingdom [24]. The difficulty here is that other influences could affect the outcome while very large groups would have to be studied in order to obtain the same power as from a randomized trial.

In considering all these approaches, it will be apparent that death is our end point, case detection is simply inappropriate because of the screening biases discussed. However, an intermediate step which has so far really only been used in the Swedish study is to assess the prevalence of advanced disease over the period in which screening operates in the screened community compared with the non-screened [23]. In the Swedish trial this approach showed that after an initial increase in the amount of advanced disease in the screened group compared with the control, there was a crossover with the amount of advanced disease accumulating less rapidly in the screened group than in the control. This, in fact, proved to be a predictor of the eventual mortality reduction in the screened group. This approach has not yet been used in other studies though it is being evaluated as a possible indication of future benefit in the National Breast Screening Study.

Results of Screening with Mammography: Review

There are basically four questions to address. The first one is, does the use of mammography result in a reduction in mortality from breast cancer? As will be seen, the answer to this is an unequivocal yes. The second one, and particularly critical is, whether mammography is better than other approaches to breast cancer screening in reducing deaths from breast cancer. The answer to this question is currently unknown though it is being evaluated in the National Breast Screening Study in Canada, and there are signs that the contribution of mammography could be less than many imagined. The third one is, does the use of mammography result also in the detection of advanced breast cancer as distinct from early breast cancer? The answer to this question is yes. The fourth one is, does the use of mammography result in a reduction of advanced breast cancer because the lesions which would have developed into advanced breast cancer (and thus considered high risk) are found earlier, thus preventing the development of advanced disease? The answer, at least from the Swedish study [23], also seems to be yes. Superimposed on these questions are queries whether mammography should be used for every age group and how often it should be used for screening. These are largely operational questions and I will address them in the final section of this chapter. I shall draw largely on the experience in the HIP study of Greater New York, the European studies, especially the Swedish study, and our own National Breast Screening Study in Canada.

HIP Study

In the 18-year results of the HIP study now available it is clear that screening by a combination of mammography plus physical examination reduces mortality from breast cancer. The reduction appears to occur in every age group included in the study, though with a delay in the reduction in mortality in women under the age of 50 of 5-8 years after screening compared with the appearance of a benefit in older women about 3 years after screening was started [22].

The difficulty with the HIP study is that it used the combination of mammography and physical examination, the mammography being relatively less efficient in detecting breast cancer than it has become subsequently. There are several indications from the study, however, that the physical examination at least contributed to the mortality reduction seen, particularly in women under the age of 50. The first is the proportion of lesions found on screening by the two modalities (Table 1). This table, based as it must be on case detection, emphasizes the important contribution of physical examination to the yield from screening. It has been calculated that this contribution might amount to as much as 70% of the mortality reduction [2, 5].

Two other observations support an inference that the reduction in mortality was due to the earlier detection of advanced disease with a major contribution from the physical examination component of the screen. The first was the early benefit seen in women over the age of 50 first detected at 3 years, a benefit that became

Table 1. Breast cancer cases histologically confirmed by modality of detection on screening, HIP study. (Source: Shapiro et al. [22])

Age at entry (years)	Total	Percentage detected by: Mammography alone	Clinical alone	Mammography and clinical
40-49	40	25	58	18
50-59	67	39	40	21
60-64	25	32	36	32
All ages	132	33	45	22

maximal 7 years after the initiation of screening [21]. This early impact of screening must mean that relatively rapidly progressive disease was affected by the screening process. Walter and Day [28], modeled the lead time distribution and found the best fit with an exponential distribution. This gave an estimate of a mean lead time of 1.7 years (20 months), corresponding to approximately 44% of cases with a duration of less than 1 year and 5% with a duration of more than 5 years. It seems unlikely that the cases with a longer than average lead time, many of which were probably identified by mammography, could have contributed to an early mortality reduction. The implication is that screening for breast cancer reduces the risk of death in patients whose disease is detected somewhat late in its natural history. The second observation which tends to confirm this is that the survival of patients with stage II disease was better in the study group than for stage II patients in the control group [21]. Although some of this survival advantage might have been due to lead time it is striking that the survival advantage seems greater for stage II than for stage I disease, whereas lead time would have been expected to have most impact on stage I disease. This seems to suggest once again that there was a real benefit from the earlier detection of advanced disease, even in those patients with large tumors and involved nodes.

Swedish and Canadian Studies

The fact that screening incorporating modern mammography will advance the point of diagnosis of patients with advanced disease was confirmed by the initial results from Sweden [23]. In the Swedish study, after the first screening rounds, more women were found to have advanced breast cancer in the study group than in the control group. That mammography, even when used in combination with physical examination, contributes to this process, has been confirmed by the results of the initial screening in the National Breast Screening Study in Canada. Table 2 illustrates this. Two things are obvious. First, more cancers are found when mammography is used, but second, in absolute number terms, more are found with involved nodes, especially in women aged 40-49. This therefore raises the possibility

Table 2. Preliminary findings for nodal involvement in breast cancers detected at the first screen in the National Breast Screening Study

Age (years)	Allocation	Number of nodes involved				Total
		0	1-3	⩾4	NA	
40-49	MX+PX	69	16	24	12	121
	PX alone	50	21	7	15	93
50-59	MX+PX	97	26	10	30	163
	PX alone	48	16	15	7	86

NA, not available; MX, mammography; PX, physical examination.

that mammography will contribute to a mortality reduction, not just by finding disease at an earlier stage before nodes are involved, but by finding the advanced disease at an earlier stage in its natural history. It is indeed possible that the tumor burden in such women will be lower than if this disease had been allowed to progress and present in the normal way. In an era when adjuvant chemotherapy will be used for such patients if they are premenopausal, and adjuvant hormonal therapy if they are postmenopausal, it is quite possible that a combination of earlier detection by screening and earlier treatment with adjuvant therapy could eventually result in an important reduction in mortality. It is too early to tell from the National Breast Screening Study in Canada whether this expectation will be realized, though a definite answer to this question should be available within a few years.

Other Screening Data

None of the other screening studies have done more than just confirm the findings from the HIP and Swedish studies. The case-control analyses of the population programs in the Netherlands and in Italy [6, 16, 27] have demonstrated that, as for the initial results in both the Swedish and HIP studies, an early effect of screening with mammography cannot be expected in women under the age of 50, but an important reduction in mortality is detectable within 5-7 years for women over the age of 50. None of these studies, however, contribute to answering the question as to whether or not mammography is adding significantly to the benefit that could be achieved by physical examination. The National Breast Screening Study is the only study designed to answer this question, but again we will have to wait for the mortality results, the next few years being critical.

There is, however, one other aspect of the use of mammography in relation to high risk lesions for which the National Breast Screening Study is helping to provide at least a partial early answer. It is well recognized that in all screening programs cancers occur between screens. These may be a result either of the continued growth of cancers which were detectable, but not detected on the previous screen, or of cancers that were growing so rapidly that they became detectable clinically in the intervals between the screens. Evaluations of the sensitivity of mammography in the National Breast Screening Study have shown over all centers a sensitivity of first-screen mammography of 75% [3]. This assessment of sensitivity of mammography capitalized on our use of a reference radiologist who was able to make an independent assessment of the extent that cancers found at the second screen or which presented as interval cancers were, in fact, detectable at the first screen. Of the total number of 76 cancers missed on mammography, 62% were found on physical examination at the first screen, but not detected on mammography.

This rather classical approach to sensitivity does not in fact fully evaluate the question of the sensitivity of mammography in preventing interval cancers. To do so requires an approach described by Day [7], capitalizing on the fact that we have a control group in the National Breast Screening Study. Very simply, as in the National Breast Screening Study we have two groups of equal size, the sensitivity of mammography in preventing interval cancers is determined by a comparison of the number of interval cancers found in the group given mammography and the number in the group in which mammography was not allocated. There were 38 interval cancers in the mammography group compared with 52 in the control. Therefore, the sensitivity of first-screen mammography in preventing interval cancers over the next 12 months was only 27%.

This confirms that there is an element of breast cancer which is rapidly progressive, which presumably is more likely to result in death, which presents as an interval cancer between screens, and which is not found by mammography. To the extent that these high risk breast cancers dominate the subsequent occurrence of deaths from breast cancer, mammography will imperfectly prevent mortality from breast cancer.

Future Prospects for Mammography

Even though mammography is not the final answer in our attempts to find a curative approach to breast cancer, there is no question that in the short term, screening by either mammography alone or with physical examination has been demonstrated to result in a significant reduction in mortality from breast cancer in all studies in women over the age of 50. So far, such benefit has been seen only after prolonged follow-up of the HIP study in women aged 40-49. This led the UICC workshop on screening to conclude that in countries where breast cancer is common and where the necessary resources are available, screening by mammography alone or mammography plus physical examination is applicable as public health policy [8]. The UICC group, a WHO group [15], and an earlier UICC group [13], have however emphasized the critical necessity for exquisite attention to detail in performance of mammography to ensure high quality examination. Indeed, as emphasized by Tabar [23], there is a danger with mammography that attention will be paid to the wrong abnormalities, so that those lesions which really are high risk will be ignored unless appropriate attention is paid to the technical aspect of mammographic screening and the radiologist is adequately trained in the perception of abnormalities as well as in their diagnosis.

In Europe, as evidenced by the policy decisions taken in Sweden and the United Kingdom [25], screening programs are now being introduced incorporating mammography alone. In the United States, the approach so far adopted is to recommend the introduction of mammography together with annual physical examination [1, 11]. However, as the UICC group have pointed out [8], the extent to which physical examination contributes to mortality reduction when both modalities are used or whether physical examination provides additional benefit over and above mammography is still a research issue. This research issue is in fact only being indirectly addressed by the National Breast Screening Study which, in women aged 50-59, is evaluating the extent to which mammography adds to a presumed benefit from physical examination and the teaching of breast self-examination (BSE). This presumption of benefit has largely come from our assessment of the results of the HIP study. Because of our design in this age group, i.e., we have no unscreened group, we will not be able to assess directly the benefit of physical examination and BSE when used alone. We will only be able to determine whether or not a significant effect of the addition of mammography is seen in a total sample size of just under 40 000 women randomized into the two groups. However, in our view this is a practical question in the context of North America, and badly needs answering.

The implications of the introduction of breast cancer screening are many. When mammography is used not only is it necessary to have the appropriate equipment for high quality mammographic screening, well-trained technicians, and highly trained radiologists to interpret the films, it is also necessary to have the expertise available to diagnose the impalpable lesions that will be found. Rowen et al. [18] described their experience with the use of needle localization biopsy in occult breast cancers detected by mammography. Much of this experience was derived from the National Breast Screening Study and has led them to be more cautious in their use of biopsy for certain classes of abnormalities identified on mammography. The availability of more modern mammography machines that permit coned-down, compression magnification mammography, will, however, facilitate the use of diagnostic mammography in reducing unnecessary biopsies and detecting infiltrating cancers. The WHO group [15] as well as the British task force [25], emphasized the importance of having such centers available. In Europe, it would be easier to ensure that all women detected on screening are referred to such centers for diagnosis. In North America, we will have to be content with a process whereby centers with experience in screening build up their expertise and therefore attract the relevant patients by referral.

Summary

Our main objective in screening is to find patients with the high risk lesions sooner. Mammography, providing it is given with the necessary skills and diagnostic facilities available, can be a major contributor to this aim. We cannot yet be certain that mammography is essential as a component of the screening process, and therefore some will wish to delay the initiation of screening policies until this aspect has been answered by the National Breast Screening Study. Many, however, will be content to go with the evidence now available, being prepared to modify their policy in the light of the evidence as it is derived from the ongoing studies in Europe and Canada. Most, as in the United Kingdom [25] will recognize as did the UICC group [8], however, that the greatest initial benefit will be obtained by concentrating screening on women aged 50-69.

References

1. American Cancer Society (1982) Mammography 1982: a statement of the American Cancer Society. CA 32: 229-233
2. Bailar JC (1976) Mammography: a contrary view. Ann Intern Med 84: 77-84
3. Baines CJ, MacFarlane DV, Miller AB (1988) Sensitivity and specificity of first screen mammography in 15 NBSS Centres. J Can Assoc Radiol 39: 273-276
4. Boyes DA, Morrison B, Knox EG, Draper GJ, Miller AB (1982) A cohort study of cervical cancer screening in British Columbia. Clin Invest Med 5: 1-29
5. Breslow L, Thomas LB, Upton AC (1977) Final reports of the National Cancer Institute Ad Hoc Working Groups on Mammography in Screening for Breast Cancer and summary report of their joint findings and recommendations. JNCI 59: 467-541
6. Collette HJA, Day NE, Rombach JJ, de Waard F (1984) Evaluation of screening for breast cancer in a non-randomized study (the Dom project) by means of a case-control study. Lancet i: 1224-1226
7. Day NE (1985) Estimating the sensitivity of a screening test. J Epidemol Community Health 39: 364-366
8. Day NE, Baines CJ, Chamberlain J, Hakama M, Miller AB, Prorok P (1986) UICC Project on screening for Cancer: report on the workshop on screening for breast cancer. Int J Cancer 38: 303-308
9. Day NE, Walter SD, Tabar L, Fagerberg CJG, Collette HJA (1987) The sensitivity and lead time of breast cancer screening: a comparison of the results of different studies. In: Day NE, Miller AB (eds) Screening for breast cancer. Huber, Toronto, (in press)
10. Fontana RS (1985) Screening for lung cancer. In: Miller AB (ed) Screening for cancer. Academic, Orlando, pp 377–395
11. Greenwald P, Sondik EJ (eds) (1986) Cancer control objectives for the nation: 1985-2000. NCI Monogr 2
12. Miller AB (1985) Principles of screening and of the evaluation of screening programs. In: Miller AB (ed) Screening for cancer. Academic, Orlando, pp 3-24
13. Miller AB, Bulbrook RD (1982) Screening detection and diagnosis of breast cancer. Lancet i: 1109-1111
14. Miller AB, Howe GR, Wall C (1981) The national study of breast cancer screening. Clin Invest Med 4: 227-258
15. Miller AB, Tsechkovski M (1987) Imaging technologies in breast cancer control: summary of a World Health Organization meeting. Am J Roentgenol 148: 1092
16. Palli D, Del Turco MR, Buiatti E, Carli S, Ciatto S, Toscani L, Maltoni G (1986) A case-control study of the efficacy of a non-randomized breast cancer screening program in Florence (Italy). Int J Cancer 38: 501-504

17. Prorok PC, Chamberlain J, Day NE, Hakama M, Miller AB (1984) UICC workshop on the evaluation of screening programs for cancer. Int J Cancer 34: 1-4
18. Rowen JP, Bassett AA, Simor IS, Brown DS (1986) Needle-guided breast biopsy for mammographic abnormalities in 561 patients. Can J Surg 29: 287-288
19. Sasco AJ, Day NE, Walter SD (1986) Case-control studies for the evaluation of screening. J Chronic Dis 39: 399-405
20. Shapiro S, Strax P, Venet L, Venet W (1972) Changes in 5-year breast cancer mortality in a breast cancer screening program. Natl Cancer Conf Proc 7: 663-678
21. Shapiro S (1982) Ten to fourteen-year effects of breast cancer screening on mortality. JNCI 69: 349-355
22. Shapiro S, Venet W, Strax P, Venet L (1988) Current results of the breast cancer screening randomized trial: the Health Insurance Plan (HIP) of greater New York study. In: Day NE, Miller AB (eds) Screening for breast cancer. Huber, Toronto. pp 3-15.
23. Tabar L, Gad A, Holmberg L, Ljungquist U (1985) Significant reduction in advanced breast cancer. Diagn Imag Clin Med 54: 158-164
24. UK Trial of Early Detection of Breast Cancer Group (1981) Trial of early detection of breast cancer: description of method. Br J Cancer 44: 618-627
25. UK Working Party (1987) Screening for breast cancer. Lancet i: 575-576
26. US Commission on chronic illness (1957) Chronic illness in the United States, vol 1. Harvard University Press, Cambridge
27. Verbeek ALM, Hendriks JHCL, Holland R, Mravunac M, Sturmans F (1985) Mammographic screening and breast cancer mortality: age-specific effects in Nijmegen project, 1975-82. Lancet i: 865-866
28. Walter SD, Day NE (1983) Estimation of the duration of a pre-clinical disease state using screening data. Am J Epidemiol 118: 865-886

Immunology

The Role of Monoclonal and Polyclonal Antibodies in Assessing Risk in Breast Cancer

J.L. Mansi and R.C. Coombes

Ludwig Institute for Cancer Research (St. George's Group - London Branch), St. George's Hospital Medical School, Tooting, London SW17 ORE, Great Britain

Introduction

In recent years the development of monoclonal antibodies has revolutionized our understanding of the fundamental nature of human tumors. Not only have they provided the pathologist with probes to study functional and structural properties of tissue, but they have also provided the clinician with further prognostic information on which to base management decisions, and more recently have been used therapeutically as modulators for drug targeting.

Since Kohler and Milstein [52] first developed the methodology of generating monoclonal antibodies, a large number of antibodies directed toward breast tumor antigens have been produced (Table 1). However, nearly all of these antibodies are tumor associated rather than tumor specific and this, of course, limits their therapeutic potential. Nevertheless, these probes have helped in identifying important biologic and biochemical differences between normal and neoplastic tissue, and in detecting metastases at an earlier stage in their evolution, at the micrometastatic stage.

In this chapter, the clinical utilization of monoclonal antibodies will be discussed, with particular emphasis on the detection of micrometastases in bone marrow of patients with primary breast cancer, and the prognostic value of detecting these tumor cells at such an early stage.

Clinical Utilization of Monoclonal Antibodies

Detection of Premalignant Breast Disease

The differentiation of proliferative but benign disease from ductal carcinoma in situ may be difficult. However, structural changes do occur and have been recognized increasingly with antisera to myoepithelial cells (myosin) [42] basement membrane (laminin and type IV collagen) [1, 77, 40], and epithelial cells (keratin) [40]. The basement membrane is intact in benign breast disease with the myoepithelial cells surrounding the lesion; however, in carcinoma in situ the myoepithelial cells become attenuated and fewer in number while the basement membrane remains intact. In invasive carcinoma fragmentation of the basement membrane occurs and

Ragaz/Ariel (Eds.), High-Risk Breast Cancer

Table 1. Monoclonal antibodies to human breast

Immunogen	Monoclonal antibody	Antigenic determinant	Reference
Milk fat globule membrane	Anti-EMA		[81]
	E29	265-400 000 gp	[19]
	HMFG1, HMFG11	High mol. wt. gp	[2, 9]
	M3, M8, M18, M24	Unknown	[34, 62]
	67-D-11	Unknown	[72]
	MAM series	High mol. wt. gp	[42]
	111 D5	42-57 000 gp	[53]
	LICR-LON-Lc28	Unknown	[78]
	LICR-LON-TW19.5	42-82 000	[78]
	LICR-LON-H10A	53-82 000	[78]
Mammary carcinoma metastases	B72-3	220-400 000 gp	[65] [12] [76]
	B6.2	90 000 gp	[12] [76]
	B1.1	180 000 gp	[13]
	DF3	330 000 gp	[54]
	NCRC 11	>400 000 gp	[28]
	LICR-LON-19.2	Unknown	[78]
Breast carcinoma cell lines	MBr1, 2, 3	Unknown	[63]
	MCF7		[58]
	MCF7 24-17-1, 2	90,100 000 gp	[83]
	MCF7 F36/22	Unknown	[67]
	MCF7 UCD/AB6.11	54,56 000 gp	[6]
	MCF7 AB/3	Unknown	[46]
	MCF7 3B18	Unknown	[92]
	MCF7 15A8	Unknown	[92]
	MCF7 LICR-LON-39.8	Unknown	[78]
	MCF7 LICR-LON-59.2	Unknown	[78]
	BT20 10-3D2	126 000 gp	[80]
	ZR751 H59	30 000 gp	[91]
Receptors	H222	Estrogen receptor	[39] [60]
	D547Sp,	Estrogen receptor	[39]
	D75P3		[70]
	Anti-EGF	Epidermal growth factor receptor	[75]
	LR-3	Laminin receptor	[43]

Table 1 (*continued*)

Immunogen	Monoclonal antibody	Antigenic determinant	Reference
	PR	Progesterone	[4]
Intermediate filaments (keratins)	CAM 5.2	52000 50,43,39000	[57]
	AE-1, 3	40-67000	[18]
Human lymph nodes	MBE 6	Unknown	[82]
	CLWH 5	Unknown	[35]

the myoepithelial cells can no longer be demonstrated [40, 27]. Of further interest is the recent development of two monoclonal antibodies, LICR-LON-59.2 and 19.2, which react with myoepithelial and basement membranes respectively. The former also reacts with the majority of breast carcinomas and the latter reacts with tumor cell lines in culture but not carcinoma cells from breast biopsies [78]. Although epithelial-directed antibodies stain both normal breast and breast carcinoma, there are several antisera that are made against breast differentiation antigens, and these appear to react differentially to benign and malignant tissues such that the deposition of the antigen is cytoplasmic in malignant cells and more membranous or luminal in most benign cells [6]; the exact significance of this is uncertain.

Monoclonal Antisera and Tumor Differentiation

While there is preliminary evidence that monoclonal antibodies will be useful in determining the state of differentiation of a particular tumor, very little information has been obtained regarding antigen expression and its relationship to metastatic spread, and to overall prognosis.

Monoclonal antibodies reactive with breast carcinoma can be categorized broadly on the basis of the immunogen used to produce the antibody, as shown in Table 1. Most of these antibodies can also be found on other carcinoma cells, but each antibody has certain distinguishing features such as the location of the antigen within the tumor cell, the proportion of positively reacting breast tumors to nonmammary tumors, and the degree of reactivity with normal tissues.

One outstanding observation is the universal heterogeneity of expression of the antigen or epitopes being detected within a tumor to a particular antibody [79, 34, 44, 25]. This phenomenon does not appear to be cell cycle dependent [26] and as yet the degree of heterogeneity has not been shown to be of prognostic significance. The intensity of staining is not generally thought to be related to prognosis, but a study using a monoclonal antibody raised against human mammary carcinoma cells, NCRC 11, has shown an association between high staining intensity and good prognosis [29]. Attempts continue to produce monoclonal antisera that have a tissue distribution confined to breast or breast tumors, and which are expressed homogeneously [78].

The presence of estrogen receptors in human breast tissue is known to provide important information regarding the likelihood that a particular patient will respond to endocrine manipulation [55], and this in turn affects the overall survival [45, 90]. The recent development of a monoclonal antibody to estrogen receptors [39], the assay of which compares favorably with the more commonly used biochemical analysis [60], has enabled a direct comparison of various histopathologic features and the presence or absence of receptors. An extensive study by Berger et al. [3] has shown a relationship between positive receptor status and well-differentiated tumors, smaller tumor cell size, lower levels of either tumor necrosis or lymphocytic infiltration, and the presence of tubular formation. Furthermore, because only small amounts of tissue are required for the immunocytochemical analysis, receptor status can be estimated on needle aspirates from the primary tumor and from accessible metastatic disease [61], thus providing important information with minimal inconvenience to the patient. Progesterone receptors also provide prognostic information, and a monoclonal antibody for their detection is currently being evaluated in our laboratory [4].

Detection of Metastases

The detection of metastases from breast cancer, either in suspected metastatic disease, such as in the presence of effusions or ascites, in lymph nodes at the time of primary surgery, or in the attempt to identify disease recurrence when the tumor load is small, can be difficult by conventional histochemical or cytochemical stains alone.

The cytodiagnosis of malignancy in serous effusions is currently based on strict morphological criteria, and depends on being able to distinguish tumor cells from reactive mesothelial cells, and also to identify rare events or tumor cells occurring singly. Various studies have confirmed the usefulness of monoclonal antibodies, including HMFG2 [31] and more recently B 72.3 [49, 59], in improving the identification of tumor cells.

It is well established that the presence of axillary nodal involvement is the most important prognostic factor in primary operable breast cancer [32, 30], and a decision on whether or not to start a particular patient on adjuvant therapy is frequently based on this information. However, it is also known that approximately 15%-20% of patients with negative nodes relapse within 10 years [74], and that while serial sections improve the detection of micrometastases no effect on survival is seen [33, 89]. Applying immunohistochemical techniques to this situation has shown that not only is the detection rate of involved nodes increased [86], but their presence is of prognostic significance [85].

Currently, biochemical markers in serum are unhelpful in predicting recurrent disease in patients with breast cancer [8, 15, 57]. The use of monoclonal antibodies to detect tumor-associated antigens in serum may eventually be helpful in the early detection of tumor masses, monitoring for disease recurrence, or monitoring therapy. Recent studies have included the evaluation of DF3 [65], HMFG1 and 2 [24, 6], and Ca antigen [37]. However, none of these are specific or sensitive enough to be of routine use, although further analyses using cocktails of monoclonal antibodies are currently being evaluated [84].

Radioimmunolocalization

A major aim in the new approach toward the staging of newly diagnosed breast cancer has been to use radioisotopes attached to monoclonal antibodies to permit noninvasive axillary staging and tumor localization. However, there are many unanswered questions regarding the use of these conjugates in the in vivo imaging. These include the use of an immunoglobulin versus the immunoreactive fragments, dose and route of administration, specific activity of the radiolabeled monoclonal antibody, the amount of antigen present on a given tumor, the depth, site, size, and degree of vascularization of the tumor, the choice of radionuclide, the metabolism and clearance of the antibody-radionuclide complex, the appearance of human immunoglobulin-specific antibodies, and the presence of circulating tumor antigen. There has been limited success so far in breast cancer, but one study by Rainsbury et al. [71] using M8 labeled with indium, confirmed the presence of skeletal metastases in ten patients with radiologically proven bone metastases. M8 labeled with indium also localized the primary tumor, but not soft tissue metastases. Progress in radioimmunolocalization in other cancers, such as ovarian [38], and colonic [64], may provide the basis for technologic advances in breast imaging.

Detection of Micrometastases in Bone Marrow of Patients with Primary Breast Cancer[1]

Introduction

Most patients with breast cancer present with apparently local disease, as measured by conventional techniques. However, within 5 years approximately 40% of these patients will relapse and die, regardless of the initial surgical procedure, or whether or not the patient receives radiotherapy. It is therefore widely believed that breast cancer is disseminated at presentation, and that our conventional staging methods are insensitive.

The skeleton is the commonest site of distant metastases from carcinoma of the breast [48], and is frequently the first organ in which metastases are detected.

[1] These studies were examined and approved by the ethical review boards of both the Royal Marsden Hospital, Sutton and Fulham Road, and St. George's Hospital, Tooting. In addition, all patients signed a form consenting to the procedure after being informed of the purpose and risks of the study.

However, only approximately 50% of lesions demonstrated at postmortem are detected radiologically, and metastases less than 1.5 cm are frequently not seen. The bone marrow is the logical site to look for early evidence of disease, but conventional cytology can detect tumor cells in marrow of patients without overt bone metastases in only about 1%, and this is only increased to about 28% in patients with overt skeletal metastases [73]. With the advent of immunocytochemistry, the ability to detect not only small foci of cells, but also single cells has been greatly increased [21, 22], such that tumor cells were found in marrow of patients with breast cancer in the absence of metastatic disease on routine staging. Furthermore, by increasing the number of marrow sites examined a higher number of tumor cells could be detected [16].

Accordingly, the study was extended to examine multiple marrow aspirates from patients with apparently local disease taken at the time of their initial surgery. The findings were related to various known prognostic factors and the subsequent course of their disease documented. In addition, in a series of patients, multiple marrow aspirates were repeated at some time after surgery, but before overt relapse, to determine the fate of these cells and the influence that adjuvant therapy may have on their presence.

The immunocytochemical probe used in all these studies was a polyclonal antibody, anti-epithelial membrane antigen (anti-EMA) which is a rabbit antiserum raised against human milk fat globule membranes [41, 66]. EMA is widely distributed in epithelial tissues and tumors derived from them, but its expression is generally absent from normal and neoplastic hematopoietic, lymphoid, osseous, and other connective tissue. Occasionally a weak nonspecific staining of normal bone marrow cells, in particular plasma cells, has been noted [22, 23, 68], however, these cells are usually easily distinguishable morphologically from tumor cells. Anti-EMA was kindly provided by Dr. M.G. Ormerod (Institute for Cancer Research, London).

Relation of Bone Marrow Micrometastases to Other Prognostic Factors

Of the 350 patients who entered the study between July 1981 and August 1987, 89 (25.4%) were found to have tumor cells in their bone marrow (Fig. 1). A relationship was found between the presence of these cells and T stage ($P < 0.001$), pathologic size ($P < 0.001$), node-positivity ($P = 0.005$), peritumoral vascular invasion ($P < 0.001$), and estrogen receptor-positivity ($P = 0.04$), but not menopausal status (Table 2). No tumor cells were found in peripheral blood taken at the same time as the bone marrow. The actual number of tumor cells found per patient showed very little relation to any of these prognostic factors.

The association of tumor cells in bone marrow and invasion by tumor cells of lymphatics and blood vessels within the primary tumor is of particular interest. Vascular invasion is known to be an independent prognostic variable, depicting a poor outlook for patients in whom it can be demonstrated [5, 20]. Invasion into these channels may represent a means of access for the tumor cells into the circulation.

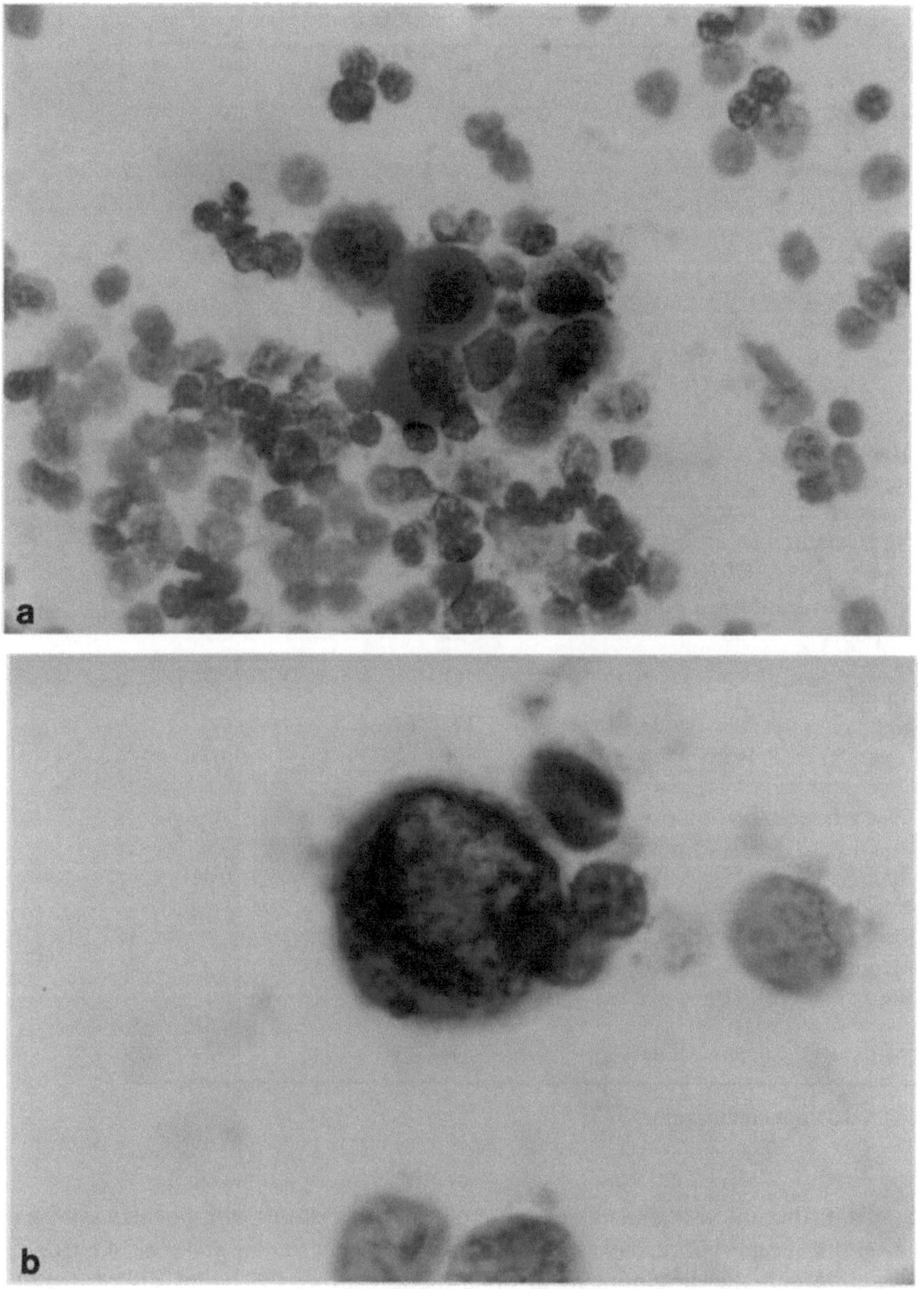

Fig. 1a, b. Anti-EMA staining of bone marrow tumor cells. The bone marrow smears have been stained by the indirect method with anti-EMA and anti-rabbit alkaline phosphatase as the secondary antibody. The reaction is visualized with the chromogen fast red, and the normal bone marrow cells are counterstained blue with hemalum. **a** Clump of anti-EMA-positive cells in bone marrow with the morphological characteristics of tumor cells, ×40. **b** Single anti-EMA-positive cell. The staining pattern is granular in appearance, a feature often seen with immunocytochemical staining, ×1760

Table 2. Relation of micrometastases to prognostic factors

	Total	Micrometastases (*n*)	(%)	No micrometastases		P^a
T stage						
T0-T2	254	48	19	206	81	<0.001
T3-T4	96	41	43	55	57	
Pathologic size (cm)						
<2	108	16	15	92	85	
2-5	204	63	31	141	69	0.01 (trend)
>5	15	4	27	11	73	
Missing values	23	6		17		
Nodal status						
−ve	170	32	19	138	81	
+ve	150	49	33	101	67	0.005
Not done	30	8		22		
Vascular invasion						
Not seen	208	33	16	175	84	
+ve	142	56	39	86	61	<0.001
Estrogen receptor						
−ve	108	36	33	72	67	
+ve	224	51	23	173	77	0.041
Not done	18	2		16		
Menopausal status						
Pre-	92	25	27	67	73	0.655
Post-	258	64	25	194	75	

[a] $P > 0.05$ not significant.

Of further interest is the association of micrometastases with positive estrogen receptors; recent reports have shown a correlation between the presence of estrogen receptors and the development of bone metastases as the initial site of distant spread [14, 90].

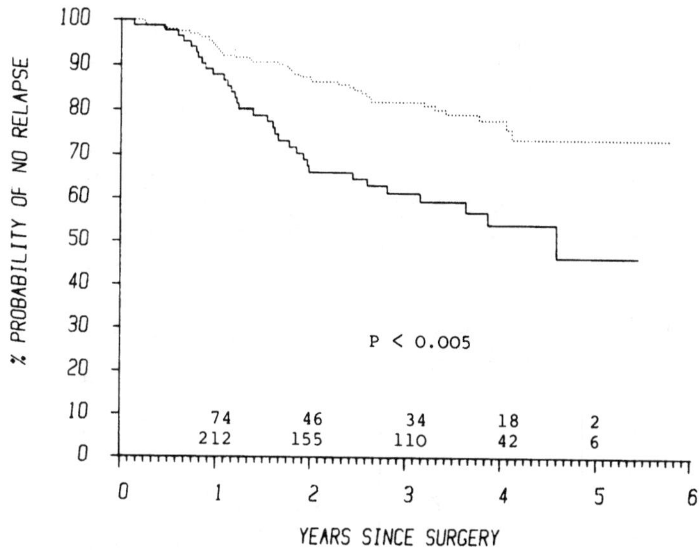

Fig. 2. Distant relapse-free interval according to the presence or absence of micrometastases at the time of initial surgery. *Full line* micrometastases-positive; *broken line* micrometastases-negative. The number of patients at risk is shown along the *x* axis

Relation of Micrometastases to Relapse and Survival

The medium duration of follow-up is 34.5 months (range 1-68 months), and there have been a total of 97 relapses. Of these relapses, 75 (77%) are at distant sites; 33 (37%) have occurred in the patients with micrometastases, and 42 (16%) in the 261 patients without. The relapse-free interval is shorter in patients with micrometastases (Fig. 2, $P < 0.005$), and this difference still exists if local as well as distant relapses are taken into account ($P < 0.005$). The number of cells stained does not appear to be useful in predicting relapse; patients with 20 or more tumor cells relapse at a similar rate to those with less than 20.

To investigate whether the presence of micrometastases is a significant predictor of relapse independent of other prognostic factors a Cox multiple regression analysis has been performed (Table 3A); pathologic size is clearly an important independent prognostic factor, but the presence of micrometastases is not.

When time to relapse in bone is considered, those patients with micrometastases relapse at a faster rate than those without (Fig. 3, $P < 0.005$). The Cox regression analysis for relapse in bone is similar for all distant relapses, but the predictive effect of micrometastases is now significant (Table 3B).

To date a total of 42 patients (12%) have died: 17/89 (19%) of the patients with micrometastases and 25/261 (10%) of the patients without micrometastases. Death was due to metastatic disease in 16 and 20 patients, respectively. This difference is significant ($P < 0.05$). However, once relapse has occurred at any distant site, the time from first relapse to death is not statistically different between the two groups.

Thus, the finding of tumor cells in bone marrow predicts a poor prognosis, and

Table 3. Cox regression analysis of time to first metastasis

Factor	Baseline	Level	Coefficient	Standard error	Hazard ratio	P
A) All distant relapses						
Pathologic size	<2 cm	2-5 cm	1.01	0.42	2.75	<0.05
	<2 cm	>5 cm	1.54	0.40	4.65	<0.01
Lymph nodes	−ve	+ve	0.79	0.29	2.21	<0.05
Vascular invasion	Absent	Present	0.39	0.28	1.48	
Micrometastases	−ve	+ve	0.43	0.27	1.55	
B) Bone relapse only						
Pathologic size	<2 cm	2-5 cm	0.83	0.69	2.30	
	<2 cm	>5 cm	1.53	0.65	4.62	<0.05
Lymph nodes	−ve	+ve	0.66	0.49	1.93	
Vascular invasion	Absent	Present	0.48	0.47	1.62	
Micrometastases	−ve	+ve	0.99	0.44	2.68	<0.05

The independent effect of each factor on relapse-free survival is assessed by modeling the effect at different levels of the factor compared with a baseline level. The coefficients obtained and the hazard ratio are given in the table. The hazard ratio estimates the ratio of the relapse rate in patients with the given level of the factor to the relapse rate in patients with the baseline level.

in particular, predicts for relapse in bone. However, failure to detect micrometastases in patients who either had a combination of poor prognostic factors or who relapsed in bone may be due to lack of sensitivity of the technique or to examination of an insufficient number of sites. To explore this further, a cytokeratin monoclonal antibody (which probably represents a more consistent tumor marker than anti-EMA [69]) has been combined with EMA in the staining protocol as a "cocktail." To date the percentage of tumor cells found has not been increased, but the initial evaluation involves only 25 patients. Increasing the number of sites

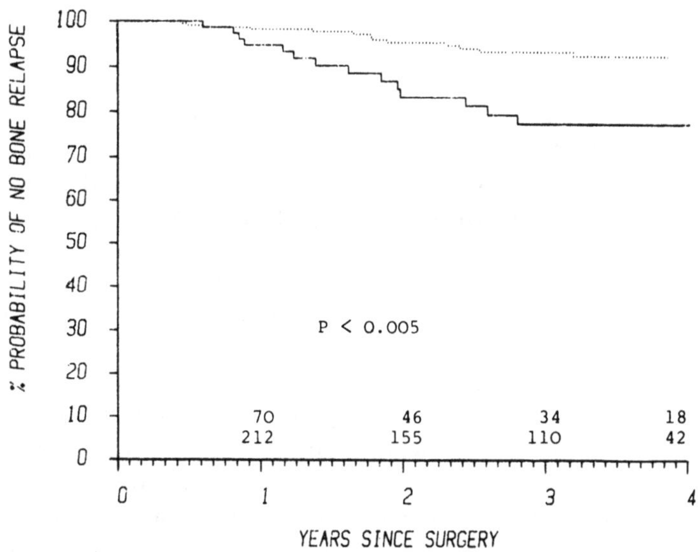

Fig. 3. Probability of first relapse in bone according to the presence or absence of micrometastases at the time of initial surgery. *Full line* micrometastases-positive; *broken line* micrometastases-negative. The number of patients at risk is shown along the *x* axis

examined from the traditional 8 to 20 has not increased either the incidence of tumor cells (about 25%) or the number of tumor cells found per patient. It is possible that the development of more specific monoclonal antibodies that can be used in the "cocktail" will improve the detection rate.

This technique thus provides a more rational strategy for preventing the evolution of symptomatic bone metastases by treatment with adjuvant chemotherapy or endocrine therapy. In addition, intensive therapy may be warranted for patients who have micrometastases, but a major concern is the possibility of reinfusing micrometastases in autologous marrow rescue procedures. A variety of techniques have been devised for depleting tumor cells from bone marrow harvested for autologous transplantation; initial experience with a monoclonal antibody toxin conjugate, LICR-LON-Fib 75/Abrin A-Chain [7] on patients with advanced breast cancer confirmed that in theory this was a possible approach in terms of comparable bone marrow recovery time in patients who received treatment and in unrelated marrow, but the relapse-free interval was not increased [17]. This suggests the method may be more applicable to patients with limited disease, such as patients with poor prognosis primary breast cancer with micrometastatic bone marrow involvement.

The Fate of Bone Marrow Micrometastases

To determine the fate of these tumor cells found at the time of initial surgery, both in patients receiving and not receiving adjuvant therapy, multiple bone marrow aspirates were repeated in 82 patients at a median time of 18 months after surgery, but prior to overt relapse. In both treated and untreated patients micrometastases were found in only 2% and 3% of patients, respectively (Table 4). However, when multiple aspirates were taken from patients with local recurrence, the incidence of micrometastases was 19%, and this rose to 30% in patients with disease at distant sites other than bone, and to 100% in patients with radiologically proven bone disease (Fig. 4).

These results suggest that many of the micrometastases from breast cancer patients are the result of "shedding" of cells from the primary tumor; some of these cells are viable with proliferative potential while others are nonviable. Thus, once the tumor is removed, the continual source of shedding cells is also removed. Subsequently, the viable tumor cells probably proliferate at a variable rate, some die and others remain at such low levels that our current techniques are not sufficiently sensitive to detect them.

Previous investigations into the fate of circulating tumor cells have been based on tumor-bearing animal models. These have shown that the development of metastases is an inefficient process in terms of cancer cell economics because the number of circulating cancer cells from many tumors is considerably higher than the resulting metastases [87, 88, 36]. This may also explain why the actual number of tumor cells found in bone marrow at the time of surgery is related neither to poor prognostic factors nor to the subsequent development of metastases. The technique, although providing valuable information regarding the natural history of breast cancer, is insufficiently sensitive to provide accurate monitoring of adjuvant therapy in breast cancer patients.

Table 4. Repeat bone marrow aspirates in untreated patients and patients on adjuvant therapy

Group	Total	Subsequently positive (*n*)	(%)
A) Adjuvant therapy			
Micrometastases +ve	11	1	9
Micrometastases −ve	34	0	0
B) Untreated			
Micrometastases +ve	10	1	10
Micrometastases −ve	27	0	0
Total	82	2	2

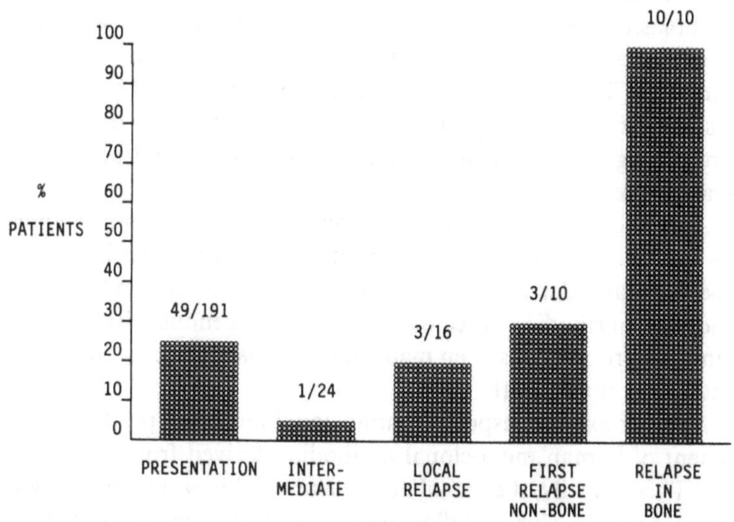

Fig. 4. The histograms show the incidence of micrometastases in patients with breast cancer at various stages of development of their disease. The percentage of patients with micrometastases who did not receive adjuvant therapy after the initial surgery is compared with the incidence of micrometastases after surgery, but before overt relapse. This in turn is compared with the incidence of micrometastases in patients with local recurrence, distant recurrence not in bone, and bony metastatic disease

Future Prospects for Therapy with Monoclonal Antibodies

The production of monoclonal antibodies directed toward the tumor cell surface gave most investigators initial hope that these agents could be used for tumor cell killing. However, as with radioimmunolocalization, numerous problems have been encountered. These include tumor cell antigenic modulation, anti-mouse antibody generation by the patient, antibody penetration to the tumor, and antigenic heterogeneity. The latter may be overcome to some degree with the use of several monoclonal antibodies used simultaneously or sequentially.

Preliminary work in model xenograft breast cancer systems with two monoclonal antibodies resulted in a rapid reduction of the tumor to 25% of the pretreatment volume, but the effect lasted only 4-30 days and regrowth of the tumor then took place [10]. More recently, in another animal study, a cocktail of monoclonal antibodies caused a very significant arrest of growth in breast carcinomas compared with nonmammary carcinomas, thus confirming the breast specificity of the cocktail. Furthermore, no toxic effects related to the administration of the antibodies were observed [11]. Clearly, their effectiveness could be improved by conjugating them with cytotoxic drugs, vegetable toxins, and/or radioactive elements.

The depletion of tumor cells from bone marrow in breast cancer patients has already been discussed. Considerable success has been achieved in patients with neuroblastoma in which a panel of monoclonal antibodies selectively binds to neuroblastoma cells in bone marrow; subsequently, microspheres coated with the secondary antibody are added to the system which bind to the antibody-coated tumor cells. The cells are then separated from the normal bone marrow constituents by samarium-cobalt magnets [50, 51]. This method has been shown to be efficient in removing tumor cells from bone marrow, and could be of use in patients with breast cancer.

Anti-idiotype monoclonal antibodies represent a novel approach to cancer therapy. This involves stimulation of the patient's own immune system with an experimentally derived anti-idiotype monoclonal antibody. The patient, in turn, produces antibodies directed against endogenous tissue-associated antigens. Although progress has been made in other malignancies, the application to breast cancer is at a very early stage.

Another exciting aspect of monoclonal antibody production lies in the development of human monoclonal antibodies derived from the patient's own tumor [47]. Theoretically, the actual advantages of this would be that less of an immune response will be elicited following repeated inoculations compared with the Fab fragment of a mouse immunoglobulin, and that they may recognize epitopes that the mouse immune system does not. Unfortunately, the technology to achieve clinically meaningful results is not yet fully developed.

Conclusions

Monoclonal antibodies are now available to aid in the understanding of the functional and structural differences between normal and neoplastic breast cells. Many have a role as probes in the detection of metastases, but as yet none are sensitive or specific enough to provide the clinician with a serum tumor marker to detect early disease recurrence. A major step forward in understanding the biology of breast cancer has been the detection of tumor cells in bone marrow of patients with primary breast cancer when taken at the time of initial surgery and stained immunocytochemically; not only are these cells associated with other poor prognostic factors, but they predict for the development of subsequent bone disease. The results of longer follow-up are awaited with interest. The future development of more specific monoclonal antibodies and technical advances in their use in radioimmunolocalization and targeting will hopefully revolutionize the management of breast cancer which remains a depressing disease to treat.

References

1. Albrechtsen R, Nielsen M, Wewer U, Engvall E, Ruoslahti E (1981) Basement membrane changes in breast cancer detected by immunohistochemical staining for laminin. Cancer Res 41: 5076-5081
2. Arklie J, Taylor-Papadimitriou J, Bodmer W, Egan M, Millis R (1981) Differentiation antigens expressed by epithelial cells in the lactating breast are also detectable in breast cancers. Int J Cancer 28: 23-29

3. Berger U, Wilson P, McClelland RA, Davidson J, Coombes RC (1987) A comparison of immunocytochemically-demonstrated estrogen receptor distribution with histopathologic features of primary breast cancer. Human Pathology 8: 1263-1267
4. Berger U, Wilson P, Thethi S, McClelland R, Greene GL, Coombes RC. Immunocytochemical assay for progesterone receptor: comparison with a biochemical method of measurement and relationship to estrogen receptor status. To be published
5. Bettelheim R, Penman HG, Thornton-Jones H, Neville AM (1984) Prognostic significance of peritumoral vascular invasion in breast cancer. Br J Cancer 50: 771-777
6. Brabon AC, Williams JF, Cardiff RD (1984) A monoclonal antibody to a human breast tumor protein released in response to estrogen. Cancer Res 44: 2704-2710
7. Buckman R, Shepherd V, Coombes RC, McIlhinney RAJ, Patel S, Neville AM (1982) Elimination of carcinoma cells from human bone marrow. Lancet ii: 1428-1430
8. Buckman R, Coombes RC, Dearnaley DP, Gore M, Gusterson BA, Neville AM (1984) Some clinical uses of biological markers. In: Breast cancer: diagnosis and management. Bonnadonna G (ed) Wiley, New York, pp 109-126
9. Burchell J, Durbin H, Taylor-Papadimitriou J (1983) Complexity of expression of antigenic determinants recognized by monoclonal antibodies HMFG1 and HMFG2 in normal and malignant human mammary epithelial cells. J Immunol 131: 508-513
10. Capone PM, Papsidero LD, Croghan GA, Ming Chu T (1983) Experimental tumoricidal effects of monoclonal antibody against solid breast tumors. Proc Natl Acad Sci USA 80: 7328-7332
11. Ceriani RL, Blank EW, Peterson JA (1987) Experimental immunotherapy of human breast carcinomas implanted in nude mice with a mixture of monoclonal antibodies against human milk fat globule components. Cancer Res 47: 532-540
12. Colcher D, Hand P, Nuti M, Schlom J (1981) A spectrum of monoclonal antibodies reactive with human mammary tumor cells. Proc Natl Acad Sci USA 78: 3199-3203
13. Colcher D, Horan Hand P, Nuti M, Schlom JA (1983) Differential binding to human mammary and non-mammary tumors of monoclonal antibodies reactive with carcinoembryonic antigen. Cancer Invest 1: 131-139
14. Coleman RE, Rubens RD (1987) The clinical course of bone metastases from breast cancer. Br J Cancer 55: 61-66
15. Coombes RC, Powles TJ, Abbott M, De Rivas L, Fort HT, McCready VR, Neville AM, Gazet JC (1980) Physical tests for distant metastases in patients with breast cancer. J R Soc Med 73: 617-623
16. Coombes RC, Dearnaley DP, Redding WH, Ormerod MG, Skilton RA, Sloane JP, Imrie S, Edwards PAW, Monaghan P, Neville AM (1983) Micrometastases in breast cancer. In: Peeters H (ed) Protides of the biological fluids, Vol 31. Pergamon, Oxford, pp 317-323
17. Coombes RC, Buckman R, Forrester JA, Shepherd V, O'Hare M, Vincebt M, Powles TJ, Neville AM (1986) in vitro and in vivo effects of a monoclonal antibody-toxin conjugate for use in autologous bone marrow transplantation for patients with breast cancer. Cancer Res 46: 4217-4220
18. Cooper D, Schermer A, Pruss R, Sun T (1984) The use of aIF, AE1 and AE3 monoclonal antibodies for the identification and classification of mammalial epithelial keratins. Differentiation 28: 30-35
19. Cordell J, Richardson TC, Pulford KAF, Ghosh AK, Gatter KC, Heyderman E, Mason DY (1985) Production of monoclonal antibodies against human epithelial membrane antigen for use in diagnostic immunocytochemistry. Br J Cancer 52: 347-354
20. Davis BW, Gelber R, Goldhirsch A, Hartmann WH, Hollaway L, Russell I, Rudenstam CM for the Ludwig Breast Cancer Study Group (1985) Prognostic significance of

peritumoral vessel invasion in clinical trials of adjuvant therapy for breast cancer with axillary node lymph node metastasis. Human Pathol 16: 1212-1218
21. Dearnaley DP, Sloan JP, Ormerod MG, Steele K, Coombes RC, Clink HMcD, Powles TJ, Ford HT, Gazet JC, Neville AM (1981) Increased detection of mammary carcinoma cells in marrow smears using antisera to epithelial membrane antigen. Br J Cancer 44: 85-90
22. Dearnaley DP, Ormerod MG, Sloane JP, Lumley H, Imrie S, Jones M, Coombes RC, Neville AM (1983) In collaboration with te Combined Breast Unit and the Department of Haematology, Royal Marsden Hospital. Detection of isolated mammary carcinoma cells in marrow of patients with primary breast cancer. J R Soc Med 76: 359-364
23. Delsol G, Gatter KC, Stein H, Erber WN, Pulford KAF, Zinne K, Mason DY (1984) Human lymphoid cells express epithelial membrane antigen: implication for diagnosis of human neoplasms. Lancet ii: 1124-1128
24. Dhokia B, Pectasides D, Self C, Habib NA, Hersham M, Wood CB, Munro AJ, Epenetos AA (1986) A low pH enzyme linked immunoassay using two monoclonal antibodies for the serological detection and monitoring of breast cancer. Br J Cancer 54: 885-889
25. Edwards PAW, Brooks IM, Monaghan P (1984) Expression of epithelial antigens in primary cultures of normal human breast analysed with monoclonal antibodies. Differentiation 24: 247-258
26. Edwards PAW, Skilton RA, Payne AWR, Ormerod MG (1988) Antigenic heterogeneity of breast cell lines detected by monoclonal antibodies and its relationship with the cell cycle. J Cell Sci 73: 321-333
27. Ekblom P, Miettinen M, Forsman L, Andersson LC (1984) Basement membrane and apocrine epithelial antigens in differential diagnosis between tubular carcinoma and sclerosing adenosis of the breast. J Clin Pathol 37: 357-363
28. Ellis IO, Robbins RA, Elston CW, Blamey RW, Ferry B, Baldwin RW (1984) A monoclonal antibody, NCRC-11, raised to human breast cancers. 1. Production and immunohistological characterization. Histopathology 8: 501-516
29. Ellis IO, Hinton CP, MacNay J, Elston CW, Robins A, Owainati AARS, Blamey RW, Baldwin RW, Ferry B (1985) Immunocytochemical staining of breast carcinoma with the monoclonal antibody NRCR 11: a new prognostic indicator. Br Med J [Clin Res] 290: 881-883
30. Elston CW, Gresham GA, Rao GS, Zebro JL, Haybittle JL, Houghton J, Kearney G (1982) The cancer research campaign (King's/Cambridge) trial for early breast cancer: clinicopathological aspects. Br J Cancer 45: 655-669
31. Epenetos AA, Canti G, Taylor-Papadimitriou J, Curling M, Bodmer WF (1982) Use of two epithelium-specific monoclonal antibodies for diagnosis of malignancy in serous effusions. Lancet ii: 1004-1006
32. Fisher B, Slack NH (1970) Number of lymph nodes examined and prognosis in breast carcinoma. Surg Gynecol Obstet 131: 79-88
33. Fisher ER, Swamidoss S, Lee CH, Rockette H, Redmond C, Fisher B (1978) Detection and significance of occult axillary node metastases in patients with invasive breast cancer. Cancer 42: 2025-2031
34. Foster CS, Dinsdale EA, Edwards PAW, Neville AM (1982) Monoclonal antibodies to the human mammary gland 11. Distribution of determinants in breast carcinomas. Virchows Arch [A] 394: 295-305
35. Glassy MC, Handley HH, Hagiwara H, Royston I (1983) UC 729-6, a human lymphoblastoid B-cell line useful for generating antibody-secreting human-human hybridomas. Proc Natl Acad Sci USA 80: 6327-6331

36. Glaves D (1983) Correlation between circulating cancer cells and incidence of metastases. Br J Cancer 48: 665-673
37. Goodall AB, Evans CJ, Trivedi D, Coombes RC, Chantler SM (1985) Detection of Ca antigen in sera from normal individuals and patients with benign and malignant breast disease. Br J Cancer 52: 177-182
38. Granowska M, Shepherd J, Britton KE, Waird B, Mather S, Taylor-Papadimitriou J, Epenetos AA, Carroll MJ, Nimmon CC, Hawkins LA, Bodner WF (1983) Proc Annu Meet Soc Nucl Med 24 (5)
39. Greene GL, Nolan C, Emgler JP, Jensen EV (1980) Monoclonal antibodies to human estrogen receptor. Proc Natl Acad Sci USA 77: 5115-5119
40. Gusterson BA, Warburton MJ, Mitchell D, Ellison M, Neville AM, Rudland PS (1982) Distribution of myoepithelial cells and basement membrane proteins in the normal breast and in benign and malignant brease diseases. Cancer Res 42: 4763-4770
41. Heyderman E, Steele K, Ormerod MG (1979) A new antigen on the epithelial membrane: its immunoperoxidase localization on normal and neoplastic tissue. J Clin Pathol 32: 35-39
42. Hikens J, Guijs F, Hilgers J, Hageman Ph, Calafat J, Sonnerberg A, Van der Volk M (1984) Monoclonal antibodies against human milk-fat globule membranes detecting differentiation antigens of the mammary gland and its tumors. Int J Cancer 34: 197-206
43. Horan Hand P, Nuti M, Colcher D, Scholm J (1983) Definition of antigenic heterogeneity and modulation among human mammary carcinoma cell populations using monoclonal antibodies to tumor-associated antigens. Cancer Res 43: 728-735
44. Horan Hand P, Thor A, Schlom J, Rao CN, Liotta L (1985) Expression of laminin receptor in normal and carcinomatus human tissues as defined by a monoclonal antibody. Cancer Res 45: 2713-2719
45. Howat JMT, Harris M, Swindell R, Barnes DM (1985) The effect of oestrogen and progesterone receptors on recurrence and survival in patients with carcinoma of the breast. Br J Cancer 51: 263-270
46. Iacobelli S, Natoli V, Scambia G, Santeusanio G, Negrini R, Natoli C (1985) A monoclonal antibody (AB/3) reactive with human breast cancer. Cancer Res 45: 4334-4338
47. Imam A, Drushella MM, Taylor CR, Tokes ZA (1985) Generation and immunohistochemical characterization of human monoclonal antibodies to mammary carcinoma cells. Cancer Res 45: 263-271
48. Jaffe HL (1968) Tumors metastatic to the skeleton. In: Jaffe HL (ed) Tumors and tumorous conditions of the bones and joints. Lea and Febiger, Philadelphia, pp 589-618
49. Johnston WW, Szpak CA, Lottich SC, Thor A, Schlom J (1985) Use of a monoclonal antibody B72.3 as an immunocytochemical adjunct to diagnosis of adenocarcinoma in human effusions. Cancer Res 45: 1894-1900
50. Kemshead JT, Treleaven JG, Gibson FM, Ugelstad J, Rembaum A, Philip T (1985) Monoclonal antibodies and magnetic micros pheres used for the depletion of malignant cells from bone marrow. In: Evans AE et al. (eds) Advances in neuroblastoma research. Liss, New York, pp 413-423
51. Kemshead JT, Heath L, Gibson FM, Katz F, Richmond F, Treleaven J, Ugelstead J (1986) Magnetic microspheres and monoclonal antibodies for the depletion of neuroblastoma cells from bone marrow: experiences, improvements and observations. Br J Cancer 54: 771-778
52. Kohler G, Milstein C (1976) Derivation of specific antibody-producing tissue culture and tumor lines by cell fusion. Eur J Immunol 6: 511-519

53. Krohn K, Ashorn R, Helle M (1985) Generation of monoclonal antisera to human milk fat globule membrane antigens, with special reference to a precipitable secretory product of breast and ovarian carcinomas. Tumour Biol 6: 13-23
54. Lundy J, Thor A, Maenza R, Schlom J, Forouhar F, Testa M, Kufe D (1985) Monoclonal antibody DF3 correlates with tumor differentiation and hormone receptor status in breast cancer patients. Breast Cancer Res Treat 5: 269-276
55. Maass H, Jonat W (1983) Steroid receptors as a guide for therapy of primary and metastatic breast cancer. J Steroid Biochem 19: 833-837
56. Makin CA, Bobrow LG, Bodmer WF (1984) Monoclonal antibody to cytokeratin for use in routine histopathology. J Clin Pathol 37: 975-983
57. Mansi JL, Earl H, Powles TJ, Coombes RC (1988) Tests for detecting recurrent disease in the follow-up of patients with breast cancer. Breast Cancer Res Treat (In press)
58. Mariani-Constantini R, Andreola S, Rilke F (1985) Tumour-associated antigens in mammary and extra-mammary Paget's disease. Virchows Arch (A) 405: 333-340
59. Martin SE, Moshiri S, Thor A, Vilasi V, Chu EW, Schlom J (1986) Identification of adenocarcinoma in cytospin preparations of effusions using Mab B72.3. Am J Clin Pathol 86: 10-18
60 McClelland RA, Berger U, Miller LS, Powles TJ, Coombes RC (1986) Immunocytochemical assay for estrogen receptor in patients with breast cancer: relationship to a biochemical assay and to outcome of therapy. J Clin Oncol 4: 1171-1176
61. McClelland RA, Berger U, Wilson P, Powles TJ, Trott PA, Gazet JC, Coombes RC (1987) Presurgical determination of estrogen receptor status using immunocytochemically stained fine needle aspirate smears in patients with breast cancer. Cancer Res 47: 6118-6122
62. McIlhinney RAJ, Patel S, Gore ME (1985) Monoclonal antibodies recognizing epitopes carried on both glycolipids and glycoproteins of the human milk fat globule membrane. Biochem J 227: 155-162
63. Menard S, Tagliabue E, Canevari S, Fossati G, Colnaghi MI (1983) Generation of monoclonal antibodies reacting with normal and cancer cells of human breast. Cancer Res 43: 1295-1300
64. Moldofsky PJ, Sears HF, Mulhern CB Jr, Hammond ND, Powe J, Gatenby RA, Steplewski Z, Koprowski H (1984) Detection of metastatic tumor in normal-sized retroperitoneal lymph nodes by monoclonal antibody imaging. N Engl J Med 311: 106-107
65. Nuti M, Teramoto YA, Mariani-Constantini R, Horan Hand P, Colcher D, Schlom J (1982) A monoclonal antibody (B72.3) defines patterns and distribution of a novel tumour-associated antigen in human mammary carcinoma cell populations. Int J Cancer 29: 539-545
66. Ormerod MG, Steele K, Westwood JH, Mazzini MN (1983) Epithelial membrane antigen: partial purification, assay and properties. Br J Cancer 48: 533-541
67. Papsidero LD, Croghan GA, O'Connell MJ, Valenzuela LA, Nemeto T, Chu LM (1983) Monoclonal antibodies (F36/22 and M7/105) to human carcinoma. Cancer Res 43: 1741-1747
68. Pinkus GS, Kurtin PJ (1985) Epithelial membrane antigen—a diagnostic discriminant in surgical pathology: immunohistochemical profile in epithelial, mesenchymal, and hematopoietic neoplasms using paraffin sections and monoclonal antibodies. Hum Pathol 16: 929-940
69. Pinkus GS, Constance MD, Etheridge CL, O'Conner EM (1986) Are keratin proteins a better tumor marker than epithelial membrane antigen? A comparative immunohistochemical study of various paraffin-embedded neoplasms using monoclonal and polyclonal antibodies. Am J Clin Pathol 85: 269-277

70. Poulsen H, Ozzello L, King WJ, Greene GL (1985) The use of monoclonal antibodies to estrogen receptors (ER) for immunoperoxidase detection of ER in paraffin sections of human breast cancer tissue. J Histochem Cytochem 33: 87-92
71. Rainsbury RM, Westwood JM, Coombes RC, Neville AM, Ott RJ, Kalirai TS, McCready VR, Gazet JC (1983) Location of metastatic breast carcinoma by a monoclonal antibody chelate labelled with indium-111. Lancet ii: 934-938
72. Rasmussen BB, Hilkens J, Hilgers J, Nielsen HH, Thorpe SM, Rose C (1982) Monoclonal antibodies applied to primary human breast carcinoma: relationship to menopausal status, lymph node status, and steroid hormone receptor content. Breast Cancer Res Treat 2: 401-405
73. Ridell B, Landys K (1979) Incidence and histopathology of metastases of mammary carcinoma in biopsies from the posterior iliac crest. Cancer 44: 1782-1788
74. Rosen PP, Saigo PE, Braun DW, Weathers E, Depalo A (1981) Predictors of recurrence in stage 1 (TINOMO) breast carcinoma. Ann Surg 193: 15-25
75. Sainsbury JRC, Farndon JR, Sherbert GV, Harris AL (1985) Epidermal growth factor receptors and oestrogen receptors on human breast cancers. Lancet i: 364-366
76. Schlom J, Greiner J, Horan Hand P, Colcher D, Inghirami G, Weeks M, Pestka S, Fisher PB, Noguchi P, Kufe D (1984) Monoclonal antibodies to breast cancer-associated antigens as potential reagents in the management of breast cancer. Cancer 54: 2777-2794
77. Siegel GP, Barsky SH, Terranova VP, Liotta LA (1981) Stages of neoplastic transformation of human breast tissue as monitored by dissolution of basement membrane components. An immunoperoxidase study. Invasion Metastasis 1: 54-70
78. Skilton RA, Earl HM, Gore ME, McIlhinney RAJ, Gusterson BA, Wilson P, Coombes RC. Characterization of monoclonal antisera reactive with normal resting, lactating, and neoplastic breast tissue. To be published
79. Sloane JP, Ormerod MG (1981) Distribution of epithelial membrane antigen in normal and neoplastic tissues and its value in diagnostic tumor pathology. Cancer (1983) 47: 1786-1795
80. Soule HR, Lunder E, Edington TS (1983) Membrane 126-kilodalton phosphoglycoprotein associated with human carcinomas identified by a hybridoma antibody to mammary carcinoma cells. Proc Natl Acad Sci USA 80: 1332-1336
81. Taylor-Papidimitriou J, Peterson JA, Arklie J, Burchell J, Ceriani RL, Bodmer WF (1981) Monoclonal antibodies to epithelium-specific components of the human milk fat globule membrane: production and reaction with cells in culture. Int J Cancer 28: 17-21
82. Teramoto YA, Mariani-Constantini R, Wunderlich D, Schlom J (1982) The immunohistochemical reactivity of a human monoclonal antibody with tissue sections of human mammary tumors. Cancer 50: 241-249
83. Thompson CH, Jones SL, Whitehead RH, McKenzie IFC (1983) A human breast tissue-associated antigen detected by a monoclonal antibody. J N C I 70: 409-419
84. Thor A, Weeks MO, Schlom J (1986) Monoclonal antibodies and breast Cancer. Semin Oncol 13: 393-410
85. Trojani M, Mascarel I, Bonchichon F, Coindre JM, Delsol G (1987) Micrometastases to axillary lymph nodes from carcinoma of the breast: detection by immunohistochemistry and prognostic significance. Br J Cancer 55: 303-306
86. Wells CA, Heryet A, Brochier J, Gatter KC, Mason DY (1984) The immunocytochemical detection of axillary micrometastases in breast cancer. Br J Cancer 50: 193-197
87. Weiss L (1980) Cancer cell traffic from the lungs to the liver: an example of metastatic inefficiency. Int J Cancer 25: 385-392
88. Weiss L (1982) Metastatic inefficiency. In: Weiss L, Gilbert HA (eds) Liver metastases. Hall Boston, pp 126-157

89. Wilkinson EJ, Hause LL, Kuzma JF, Rothwell DJ, Donegan WL, Clowry LJ, Almagro UA, Choi H, Rimm AA, Hoffman RG, Latarocco R, Cafaro AF, Batayias GE (1981) Occult axillary lymph node metastasis in patients with invasive breast carcinoma. Lab Invest 44: 83A
90. Williams MR, Todd JH, Ellis IO, Dowle CS, Haybittle JL, Elston CW, Nicholson RI, Griffiths K, Blamey RW. (1987) Oestrogen receptors in primary and advanced breast cancer: an eight year review of 704 cases. Br J Cancer 55: 67-73
91. Yuan D, Hendler FJ, Vitetta ES (1982) Characterization of a monoclonal antibody reactive with a subset of human breast tumors. J N C I 68: 719-728
92. White CA, Dulbecco R, Allen R, Bowman M, Armstrong B (1985) Two monoclonal antibodies selective for human mammary carcinoma. Cancer Research 45: 1337-1349

A Review of the Role of Immune Reactants in Patients with High-Risk Breast Carcinoma

F. A. Salinas

Advanced Therapeutics Department, Cancer Control Agency of British Columbia
and Department of Pathology, University of British Columbia,
600 West 10th Avenue, Vancouver, B.C. V5Z 4E6, Canada

Introduction

The antigenic heterogeneity that is known to occur on the surface of breast carcinoma cells is reflected by the immunological reactions observed and reported in patients with breast carcinoma [14, 24, 47, 62, 65]. As a result of these observations, both free and immune complex-bound tumor-immune reactants have been detected [56, 57, 59–63, 65, 66, 69]. Examples of these tumor- and host-interactive immune components include: breast carcinoma-associated antigens, tumor-associated antibodies, and their respective immune complexes. Subsequent advances in technology, including the determination of circulating immune complexes, the extraction of tumor-associated antigens from circulating immune complexes, and the use of monoclonal antibodies have made possible the detection, isolation, and characterization of human mammary-epithelial antigens in patients with benign and malignant breast disease [56, 61, 63 and F. A. Salinas, Ragaz, and R.L. Ceriani, unpublished results]. Monoclonal antibodies have been produced against breast carcinoma-associated antigens, breast tumor cell lines, membrane-enriched extracts of breast carcinoma metastases, and mammary tissue-specific antigens [11, 24, 26, 38, 50, 51, 78]. Subsequent use of monoclonal antibodies in therapy [8], immunodetection, diagnosis [50, 66], prognosis [4, 13, 61, 66], and other clinical applications in breast carcinoma have been recently reviewed [40, 66].

The relationship of tumor burden to circulating immune complexes has also demonstrated useful clinical correlations, both in breast carcinoma and in other solid tumor types [9, 61, 66 and F.A. Salinas, J. Ragaz, and R.L. Ceriani, unpublished results]. Efforts have been made to explain the apparent lack of consistency in relating immune complex concentration to clinical status and to further clarify the immunopathogenetic and modulatory roles of both free and bound immune complexes in cancer patients [56, 62, 67 and F.A. Salinas, J. Ragaz and R.L. Ceriani, unpublished results]. The following paragraphs will highlight the impact that circulating immune complexes have as tumor markers in the clinical assessment of cancer patients at high risk for recurrence, in the evaluation of postsurgical follow-up and in the monitoring of tumor burden changes. Ceriani et al. [11, 12], Taylor-Papadimitriou et al. [78] and, more recently, Salinas et al. [61] have characterized differentiating human mammary-epithelial antigens and have

Ragaz/Ariel (Eds.), High-Risk Breast Cancer

demonstrated their heterogeneity. Use of monoclonal antibodies prepared against human mammary-epithelial antigens of milk fat globule membrane has enabled detailed analysis of antigenic heterogeneity and quantitative reactive similarities of breast carcinoma-associated antigens detected in sera and in circulating immune complexes from breast carcinoma patients [56, 60]. Using a solid-phase assay we have recently demonstrated that these antigens are related to the extent of tumor burden and to the size and concentration of circulating immune complexes in the serum of patients with benign and malignant breast disease. The solid-phase assay also facilitated demonstration of differential expression of several breast carcinoma-associated antigens even within a tumor mass [1, 16, 26, 78]. These observations indicate that measurement of breast carcinoma-associated antigens to monitor the course of disease is a method that shows great promise, particularly if changes in their levels, as shown by solid-phase assay, prove to antedate objective clinical evidence of tumor burden changes [56, 61].

In a retrospective study, 159 patients with histopathological confirmation of breast carcinoma were assigned to groups on the basis of objective evaluable tumor burden, as previously described [66]. Group 1 included 65 patients with no evidence of residual disease at 4–6 weeks after surgical excision of all known carcinoma; group 2 comprised 43 patients with limited recurrent disease confined to the chest wall with a tumor mass estimated at less than 5 g; group 3 consisted of 46 patients known to have advanced regional or distal metastatic disease, with estimated tumor mass of more than 5 g. Serial sample determinations were performed on 36 patients selected on the basis of known objective clinical episodes of tumor burden changes.

All patients were participants in the breast carcinoma program of the Cancer Control Agency of British Columbia. They were evaluated at 1- to 3-monthly intervals for objective evidence of tumor burden reduction, stabilization, or increase according to criteria reported elsewhere [56, 61]. Assessment of response was done independently from results of immune reactants. The results from 40–60 sera per each tumor burden group were analyzed and compared.

Such assessment was performed using an independent paired difference rank analysis, Mann-Whitney – test, or χ^2 analysis [72]. In addition, 55 patients who had benign breast disease with biopsy-proven diagnosis of fibrocystic disease or fibroadenoma were similarly evaluated. For comparison, 70 control serum samples from healthy nonhospitalized volunteers (35 males, 35 females) with no known medical illness were selected from the serum bank maintained at the Cancer Control Agency of British Columbia. Also included were serum samples from pretested patients with malignant melanoma, osteosarcoma, and colon and ovarian carcinoma.

In view of the reported advantages of evaluating multiple serum markers, and in order to examine how they relate to breast carcinoma-associated antigen, patients were monitored concurrently with a panel of markers including carcinoembryonic antigen, anti-xenogeneic oncofetal antigens (XOFA) by isotopic antiglobulin test [57, 60, 67] and circulating immune complexes by fetal liver cell, Raji, or SC1Q radioimmunoassays (See Appendix) [56, 62, 68]

Clinical Role of Immune Reactants in Benign Breast Disease

Breast carcinoma has a long natural history and thus any attempt to define the role of a given marker will be seriously limited by the length of follow-up required to monitor the outcome in patients with benign breast disease.

It is well known that the distinction between benign breast disease and minimal breast cancer is not always clearly detected. Minimal breast carcinoma refers to a definite group of intraductal, lobular *in situ* or invasive cancers 0.5 cm or less in diameter [83]. Structural changes occurring during the transition from benign to malignant include changes in the basal membrane and in the quantity and density of myoepithelial cells [20]. The incidence of breast cancer in women with histologically confirmed benign breast disease is 2-3 times greater than the general population [30]. Hence, women who have undergone a breast biopsy for benign disease have an increased risk of breast carcinoma.

Extensive studies concerning risk factors for breast cancer in women with benign breast disease have been conducted by the Vanderbilt University Group [19, 49]. Their results, based on more than 10000 reevaluated breast biopsies, indicated that women having proliferative disease without atypical hyperplasia had twice the risk of women with non-proliferative lesions. The risk in women with atypical hyperplasia (atypia) was 5 times that in women with non-proliferative lesions, while in women with atypia associated with a family history of breast cancer the risk was found to be increased 11 times. In addition, and contrary to established findings, this study demonstrated that the majority of women (70%) who undergo breast biopsy for a benign condition without proliferative disease are not at increased risk of cancer [19].

An evaluation of serum markers was performed in patients with benign breast disease in order to estimate their role in predicting the risk of breast carcinoma [60]. Among the markers, selected serum immune reactants played a prominent role. The concentration, size, and composition of associated circulating immune complexes and antibodies has been determined in single sample sera of 55 patients with benign breast disease, and in 159 breast carcinoma patients grouped according to objective measurable tumor burden [58, 66 and F.A. Salinas, J. Ragaz, and R.L. Ceriani, unpublished results].

Significant correlations ($P<0.01$) with tumor burden in patients with breast carcinoma were also detected when FLC, Raji, and SC1Q assays for determination of circulating immune complexes were compared. Each of the three circulating immune complex evaluation assays discriminated between sera from breast cancer patients and normal control sera ($P<0.01$) and between breast cancer patients and 55 patients with biopsy-proven fibrocystic disease or fibroadenoma. Sucrose gradient fractionation demonstrated a large (25S) peak size of circulating immune complexes, similar in patients with benign breast disease and in group 1 breast cancer patients (no residual disease) [55, 60, 65, and F.A. Salinas, J. Ragaz, and R. L. Ceriani, unpublished results]. Furthermore, in our recent update, 20 of 35 (57%) samples of the patients with benign breast disease had a significant ($P<0.04$) increase in free breast cancer-associated antigen levels as compared with background levels (20 ng/ml) observed in 70 normal controls [56, 61].

In summary, evidence using immunological approaches in addition to morphologic, biochemical and epidemiological methods is accumulating which may clarify the transition from "late" benign to 'initial" malignant breast disease. This renewed emphasis will result in increased knowledge about the biology of breast disease as well as a better understanding and improved management of high risk benign breast disease.

Significance of Immune Reactants in Established Invasive Breast Carcinoma

In previous reports we emphasized the need to develop clinically reliable tumor markers to monitor tumor burden, in particular to predict disease recurrence and response to treatment [56, 63, 66, 67]. In a recent discussion by Hellman and Harris it was noted that "perhaps the most important problem facing clinical breast cancer research at this time is the development of more sophisticated markers within the primary tumor which predict for metastatic spread and which allow the appropriate treatment for the individual patient" [26]. In this regard, the measurement of breast carcinoma-associated antigens in the patients' serum by the use of single or a mixture (cocktail) of monoclonal antibodies has recently shown itself to be of use in early detection and even prediction of tumor metastasis [17, 23, 61, 81]. While successful clinical validation of any single such marker appears to be elusive, at present the use of two or more markers in combination appears to be a prevailing trend. Some of the efforts of clinical research in this area will be reviewed in the following paragraphs.

Correlation of Circulating Immune Complexes with Tumor Burden

The frequency and extent of elevation of circulating immune complexes varied for each test performed, but proved to be significantly different from the 5% noted for normal controls and the 4% elevation observed in samples of patients with benign breast disease. In fact, each of the three assays for circulating immune complexes discriminated between cancer patients and normal controls ($P<0.01$, Mann-Whitney U test), and notably between patients with breast cancer and benign disease ($P<0.01$).

To further understand the observed relationship between levels of circulating immune complexes and tumor burden, retrospective serial determinations were performed on 57 patients with breast cancer, with a follow-up of 11-48 months (median 35). Of these 57 patients, 39 were receiving standard adjuvant chemotherapy (consisting of cyclophosphamide, methotrexate and 5-fluorouracil), while the remaining 18 were receiving radiotherapy and/or hormonal therapy in line with institutional treatment policies. The results showed an overall inverse trend with tumor burden: while fluctuating decreased levels of circulating immune complexes correlated with increasing tumor burden, the levels were unchanged for patients who remained clinically stable, were increased moderately (three-fold) for those achieving objective responses, and reduced maximally (more than six-fold) for those who progressed from limited tumor burden to advanced disease. Overall, the magnitude of changes in the level of circulating immune complexes reflected the tumor burden: greater changes in level antedated larger increases in tumor burden.

Further analysis of extracted breast cancer-associated antigens and of monoclonal antibodies Mc 3 and Mc 8 showed the following interactions with tumor burden in sera from breast carcinoma patients. Immune complexes of patients from Group 3 were close to or at antigen:antibody equivalence; in Group 2, there was relative antigen excess, while in Group 1, relative antibody excess was observed [56, 61, 65].

Correlation of Breast Cancer-Associated Antigen with Tumor Burden

Sera of 135 patients with breast cancer, 20 each with osteosarcoma and malignant melanoma, 10 with colon carcinoma, 10 with ovarian carcinoma, 35 with benign breast disease and 70 controls were evaluated for circulating breast cancer-associated antigen concentration by use of a three-step radioligand assay. The results using monoclonal antibody Mc 8 as the detection agent showed significantly elevated values (mean 105 ng/ml, $P<0.001$) of breast cancer-associated antigen in 102 of 135 (76%) patients with breast cancer compared to background levels in each of 20 patients with sarcoma and malignant melanoma and in 70 normal control subjects. Levels of this antigen were also significantly elevated ($P<0.04$) in 20 of 35 (57%) tested samples of patients with benign breast disease. Conversely, minimal increases were observed in samples of patients with solid tumors other than breast cancer.

In an analysis of samples grouped by tumor burden, patients with breast cancer showed elevated antigen concentration (mean = 197 ng/ml) in 95% of instances in Group 2, three-fold higher values than that observed in Group 1 patients (65% elevation), and four-fold higher values than that observed in patients from Group 3 (65% elevation) [56, 61].

Role of Immune Complexes in Prognosis of Breast Cancer

As circulating immune complexes have been shown to be a sensitive monitor of tumor burden, our group has examined their potential predictive value for disease-free and overall survival. Follow-up time in 57 patients with breast cancer was 1–4 years (median 3 years) [59]. Prognostic variables used in the analysis at diagnosis and during follow-up included age, parity and performance status, tumor burden, carcino embryonic antigen, anti-XOFA antibody, sialic acid, number of axillary lymph nodes involved, estrogen receptor status, and length of both disease-free interval and overall survival. The results confirmed that changes in immune complexes antedated clinical objective increase or reduction in tumor burden. Conversely, immune complex levels were unchanged in patients who remained clinically stable. Furthermore, using a univariate analysis circulating immune complexes proved to be significant predictors, at diagnosis, of disease-free interval ($P<0.009$) and overall survival ($P<0.009$). In addition, using a multivariate analysis during patients' follow-up, tumor burden and immune complex levels proved to be independent predictors of disease-free interval ($P<0.026$) and overall survival ($P<0.048$). Hence, in addition to more frequently used prognostic factors, circulating immune complexes may also be important markers of risk in patients with breast cancer.

Role of Breast Cancer-Associated Antigens in the Prediction of Relapse and Disease Recurrence

As breast carcinoma-associated antigens have been shown to be a sensitive marker for tumor burden changes in breast cancer patients, further studies on these antigens' potential predictive value for the assessment of disease-free interval and overall survival were performed. Such an evaluation of breast carcinoma-associated antigens with emphasis on its predictive value for disease recurrence and relapse was conducted in a retrospective study [58, 61]. Other variables under study which were considered at diagnosis included: age, parity status, performance status, tumor burden, carcinoembryonic antigen (CEA), circulating immune complexes, sialic acid, anti-XOFA, axillary lymph nodes involved, estrogen receptors, disease-free interval, overall survival and survival status. In total, 60 eligible breast carcinoma patients were included, 41 undergoing adjuvant chemotherapy and 19 receiving hormonal therapy and/or radiotherapy. Results from a univariate analysis of the 19 factors considered demonstrated that tumor burden was the only significant predictor of disease-free interval ($P<0.009$) and of overall survival ($P<0.009$) as assessed at diagnosis. A similar analysis performed during follow-up identified breast carcinoma-associated antigens and circulating immune complex as the only predictors of disease-free interval ($P<0.0061$) and overall survival ($P<0.00001$). Using a multivariate analysis that allows for control of selected variables, further analysis of the prognostic role of breast carcinoma-associated antigens was performed. During patient's follow-up, circulating immune complexes, tumor burden and breast carcinoma-associated antigens were the only independent predictors of disease-free interval ($P<0.0031$) and overall survival ($P<0.0033$). In summary, the tumor marker role of circulating immune complexes, tumor burden and breast carcinoma-associated antigens emerged as a latent valuable clinical tool for predicting metastatic spread. These markers appears also to be of benefit in both selecting appropriate treatment for individual patients and identifying risk groups during clinical trials.

Diagnostic Aspects of Monoclonal Antibodies: Radioimmunolocalization

The clinical utilization of monoclonal antibodies (MAb) in breast and other cancer types has also included the following approaches: (a) assessment of the transition from benign to malignant breast disease, (b) determination of hormonal receptor status from a small sample of breast tissue obtained by fine needle aspirate procedure, and (c) radioimmunodetection of micrometastasis, including localization of tumor cells in bone marrow aspirates.

The early *in situ* detection and therapy of carcinoma lesions remains one of the goals of MAb clinical application. The detection of metastasis and noninvasive staging of lymph node involvement in the management of breast carcinoma and other tumor types by use of radiolabeled MAb directed to tumor-associated antigens are presently being studied in ongoing clinical trials [6, 14–16, 29, 33, 41, 52, 68, 74]. In recent years this technique has evolved into an effective methodology for cancer imaging by scintigraphy. Selection of the optimal imaging agent requires consideration of the isotope and structural form of the antibody in addition to specificity to be taken into account. It is not clear whether radioiodine, ^{111}In, or ^{99}Tc attached to MAb will be the optimal agent for diagnosis in a given clinical situation [6]. The detection of MAb with a differential ratio of uptake in tumor versus a range of normal tissue is difficult to obtain in some unresected lesions. These data are needed for the dosimetry calculations which would be required if radiolabeled MAb were to be used therapeutically. The fact that no one MAb detects all carcinoma lesions indicates that a mixture of several may be more efficacious in both *in situ* detection and therapy trials [15]. Other points of importance include the amount of free and bound antigen, the clearance and pharmacokinetics of the MAb isotope involved, and the route, dose, and specific activity of the labeled MAb used. Whether intact MAb have better pharmacokinetic properties than do proteolytic fragments for radioimmunodiagnosis and biolocalization appears to depend on the intended use [6, 10]. Most studies until now have concentrated on assessing the different variables involved in achieving optimal localization profiles by use of athymic mice bearing human tumor models. The clinical phase I trials of radioimmunolocalization presently using radiolabeled MAb directed against human tumor-associated antigen include ovarian, breast and gastrointestinal tumors [21, 22, 25, 27, 80], malignant melanoma [6, 34], and colon carcinoma [42, 45].

Therapeutic Role of Immune Reactants

The objective of the manipulation of immune reactants in therapy has been to reinstate an effective immunity in the tumor-bearing host. It has become clear that the complexities of the deranged immune regulatory factors involved are yet to be fully clarified. Therapeutic approaches to be reviewed here include the removal of circulating immune complexes and the multiple use of monoclonal antibodies in cancer therapy.

Circulating Immune Complexes

Many approaches to remove specific and nonspecific blocking factors from patients' sera have been directed toward removal of circulating immune complexes. The use of plasmaphoresis [31, 57, 66, 71] and/or immunoabsorption of extracorporeal protein A have resulted in subjective and objective clinical responses in tumor-bearing patients and in experimental animals. These attempts stimulated clinical trials for cancer therapy in animals [28, 32, 63, 78, 83] and in humans [2, 3, 37, 38, 39, 43, 53, 78] with advanced carcinomas including breast, colon, lung and other types.

Main side effects on immunoabsorption treatment as evaluated by Phase I studies ranged from lethal [43] to severe but manageable [38, 39, 53, 54, 79]. The most frequently noted side effects included fever, chills, hypotension, tachycardia, and bronchospasm. Reported response rates ranged from 0% [43] to 60% [79] in series involving five or more breast cancer patients.

The removal of circulating immune complexes and other factors that inhibit the host anti-tumor immunity appears to be a promising approach to cancer therapy. Several groups have documented *in vitro* and *in vivo* tumor response to protein A-bearing material in a variety of experimental and clinical approaches. Whether the demonstrated *in vivo* and *in vitro* tumor responses are effects of the protein A materials used during the immunoabsorption procedures, or are due to the removal of blocking factors, complement activation, or action of additional bioreacting components, remains to be determined. As yet, plasma immunoabsorption in clinical human cancer patients has not achieved the beneficial effects noted in animal studies. Data from feline leukemia studies have provided a clear-cut correlation between lowered circulating immune complex levels and clinical response. Although some provocative results have been documented in humans [66], the value of and mechanisms involved in this form of therapy still remain to be validated.

Monoclonal Antibodies

Until recently, the most important limitation on the use of antibodies as therapeutic agents was their impurity and heterogeneity. During the last decade, however, the advent of novel MAb technology has accelerated the development of unlimited quantities of homogeneous antibodies of defined specificity, thus eliminating a major precluding obstacle to new attempts to explore the potential of antibody therapy. The list of problems to be encountered in immunotherapy of cancer with MAb include: lack of specificity, *in vivo* deposition, class and fragments, coupling and delivering, circulating free antigen and antibody, antigenic modulation, and host response to foreign antibody [35]. As progress in the clinical setting has evolved, the relevance of these problems to a successful therapy has become quite evident.

Because most of the MAb against human tumor-cell antigens have been made in mice, host reaction to foreign antibodies is an important problem encountered in patients. A review of the MAb prepared against breast carcinoma demonstrated that most of them are directed towards breast cancer-associated antigens or tissue differentiation antigens. While there are many problems involved in the use of mouse immunoglobulins as therapeutic agents in man, the knowledge gained from mouse monoclonal mechanisms has provided valid essential insight into their clinical therapeutic application. These preliminary steps may prove a valuable means to accruing information while we await the forthcoming human–human MAb. While each of the reagents listed below carried its own therapeutic capabilities as well as its own intrinsic toxicity, the testing of MAb alone or conjugated to radioisotopes, toxins, or chemotherapeutic drugs has proceeded in clinical trials. The results have demonstrated limited toxicity accounted for by doses of up to 1500 mg of mouse MAb administered to humans. Previous reviews with detailed information concerning the assessment of MAb therapy in animal tumor models are available [22, 34, 35, 48].

Earlier clinical trials have been conducted mainly with leukemia and lymphoma patients, including a few studies testing patients with solid tumors (malignant melanoma and gastro-intestinal carcinomas) [7, 18, 45, 55, 70, 75, 77, 85]. MAb have been used as therapeutic agents either alone or as carriers of isotopes, toxins, chemotherapeutic agents, or a combination of these. The bulk of research in this area is at the stage of phase I clinical trial. Most of the clinical studies of solid tumors have concentrated on MAb prepared against gastrointestinal tumors [70], colon and gastric carcinomas [18], malignant melanoma [45, 77, 82], cutaneous T-cell lymphomas (55) and small-cell carcinoma of the lung [75]. So far, breast carcinoma has not been frequently selected for clinical immunotherapy trials [7].

Immunotoxins

The basic rationale of the immunotoxin approach to therapy is to link a toxic agent to a MAb in an attempt to destroy targeted cancer cells but leave normal cells unharmed. The term "immunotoxin" has been used to refer to a cell-binding antibody or antigen covalently bound to a plant or bacterial toxin. The toxin may be the whole molecule or a polypeptide portion carrying the toxic activity [84]. The most commonly used plant toxin is ricin. Other toxin moieties in use are ricin-R, ricin-R A chain, diphtheria toxin, abrin, and gelonin. In order for an immunotoxin to be effective, antitumor antibodies must promote the delivery of a toxin to sites of biological activity specifically within the cell [84, 85]. For a detailed description of the mechanisms of action, the preparation, testing of efficacy, induction of specific immunologic unresponsiveness, and other possibilities for modulating the immune response, the readers are referred to reviews on the topic [82, 84]. From the point of view of more direct clinical applications, the use of immunonotoxins *in vitro* to purge or eradicate either tumor cells from bone marrow or T cells from allogeneic marrow before marrow transplantation represents a novel approach to cancer therapy [45, 72]. In addition to conjugation of a toxin to an antibody, it is also possible to encapsulate the toxin in a liposome for delivery across the cell membrane [36].

The therapeutic potential of immunotoxin (anti-DNP antibody–ricin A chain conjugate) treatment in conjunction with chemotherapy (doxorubicin, cyclophosphamide) is indicated by an antineoplastic synergistic effect reported in experimental leukemia [73]. The suitability of a conjugate of MAb WT1 and ricin A chain has been tested for purging bone marrow of leukemic T cells during autologous transplantation in T-cell acute lymphocytic leukemia. The results indicated that under conditions rendering maximal killing of leukemic cells, there was no toxicity to multipotential progenitors in normal human bone marrow [46]. Problems still to be solved in this area included the relative organ toxicity (intestine and reticuloendothelial system), the problem of cross-reaction with normal antigen, and adequate access of immunotoxins to the cells of solid tumors [85]. Other problems requiring attention are tumor cell heterogeneity and antigen modulation, and the concentration of antigen in circulation (antigenemia) as discussed earlier [84].

In summary, tumor-reactive antibodies conjugated to toxins have been used to eradicate tumor cells in vitro and in vivo. These immunotoxins proved to be effective in killing experimental leukemic cells in infiltrated bone marrow. Selective use of immunotoxins, with or without liposome encapsulation, should be regarded as an effective way of improving chemotherapy regimes. Preliminary results from clinical trials presently in progress are forthcoming in the near future.

Perspectives for the Future

As the advances in technology are being further transferred into the clinical setting, there is an increased potential for immune reactants to be used as therapeutic tools in the clinical management of cancer patients. The utilization of tumor-associated antigens, measured alone or in cocktail combinations, is likely to be useful in the monitoring of high-risk patients with benign breast disease or cancer patients at high risk of relapse. Another area of application for monitoring both antigen and immune complex concentration in patients' sera is related to their role in neutralizing of MAb alone or infused as a form of immunotherapy. Long-range goals for the parenteral use of immunotoxins include the killing of cancer cells *in vivo* and the modulation of the immune response for therapeutic purposes [36, 84]. Insofar as imaging, immunodetection, and immunotherapy are concerned, it is likely that in the future these procedures will be performed more frequently, and using metal chelates. A relative advantage of the metal chelates compared to the large number of isotopes to be used is their stability, which makes them well suited to commercially available kit production. The refinement of human–human monoclonal antibodies against human tumor-associated antigens will undoubtedly be advantageous to the full establishment of this modality as an element of treatment for cancer in most sites.

Detailed findings from ongoing clinical trials concerning the therapeutic value, mechanisms of action, and idiosyncrasies of each treatment must be awaited before any of these modalities can be fully accepted as effective against cancer.

Appendix: Background and Techniques for Evaluating Immune Reactants

A brief description of the methodology used is listed below; references for a full account of each technique are cited.

Aggregated Human Gamma Globulin (AHG) and Monomeric IgG. Human IgG was prepared by DEAE-52 cellulose fractionation as reported earlier [64]. A WHO standard-reference preparation of AHG, kindly provided by Dr. P. Spath, WHO, Berne, Switzerland, was used for standardization of the circulating immune complexes standard curve.

Characterization of Immune Reactants by Sodiumdodecylsulfate Polyacrylamide Gel Electrophoresis (SDS-PAGE): Tube Gel Procedure. Duplicate samples of radioiodinated circulating immune complexes and breast carcinoma-associated antigens were analyzed on 3%–10% gradient (w/v) polyacrylamide gels with and without 2-mercaptoethanol as described earlier [58]. Gels were either evaluated by autoradiography, using Kodak XARS X-ray film, staining with Coomassie brilliant blue, and scanning with a model 620 densitometer (Bio-Rad Laboratory), or sliced a 1-mm intervals for determination of radioactivity using a gamma-ray spectrometer.

Slab Gel Western Blot Analysis. Slab gels SDS-PAGE were performed essentially as reported [58, 61, 66]. Briefly, treated samples were applied to a 4% (w/v) stacking gel over a 10% (w/v) slab gel. After electrophoresis, transfer of breast carcinoma-associated antigens from gel to nitrocellulose paper was achieved by use of Bio-Rad Trans-Blot Cell according to manufacturers' instructions. Thereafter, 1 ml serially diluted Mc 3 or Mc 8 was added to samples, which were then washed, followed by peroxidase-conjugated goat anti-mouse IgG enzyme-linked immunodetection.

The resulting band intensities were measured by densitometer, Model 620 (Bio-Rad).

Quantitation of Circulating Immune Complexes. Determination of circulating immune complexes was performed by the fetal liver cell radioimmunoassay (FLC-RIA), the Raji cell radioimmunoassay (RAJI-RIA), and the solid-phase C1Q radioimmunoassay (SC1Q-RIA), essentially as described earlier [61, 64, 66]. The uptake of an optimal amount of ^{125}I-labeled anti-human IgG was referred in each case to an AHG standard curve. The concentration of immune complexes was expressed as microgram AHG equivalents per milliliter (μg AHG/ml) of serum. A doubling of the level of circulating immune complexes was considered to be a significant change. This figure was chosen on the basis of our reported combined inter- and intra-assay coefficient of variation = 5.5% [64], analyzed using the technique of Statland et al. [76] to minimize the cost of misclassifications.

Determination of Circulating Immune Complex Size. Circulating immune complex size was determined by use of a 5%–35% (w/v) isopyknic sucrose gradient in phosphate buffer saline, pH 7.2, formed in 5 ml cellulose nitrate tubes as described earlier [64]. Fractions containing circulating immune complex aggregates with an estimated size of 7-9S, 10-17S, 18-20S, 21-24S, 25-27S, and >28S were pooled for analysis. Subsequent evaluation of immune complexes in collected fractionated samples provided an indication of the size range of the complexes occurring, and an estimation of their respective Ag:Ab composition [65].

Techniques for the Isolation of Breast Carcinoma-Associated Antigens. Breast carcinoma-associated antigens have been isolated as free or bound forms from the sera of selected breast carcinoma patients in order to achieve further discriminatory capacity. Free circulating antigens have been isolated by use of MAb coated immunobead procedure. Circulating immune complex-bound breast carcinoma-associated antigens have been isolated by the polyethylene glycol and the Raji cell techniques from sera with increased (three- to five-fold above normal control sera) circulating immune complex concentration [55, 61].

In Vitro Model of Tumor Burden Change. The interaction of Mc 3, Mc 8, or isolated breast carcinoma-associated antigen with sera from selected breast carcinoma patients was studied by use of an *in vitro* test. This procedure is also that used to generate and dissociate immune complexes [61, 64]. Using this model, changes in the size of circulating immune complexes were examined by titration of either Mc 3 or Mc 8 with sera from selected Group 1, 2, and 3 patients followed by circulating immune complex determination. Furthermore, this in vitro test was used to simulate defined increases in tumor burden by addition of breast carcinoma-associated antigen to autologous (self) or allogeneic (non-self) patients' sera. The in vitro test consisted of incubating 50 μl of selected patients' sera (diluted 1:8 with PBS) with isolated ^{125}I-labeled breast carcinoma-associated antigen (1 μg) for 17 h at 4°C. In preliminary experiments this concentration of antigen was determined to render maximal immune complex size changes [64, 68]. The reaction mixture was analyzed for changes in circulating immune complex size by SDS-PAGE.

Three-Step Radioligand Assay. This radioimmunoassay was performed essentially as previously described [61, 62]. Purified breast carcinoma-associated antigen was used as standard antigen at 1-100 ng in 50 μl of normal control sera. Test sera from cancer patients and controls were similarly prepared (50 μl, undiluted) and incubated with packed MAb coated Sepharose 4B immunobeads (100 μl; Pharmacia, Uppsala, Sweden). Immunobeads were then washed and reacted with biotin-conjugated Mc 8. The beads were washed again, incubated with ^{125}I-labeled avidin, and after further washings their radioactivity was determined. The least detectable concentration of breast carcinoma-associated antigen was 10 ng/ml serum with a combined intra- and interassay coefficient of variation of 9%. The cut-off value (< 20 ng/ml serum) used for classification of results as either normal or elevated was selected on the basis of preliminary results as analyzed by the Statland et al. [76] technique to minimize the cost of misclassifications.

Acknowledgements. I acknowledge and thank Dr. P. Rebbeck and St. Vincent's Hospital for supplying serum samples from patients with benign breast disease; K Wee for technical assistance; Dr. A. Coldman, Division of Epidemiology, Biometry and Occupational Oncology, CCABC, for assistance in statistical analysis; and T. Neyten, Bio-Rad Laboratories, Canada Limited, for assistance in densitometer determinations.

References

1. Adams DJ, Hajj G, Edwards DP, Bjercke RJ, McGuire WL (1983) Detection of a M_r 24,000 estrogen-regulated protein in human breast cancer by monoclonal antibodies. Cancer Res 43: 4297-4301
2. Bansal SC, Bansal BR, Thomas HL, Siegel PD, Rhoads JE, Cooper DR, Terman DS, Mark R (1978) Ex vivo removal of serum IgG in a patient with colon carcinoma. Cancer 42: 1-18
3. Bensinger WI, Kinet JB, Hennen G, Franckenne F, Schaus C, Saint-Remy M, Holyoux P, Mahieu P (1982) Plasma perfused over immobilized protein A for breast cancer. N Engl J Med 306: 935-936
4. Berry N, Jones DB, Smallwood J, Taylor I, Kirkham N, Taylor-Papadimitriou J (1985): The prognostic value of monoclonal antibodies HMFG-1 and HMFG-2 in breast cancer. Br J Cancer 51: 179-186
5. Bjor MJ, Ring D, Frankel A (1985) Evaluation of monoclonal antibodies for the development of breast cancer immunotoxins. Cancer Res 45: 1214-1221
6. Brown BA, Comeau RD, Jones PL, Liberatore FA, Neacy WP, Sands H, Gallagher BM (1987) Pharmacokinetics of the monoclonal antibody B72.3 and its fragments labelled with ^{125}I or ^{111}In. Cancer Res 47: 1149-1154
7. Buckman R, Shepherd V, Coombes RC, MacIlhinney RA, Patel S, Neville AM (1982) Elimination of carcinoma cells from human bone marrow. Lancet ii: 1428-1430
8. Capone PM, Papsidero LD, Croghan GA, Ming Chu T (1983) Experimental tumoricidal effects of monoclonal antibody against solid breast tumor. Proc Natl Acad Sci USA 80: 7328-7332
9. Carpentier NA, Miescher PA (1983) The clinical relevance of circulating immune complexes in cancer, kidney transplantation and pregnancy. In: Ray PK (ed) Immunobiology of transplantation, cancer and pregnancy. Pergamon, New York, pp 375-408
10. Carrasquillo JA, Krohn KA, Beaumier P, McGuffin RW, Brown JP, Hellstrom KE, Hellstrom I, Larson SM (1984) Diagnosis of and therapy for solid tumor with radiolabelled antibodies and immune fragments. Cancer Treat Rep 66: 317-328
11. Ceriani RL, Sasaki M, Sussman H, Wara WM, Blank EW (1982) Circulating human mammary epithelial antigens in breast cancer. Proc Natl Acad Sci USA 79: 5420-5424
12. Ceriani RL, Peterson JA, Lee JY, Moncada R, Blank EW (1983) Characterization of cell surface antigens of human mammary epithelial cells with monoclonal antibodies prepared against human milk fat globule. Somatic Cell Genet 9: 415-427
13. Ceriani RL, Peterson JA, Blank EW (1984) Variability in surface antigen expression of human breast epithelial cells from normal breast, normal tissue peripheral to breast, and breast carcinoma. Cancer Res 44: 3033-3038
14. Colcher D, Zulutsky M, Kaplan W, Kufe D, Austin F, Schlom J (1983) Radiolocalization of human mammary tumors in athymic mice by a monoclonal antibody. Cancer Res 43: 736-742
15. Colcher D, Esteban JM, Carrasquillo JA, Sugarbaker P, Reynolds JC, Bryant G, Schlom J (1987) Quantitative analysis of selective radiolabelled monoclonal antibody localization in metastatic lesions of colorectal cancer patients. Cancer Res 47: 1185-1189
16. Colcher PM, Horan PH, Wunderlich D, Nuti M, Teramoto YA, Kufe D, Schom J (1984) Potential diagnostic and prognostic applications of monoclonal antibodies to human mammary carcinoma. In: Wright GI (ed) Monoclonal antibodies in cancer. Dekker, New York, pp 121-159
17. Dhokia B, Pectasides D, Self C, Habib MA, Hersham M, Wood CB, Munro AJ, Epenetos AA (1986) A low pH enzyme linked immunoassay using two monoclonal

antibodies for the serological detection and monitoring of breast cancer. Br J Cancer 54: 885-889
18. Dillman RO, Beauregard JC, Halpern SE, Clutter M (1986) Toxicities and side effects associated with intravenous infusions of murien monoclonal antibodies. J Biol Response Mod 5: 73-84
19. Dupont WD, Page DI (1985) Risk factors for breast cancer women with proliferative breast disease. N Engl J Med 312: 146-151
20. Ekblom P, Miettinen M, Forsman L, Anderson LC (1984) Basement membrane and apocrine epithelial antigens in differential diagnosis between tubular carcinoma and sclerosing adenosis of the breast. J Clin Pathol 37: 357-363
21. Epenetos AA, Matler S, Granowska M, Nimmon CC, Hawkins LR, Briton KE, Sheperd J, Taylor-Papadimitriou J, Durban H, Malpas JS, Bodmer WF (1982) Targetting of ^{123}I labelled tumor associated monoclonal antibodies to ovarian, breast and gastrointestinal tumors. Lancet ii: 999-1004
22. Foon KA, Berbhard MI, Oldham RK (1982) Monoclonal antibody therapy: assessment by animal tumor models. J Biol Response Mod 1: 277-304
23. Goodall AB, Evans CJ, Trivedi D, Coombes RC, Chantler BM (1985) Detection of Ca antigen in sera from normal individuals and patients with benign and malignant breast disease. Br J Cancer 52: 177-182
24. Hand PH, Nuti M, Colcher D, Schlom J (1983) Definition of antigenic heterogeneity and modulation among human mammary carcinoma cell populations using monoclonal antibodies to tumor associated antigens. Cancer Res 43: 728-735
25. Hayes DF, Sekine H, Ohno T, Abe M, Keefe K, Kufe DW (1985) Use of murine monoclonal antibody for detection of circulating DF3 plasma antigen levels in breast cancer patients. J Clin Invest 75: 1397-1402
26. Hellman S, Harris JR (1987) The appropriated breast cancer paradigm. Cancer Res 47: 339-342
27. Hilkens J, Bouijs F, Hilgers J, Hageman PH, Calafat J, Sonnenberg A, Vaan der Valk M (1984) Monoclonal antibodies against human milk-fat globule membranes detecting differentiation antigens of the mammary gland and its tumor. Int J Cancer 34: 197-206
28. Holohan TV, Phillip TM, Bowles C, Deisseroth A (1982) Regression of canine mammary carcinoma after immunoadsorption therapy. Cancer Res 42: 3663-3668
29. Houghton AN, Mintzer D, Cordon-Cardo C, Welt S, Fliegel B, Vadhan S, Carswell E, Melamed MR, Oettgen HF, Old LJ (1985) Mouse monoclonal IgG3 antibody detecting Gd3 ganglioside: a phase I trial in patients with malignant melanoma. Proc Natl Acad Sci USA 82: 1242-1246
30. Hutchinson WB, Thomas DB, Hamlin WB, Roth GJ, Peterson AV, Williams B (1980) Risk of breast cancer in women with benign breast disease. J Natl Cancer Inst 65: 13-20
31. Isbister WH, Noonan FP, Halliday WJ, Clunie G (1975) Human thoracic duct cannulation: manipulation of tumor-specific blocking factors in a patient with malignant melanoma. Cancer 35: 1465-1471
32. Jones FR, Yoshida LH, Ladiges WC, Kennedy MA (1980) Treatment of feline leukemia and reversal of FeLV by ex vivo removal of IgG: a preliminary report. Cancer 46: 675-684
33. Larson SM, Brown JP, Wright PW, Carrasquillo JA, Hellstrom I, Hellstrom KE (1983) Imaging of melanoma with ^{131}I-labelled monoclonal antibodies. J Nucl Med 24: 123-129
34. Levy R (1987) Will monoclonal antibodies find a place in our therapeutic armamentarium? J Clin Oncol 5: 527-529
35. Levy R, Miller RA (1983) Tumor therapy with monoclonal antibodies. Fed Proc 42: 2650-1656

36. Lopez-Berestein G (1985) Prospects for liposomes as a novel drug delivery system. Cancer bull 37: 203-206
37. Mariani-Constantini R, Barbanti P, Colnaghi MI, Menard S, Clemente C, Rilke F (1984) Reactivity of monoclonal antibody with tissues and tumors from human breast. Am J Pathol 115: 47-56
38. MacKintosh FR, Bennett K, Hall SW (1985) Trials of staphylococcal protein A-treated plasma infusions in cancer therapy: clinical effects and implications for mode of action. In: Salinas FA, Hanna MG (eds) Immune complexes and human cancer. Plenum, New York, pp 239-256
39. MacKintosh FR, Bennett K, Schiff S, Hall SW (1983) Treatment of advanced malignancy with plasma perfused over staphylococcal protein A. West J Med 139: 36-42
40. McDougal SJ, Kennedy SM, Hubbard M, Browning SW, Tsang VCW, Winton EF, McDuffie FC (1986) Antigen detection in immune complexes by a modified staphylococci binding assay and Western blot analysis. Clin Immunol Immunopathol 38: 184-197
41. Mach JP, Chatal JT, Lumbroso JD, Buchegger F, Forni M, Ritschard J, Berche C, Dorillard JY, Carrel S, Herlyn M, Steplewski Z, Koprowski H (1983) Tumor localization in patients by radiolabelled monoclonal antibodies against colon carcinoma. Cancer Res 43: 5593-5600
42. Masserschmidt GH, Bowles CA, Henry DH, Deisseroth A (1984) Clinical trials with staphylococcus aureus and protein A in the treatment of malignant disease. J Biol Response Mod 3: 325-358
43. Masserschmidt GH, Bowles CA, Dean D, Parker M, Lester R, Dowling R, Holohan T, Osborn L, Schaff BF, McCormack K, Corbitt R, Phillip T, Glasstien E, Diesseroth A (1982) Phase II trial of *S. aureus* Cowan I immunoperfusion. Cancer Treat Rep 66: 2027-2031
44. Moldofsky PJ, Powe J, Mulhern CB, Hammond N, Sears HF, Gatenby RA, Steplewsky Z, Koprowsky H (1983) Metastatic colon carcinoma detected with radiolabelled $F(ab')_2$ monoclonal antibody fragments. Radiology 149: 549-555
45. Murray JL, Rosenblum MG, Lamki L, Haynie TP, Blen HJ, Plager CE, Unger MW, Carlo DJ, Hersh EM (1987) Radioimmunoimaging in malignant melanoma patients with the use of Indium-111-labelled antimelanoma monoclonal antibody (ZME-018) to high molecular-weight antigen. NCI Monogr 3: 3-9
46. Myers CD, Thorpe PE, Rose WC, Cumber AJ, Katz FE, Tax W, Greaves MF (1984) An immunotoxin with therapeutic potential in T cell leukemia: WT1-ricin A. Blood 63: 1178-1185
47. Nordquist RE, Schafer FB, Manning NE, Ishmael DR, Hoge AF (1977) Antitumor antibodies in human breast cancer sera as detected by fixed cell immunofluorescence assays. J Lab Clin Med 89: 257-261
48. Oldham RK (1983) Monoclonal antibodies in cancer therapy. J Clin Oncol 1: 582-590
49. Page DL, Dupond WD, Rogers LW, Rados MS (1984) Atypical hyperplastic lesions of the female breast: a long-term follow-up study. Cancer 55: 2698-2708
50. Papsidero LD, Croghan BA, O'Connell MJ, Valenzuela LA, Nemoto T, Ming Chu T (1983) Monoclonal antibodies (F32/22 and M7/105) to human mammary carcinoma. Cancer Res 43: 1741-1747
51. Papsidero LD, Nemoto T, Croghan BA, Ming Chu T (1984) Expression of ductal carcinoma antigen in breast cancer sera as defined using monoclonal antibody. Cancer Res 44: 4653-4657
52. Rainsbury RW, Westwood JM, King WJ, Grene GL (1983) The use of monoclonal antibodies to estrogen receptors (ER) for immunoperoxidase detection of ER in paraffin sections of human breast cancer tissue. J Histochem Cytochem 33: 67-92

53. Ray PK, Idiculla A, Mark R, Rhods JE, Thomas H, Bassett JG, Cooper DR (1982) Extracorporeal immunoadsorption of plasma from a metastatic colon carcinoma patient by protein A-containing nonviable *S. aureus*. Cancer 49: 1800-1809
54. Ray PK (1985) Immunosuppressor control as a modality of cancer treatment: effect of plasma adsorption with *Staphylococcus aureus* protein A. In: Salinas FA, Hanna MG (ed) Immune complexes and human cancer. Plenum, New York, pp 147-211
55. Rosen ST, Zimmer M, Goldman-Leikin R, Gordon LI, Kazikiewicz JM, Kaplan EH, Variakojis D, Marder RJ, Dykewicz MS, Piergies A, Silvertein EA, Rosnigk HH, Spies SM (1987) Radioimmunodetection and radioimmunotherapy of cutaneous T cell lymphomas using an ^{131}I-labelled monoclonal antibody: an Illinois Cancer Council Study. J Clin Oncol 5: 562-573
56. Salinas FA (1987) Advances towards clinical relevance of breast carcinoma associated antigens. In: Ceriani RL (ed) Immunological approaches to the diagnosis and therapy of breast cancer. Plenum, New York, pp 69-82
57. Salinas FA, Silver HK, Grossman L, Thomas JW (1981) Plasmaphoresis: A new approach in the management of advanced malignant melanoma. In: Serrou B, Rosenfeld C (eds) Immune complexes and plasma exchanges in cancer patients. Elsevier North-Holland, Amsterdam, pp 253-270
58. Salinas FA, Silver HK, Sheikh KM, Chandor SB (1978) Natural occurrence of human tumor associated antifetal antibodies during normal pregnancy. Cancer 42: 1653-1659
59. Salinas FA, Wee KH (1986) Prognostic and pathogenetic implications of immune complexes in human cancer. In: Ray PK (ed) Advances in immunity and cancer therapy. Springer-Verlag, New York, pp 189-209
60. Salinas FA, Wee KH, Ceriani RL (1986) Breast carcinoma associated antigens: role in benign and malignant breast disease (abstract). Proc Am Assoc Cancer Res 27: 325
61. Salinas FA, Wee KH, Ceriani RL (1987) Significance of breast carcinoma associated antigens as a monitor of tumor burden: characterization by monoclonal antibodies. Cancer Res 47: 907-913
62. Salinas FA, Wee KH, Ragaz J, Silver HK (1983) Correlation of tumor burden to antigen, antibody and immune complexes in breast carcinoma (abstract). Breast Cancer Res Treat 3: 303
63. Salinas FA, Wee KH, Ragaz J, Silver HK, Ceriani RL (1984) Analysis of differential expression of breast carcinoma associated antigens (BCAA) concentration in patients' sera (abstract). Proc Am Soc Clin Oncol 3: 49
64. Salinas FA, Wee KH, Silver HK (1981) Immune complexes and human neoplasia: detection and quantiation of circulating immune complexes by the fetal liver cell assay. Cancer Immunol Immunother 12: 11-19
65. Salinas FA, Wee KH, Silver HK (1984) Tumor burden and its relationship to antigen, size and composition of immune complexes. In: Peeters H (ed) 31st Colloquium Prot Biol Fluids. Pergamon, Oxford, pp 749-752
66. Salinas FA, Wee KH, Silver HK (1985) Clinical evidence of immune complexes, associated antigen and antibody in cancer. In: Salinas FA, Hanna MG (eds) Immune complexes and human cancer. Plenum, New York, pp 55-109
67. Sasaki M, Barber S, Ceriani RL (1985) Breast cancer markers: comparison between salyltransferase and human mammary epithelial antigens (HMEF-Ags) for the detection of human breast grafted in nude mice. Breast Cancer Res Treat 5: 51-56
68. Schroff RW, Woodhouse CS, Foon KA, Oldham RK, Farrel MM, Klein RA, Morgan AC (1985) Intratumor localization of monoclonal antibody in patients with melanoma treated with antibody to a 250, 000 dalton melanoma-associated antigen. J Natl Cancer Int 74: 299-306

69. Schlom SS (1986) Basic principles and applications of monoclonal antibodies in the management of carcinomas. Cancer Res 46: 3225-3228
70. Sears HF, Mattis J, Herlyn D, Stepewsky Z, Koprowsky H (1982) Phase I clinical trial of monoclonal antibody in treatment of gastrointestinal tumors. Lancet i: 762-765
71. Serrou B, Rosenfeld C (eds) (1981) Immune complexes and plasma exchanges in cancer patients. Elsevier-North Holland, Amsterdam
72. Siegel SS (1957) Nonparametric statistics for the behavioral sciences. McGraw-Hill, New York
73. Siroti M, Canegrati MA, Romano M, Vecchi A, Spreafico F (1984) Chemotherapy-increased antineoplastic effects of antibody-toxin conjugates. Cancer Treat Rep 68: 643-645
74. Sharkey RM, Primus FJ, Goldenberg DM (1984) Second antibody clearance of radiolabeled antibody in cancer immunodetection. Proc Natl Acad Sci USA 81: 2843-2846
75. Stahel RA, Mabry M, Skarin AT, Speak J, Bernal SD (1985) Detection of bone marrow metastasis in small cell lung cancer by monoclonal antibody. J Clin Oncol 3: 455-461
76. Statland BE, Winkel P, Burke MD, Golen RS (1979) Quantitative approaches used in evaluating laboratory measurements and other clinical data. In: Henry JB (ed) Clinical diagnosis and management by laboratory methods. Saunders, Philadelphia, pp 525-534
77. Taylor A, Milton W, Eyre H, Wu FP, Christian P, Alazraki N, Datz F, Unger MW (1987) Radioimmunodetection of human melanoma with indium-111-labelled monoclonal antibodies. NCI Monogr 3: 25-31
78. Taylor-Papadimitriou J, Peterson JA, Arkie J, Burchell J, Ceriani RL, Bodmer WF (1981) Monoclonal antibodies to epithelial-specific components of the human milk fat globule membrane: production and reaction with cells in tissue culture. Int J Cancer 28: 17-21
79. Terman DS, Young JB, Shearer WT, Ayus C, Matioli C, Lehane D, Espada R, Howell JF, Yamamoto T, Zeleski HI, Feldman L, Miller L, Frommer P, Tilquist R, Cook G, Daskal Y (1981) Preliminary observations of the effects on breast carcinoma of plasma perfused over immobilized protein A. N Engl J Med 305: 1195-1200
80. Thor A, Weeks MD, Schlom J (1986) Monoclonal antibodies and breast cancer. Sem Oncol 13: 939-410
81. Thurin J, Thurin M, Kimoto Y, Herlyn M, Lubeck MD, Elder DE, Smereczynska M, Karlsson KA, Clark WM, Stpewsky Z, Korowsky H (1987) Monoclonal antibody-defined correlations in melanoma between levels of Gd2 and Gd3 antigens and antibody cytotoxicity. Cancer Res 47: 1229-1233
82. Uhr JW (1984) Immunotoxins: harnessing nature's poisons. J Immunol 133: i-x
83. Unzeitig GW, Frankl G, Ackerman M, O'Connell X (1983) Analysis of the prognosis of minimal and occult breast cancers. Arch Surg 118: 1403-1404
84. Vitella Es, Krolick KA, Miyama-Inaba M, Crushley W, Uhr JW (1983) Immunotoxins: A new approach to cancer therapy. Science 219: 644-650
85. Wetman JK, Pedroso P, Johnson SA, Davignon D, Fast JD, Leone LA (1987) Rapid screening with indirect immunotoxin for monoclonal antibody against human cell lung cancer. Cancer Res 47: 5552-5556

General

Growth Regulation of Breast Cancer

D. Yee and M.E. Lippman

Medical Breast Cancer Section, Medicine Branch, National Cancer Institute, National Institutes of Health, Bethesda, MA 20892, USA

Introduction

The normal proliferation of breast epithelium at the time of puberty is dependent on increasing ovarian estrogen concentrations. Breast cancers also appear to be regulated by estrogens. Approximately 60% of metastatic breast tumors express estrogen receptors (ERs), and 50% of these can be treated effectively with hormonal manipulation. Risk factors for breast cancer include early menarche, nulliparity, increased height or weight, and late menopause, all suggestive that prolonged estrogen exposure unopposed by progesterone may be important in breast cancer development [122].

Although estrogens have been implicated as the most significant epidemiologic risk, clearly other factors have been linked to an increased risk of breast cancer. Racial differences, environmental factors, and dietary habits are associated with varying rates of breast cancer. Asian women have a lower incidence of breast cancer when compared with women in the United States, but this difference is substantially decreased in first-generation daughters raised in the United States, perhaps owing to dietary or environmental factors [124]. Dietary fat, hair dyes, and alcohol consumption have been linked to an increased incidence of breast cancer [131, 84, 171, 208, 141, 210]. These factors may be directly carcinogenic, however it is possible that they may act via direct or indirect estrogen effects. It also seems possible that other important growth-regulatory factors are perturbed by these environmental factors.

At the time of diagnosis, ERs cannot be found in 30%–40% of breast cancers and these are not growth regulated by hormonal manipulation. These ER-negative tumors are generally the more aggressive [24, 110, 130]. This observation is paralleled by studies performed on human breast cancer cells in vitro. Most cell lines have been established from metastatic sites, and some express the ER. Some of these ER+ lines require estrogen to survive in culture and to form tumors in athymic mice, and can be inhibited by antiestrogens [123, 145, 48, 37, 181, 119, 152, 105, 34]. Other cell lines are ER− and can grow in culture and in athymic mice without added estrogens. These cells cannot be growth inhibited by antiestrogens [65]. Presumably breast cancers, and cell lines derived from metastatic breast cancers, originally arose from normal breast epithelium that was growth responsive to estrogens. During the events that lead to malignant transformation, some cancers

Ragaz/Ariel (Eds.), High-Risk Breast Cancer

continue to be responsive to estrogens. However, other cancers lose this responsiveness, perhaps by constitutively expressing estrogen-induced growth-regulatory factors, or are transformed by events that bypass estrogen-induced pathways.

Therefore, estrogens are important in normal breast development and are implicated in the pathogenesis of breast cancer. Several hypotheses involving estrogens as a growth-regulatory factor in breast cancer can be made:

1. Estrogens directly stimulate growth of normal breast epithelium and cancer. Estrogens, either acting alone or in concert with other factors, can initiate and maintain the malignant phenotype. Estrogens stimulate transcription of genes that are important in maintenance of the malignant state.
2. Once cancer is established, estrogens continue to stimulate cell growth, in part via proteins that act in an autocrine or paracrine fashion to cause stimulation of quiescent cells and continued proliferation of cells that are already in cycle.
3. Hormone-responsive cancer may be converted to hormone-unresponsive cancer by constitutive expression of some of these autocrine or paracrine growth factors.
4. During normal breast development, breast epithelium reaches maturity, and does not continue to proliferate uncheked, despite continued systemic exposure to estrogen. This suggests that expression of negative regulatory factors may be important in establishement of the normal mammary gland. Estrogen stimulation may overwhelm or cause the loss of these negative regulatory factors.

Several model systems may be used to examine these hypotheses. Epidemologic studies in human populations have identified risk factors important in the development of breast cancers. Identifying a cause-and-effect relationship from these kinds of data, however, is impossible. Spontaneous breast cancers and chemically induced breast cancers can be studied in animal systems. Many basic observations on breast cancer regulation have been made in the rodent system. For example, rodent mammary cancer can be initiated by injections of methylnitrosourea (an alkylating agent) or by a single feeding of dimethylbenzanthracene (a polycyclic hydrocarbon). These tumors express ERs and respond to estrogens and antiestrogens in a fashion analogous to human cancer. Therefore, this carcinogen-induced system can be used to study the effects of pharmacologic agents, hormonal manipulation, and environmental factors on the growth of breast cancer. However, carcinogen-induced rodent breast cancers are predominantly prolactin dependent, while human cancers are generally estrogen dependent. While rodent breast cancers may be an extremely useful system to study, they may be in many aspects different from breast cancer development and growth regulation in the human [100, 205].

One way to identify and characterize the proposed growth factors and events is to examine the hormone-responsive and hormone-unresponsive human breast caner cell lines in vitro. With this system, many valid observations have been made on the growth regulation of breast cancer. However, there is variety of limitations to this system, and the results must be interpreted carefully. The breast cancer cell lines have been derived primarily from metastatic sites and carried in culture for many years. When the cells are first placed in culture most go through a "crisis" and the majority of cells die. The surviving cells are therefore a subclone of cells from the original cancer that have been selected for their ability to grow in vitro, and may not be representative of the growth characteristics of the entire tumor. It is also possible that prolonged tissue culture induces phenotypic and/or genotypic changes in the cell line. Although the cell lines vary in their ability to form tumors and to metastasize in the athymic mouse, they all possessed these characteristics in their human host. Therefore, it is likely that the biology of cell lines in culture is only an approximation of human tumor biology.

When a tumor is placed in culture, it is removed from its stromal influences. It is becoming increasingly clear that stromal factors modulate some aspects of the malignant and normal cell [75, 137]. For example, in the mouse system, isografting of fetal salivary mesenchyma into adult mammary glands resulted in the outgrowth of nodules that are morphologically similar to salivary glands. In addition, the salivary gland mesenchyma accelerated the formation of cancers induced by carcinogens or by virus [165]. These mesenchyma–epithelium interactions have also been demonstrated in the gastrointestinal tract. Mouse stomach epithelia grown in contact with intestinal mesenchyma in an intact animal causes the stomach to take on many characteristics of the normal intestinal epithelium [164]. Therefore, it is clear that stromal factors influence the development of their overlying epithelium, and these interactions cannot be studied in a culture system utilizing only malignant epithelium.

Despite these caveats, the in vitro tissue culture system can be utilized to isolate malignant human breast cancer cells and examine their growth regulation. This chapter will review some of the steroidal and polypeptide growth-regulatory factors, as well as potential therapeutic benefits based on manipulation of these factors.

Estrogen and Estrogen Receptor

The effects of estrogen are mediated through the intracellular ERs [184, 97]. ERs are localized in the nucleus and exist there in both unoccupied and occupied forms [215, 61, 108, 206]. When the receptor binds to its ligand, the complex probably interacts with DNA and chromatin, but this interaction is poorly understood [149, 11]. Recent cDNA cloning of the ER from MCF-7 show that the putative DNA-binding region of the ERs shares strong homology with glucocorticoid and thyroid hormone receptors, the latter of which is the cellular homolog of an acutely transforming avian erythroblastosis virus (v-*erb*-A) [202, 73, 74].

Through the interaction of estrogen with its receptor, a large variety of biochemical events are induced. Estrogen is a mitogen for breast cancer cells and many enzymes involved in DNA synthesis are induced, including DNA polymerase, thymidine and uridine kinases, thymidylate synthetase, carbamyl phosphate synthetase, aspartate transcarbamylase, dihydroorotase, and dihydrofolate reductase [62, 3, 4]. There is evidence that both thymidine kinase and dihydrofolate reductase are regulated at the mRNA level [45, 103]. The net effect of these induced enzymes is to stimulate DNA synthesis as measured by thymidine incorporation [2], by both de novo and scavenger pathways.

Estrogens also cause an induction of secreted peptides, including some well-characterized proteins such as plasminogen activator and collagenolytic enzymes [35, 101]. Induced proteases and collagenases may be important in allowing the cancer to digest its surrounding stroma, thereby increasing the cancer's invasive and metastatic potential. It also seem possible that the proteases serve to process growth factor precursors (such as prepro-IGF-I) or to release other growth factors from their binding protein.

Estrogens also increase the expression of laminin receptor on the surface of the hormone-responsive cell line MCF-7. Laminin is a component of the basement membrane and laminin receptors mediate the attachment of the cells to the basement membrane. This interaction is likely to be important in invasion of the cancer. Estrogen-treated cells showed greater binding to laminin, increased migration toward laminin, a greater ability to proliferate in an artificial basement membrane matrix, and an increased ability to traverse an artificial basement membrane [6]. Estrogens induce changes in the cytoskeleton and adhesion structures of breast cancer cells as well as cell ruffling, as noted by scanning electron microscopy [168]. These findings suggest that estrogen can induce increased cell-basement membrane interactions with a resultant increase in invasiveness.

Other secreted proteins are less well characterized, but include a 24 K dalton protein described by McGuire [41, 1], 52 K and 160 K dalton glycoproteins described by Rochefort [207, 157], a 39 K dalton glycoprotein complex [32], and a 7 K dalton protein [95] identified by Chambon by analyzing estrogen-induced mRNA species (pS2). The 52 K dalton glycoprotein appears to have cathepsin D-like activity and is mitogenic for MCF-7; it will be discussed in a later section [36, 199, 157]. The level of expression of the 24 K dalton protein correlates well with the presence of ER [1], however its function is not known. The pS2 expression is restricted to breast cancer cells, and its transcription is induced by estrogens in MCF-7, although it does not share nucleotide sequence homology with other estrogen-responsive genes [38]. The functions of the 160 K, 39 K, and 7 K dalton proteins are not understood. However, expression of the 160 K and 7 K dalton proteins is not tightly coupled to growth regulation as suggested by experiments with antiestrogen-resistant MCF-7 clones [30, 33]. In these cells, the two proteins are equally decreased by antiestrogen in both antiestrogen-sensitive and antiestrogen-insensitive cells. In addition, both proteins are induced by estrogen in an MCF-7 variant that is growth arrested by estrogen [49]. Therefore, the expression of these proteins is regulated by estrogen, but it does not appear that this regulation is important in the regulation of growth.

Although estrogens induce a plethora of effects in breast cancer cells, it is not clear which, if any, of these are the proximal event in malignant transformation, or if the events are critical to the maintenance or progression of the malignant phenotype. One experimental approach to this problem utilizes isolation and characterization of estrogen-induced factors in a defined serum-free in vitro system. This has produced some evidence which suggests that hormones other than estrogens are also important in growth regulation. First, many other trophic substances can be growth-stimulatory for breast cancer in culture, and their specific receptors are expressed. These include glucocorticoids, androgens, progestins, thyroid hormone, vitamin D, retinoids, epidermal growth factor, insulin-like growth factor I and II, calcitonin, and prolactin [121, 63, 71, 136]. Second, the initial growth rate of breast cancer cells in culture is proportional to the number of cells plated, suggesting that these cells may produce autostimulatory substances [94]. Third, in vitro estrogen-dependent cell lines can be made to grow without estrogen if the medium is supplemented with optimal concentrations of other growth hormones or conditioned media from estrogen-treated cells [92, 58, 200]. Fourth, in vivo estrogen does not have to be systemically released to be effective. When athymic mice are injected with human breast cancer cells that require estrogen for tumor formation, estrogen released locally from a pellet can substitute for systemic estrogen [90]. This suggests that tumor formation does not necessarily require systemically derived estrogen-induced growth factors. One interpretation of this experiment is that locally released estrogen stimulates the production of autocrine or paracrine growth factors. If these factors are indeed secreted by the breast cancer cells in response to estrogen, then it would be possible to isolate them from media conditioned by isolated cells.

For these reasons, our laboratory has examined serum-free conditioned medium from MCF-7 cells in order to identify proteins secreted by the cells in response to estrogen [7]. When this medium is harvested, filtered, dialyzed against 1 *M* acetic acid, lyophilized, and reconstituted in phosphate-buffered saline, 99.98% of the estrogen is removed. The medium however remains growth-stimulatory in vitro. Concentrated medium infused into ovariectomized athymic mice can partially replace estrogen in causing tumor formation by MCF-7. This effect is probably not due to estrogen, as the uterine weights of the mice did not change. The tumors induced by conditioned medium were smaller than those stimulated by estrogen, and tended to regress, while those that were estrogen-stimulated continued to grow in size [60].

These observations suggest that conditioned medium contains factors other than estrogen that can stimulate tumor formation. Column chromatography and radioimmunoassay have shown that a variety of polypeptide hormones are secreted into the media, including IGF-I-related activity, TGF-α, PDGF, and TGF-β. These and other factors will be discussed in the next few sections.

Transforming Growth Factor α

TGF-α is a 7 K dalton polypeptide protein initially isolated from fibroblasts transformed by Moloney murine sarcoma virus [52]. The murine form shares 40% amino acid homology with epidermal growth factor, and both EGF and TGF-α apparently act through EGF receptor, as media conditioned by murine sarcoma virus-transformed cells will compete with ^{125}I-labeled EGF for binding to a common cell surface receptor [126, 125, 188, 53, 56]. Normal rat fetal tissues, placenta, and bovine anterior pituitary produce TGF-α [185, 155, 129, 193, 111]. The normal functions of TGF-α and EGF are similar. They are both mitogenic for human epidermal cells and fibroblasts, cause precocious eyelid opening in newborn mice, and cause cell ruffling [53, 127]. However TGF-α is a more potent mediator of bone resorption, calcium release from bone, and neovascularization than EGF [173, 91].

TGF-α is synthesized as a 19 K dalton transmembrane precursor protein and inserted into the endoplasmic reticulum. While there, the molecule is cleaved by proteases in several different sites to release mature TGF-α into the secretory vesicles to be released into the extracellular space. Glycosylation also occurs in the endoplasmic reticulum, but it is unclear if this is important in secretion. Because of the differential protease cleavage and glycosylation, a larger glycosylated form and a smaller species can be found in conditioned media. The intracellular portion is palmitoylated and stays associated with the plasma membrane, its function may be to serve as an anchor for the entire protein [29].

Several human tumors have been reported to express TGF-α [169, 57, 54], and TGF-α activity can be found in the urine and serum of cancer patients [175, 106, 192, 107]. TGF-α cDNA, under the influence of SV40 promotor, can transform murine fibroblasts and cause tumor formation in athymic mice (this occurs presumably because of the creation of an autocrine loop) [159]. However, anti-EGF receptor antibodies have been unable to block growth of a TGF-α-secreting melanoma line [114]. This may be due to the low level of EGF receptor expression on the surface of these cells.

TGF-α activity can be assayed by its ability, together with TGF-β, to cause anchorage-independent growth in normal rat kidney (NRK) cells. [189] Conditioned media obtained from estrogen-treated MCF-7 and other breast cancers contain TGF-α activity in the NRK assay [167, 147, 197]. MCF-7 acid-treated conditioned medium contains two principal peaks of activity that correspond to 30 K and 7 K dalton species. Each of the peaks contains TGF-α activity as determined by NRK colony assay. Radioreceptor assay with A431 squamous carcinoma cells, a rich source of EGF receptor, shows that conditioned media from estrogen-treated MCF-7 cells produce binding activity. In addition, a radioimmunoassay using a TGF-α-specific antibody demonstrates the presence of the ligand in conditioned media. Immunoprecipitation with a polyclonal antibody of metabolically labeled conditioned media shows that there are multiple immunoreactive species at 30 K dalton, and these species are lost when incubated with unlabeled 7 K dalton TGF-α. However, the 30 K dalton form is significantly larger than the mature purified human 7 K dalton species or the 17 K–19 K dalton precursor protein. It is unclear if this 30 K dalton protein represents a product obtained by alternative mRNA splicing, posttranscriptional modification, or perhaps a novel TGF-α-related protein [13].

Estrogen treatment induces the 30 K dalton protein in the ER+ lines MCF-7, T47-D, and ZR-75-1 by 2- to 8-fold, depending on the culture conditions [13]. The induction of TGF-α by estrogen has been confirmed by radioreceptor assay [12].

The 4.8 kilobase (kb) mRNA species is found in MCF-7 and some other breast cancer cell lines. There is also a less abundant 1.6 kb message of uncertain origin. The mRNA abundance is increased 2-6-fold by estrogen in ER cell lines. This induction occurs as early as 6 h after estrogen exposure and remains stable over 6 days. ER- cell lines also express the mRNA although the message was undetectable in the carcinosarcoma cell line, Hs578T. In vivo estrogen regulation of mRNA levels has been shown with MCF-7 xenografts implanted in nude mice. Withdrawal of estrogen in this system causes a decrease in the TGF-α message. After withdrawal for 10 days, mRNA levels were 2.5-fold less than in estrogen-treated MCF-7 xenografts. mRNA obtained from human breast cancer shows that 70% of specimens contain detectable message. This did not apparently correlate with ER status [12, 14]. Normal rapidly proliferating breast epithelial cells also express TGF-α, while nonproliferating tissue expresses low levels. This suggests that TGF-α is important in proliferation of both normal and malignant tissue [197].

Since TGF-α probably acts via EGF receptor, it seems possible that TGF-α-EGF receptor interactions could be the basis for an autocrine loop. The EGF receptor is a 170 K dalton glycoprotein that, like other growth factor receptors, has tyrosine kinase activity in its intracellular domain [44, 196]. It has been detected in human and rodent breast cancer biopsies, malignant cell lines, and normal cells [66, 50, 144]. Antibodies directed against EGF receptor can cause a decrease in MCF-7 estrogen-stimulated monolayer growth during the first 5 days of treatment. This inhibition, however, is lost with longer culture intervals; it is also lost when TGF-α is added to the anti-EGF receptor antibody. Anti-TGF-α antibody can inhibit MCF-7 colony formation.

Therefore, some breast cancers and breast cancer cell lines secrete a 30 K dalton protein that has TGF-α-like activity and EGF receptor is expressed in these cell lines. Tumors, tumor cell lines, and normal breast epithelial cell lines express TGF-α mRNA. Estrogen regulates mRNA level and subsequent protein secretion in the ER + MCF-7 cell line. Since these cell lines also express low levels of EGF receptor, one interpretation of the data is that TGF-α behaves as an estrogen-induced autocrine growth factor for breast cancer. However, the interruption of this putative autocrine loop by anti-TGF-α antibody and anti-EGF receptor antibody is not completely growth-inhibitory, implying the existence of other factors important in growth regulation. In addition, normal proliferating breast epithelium expresses high levels of TGF-α mRNA. There is also no consistent relationship between expression of TGF-α mRNA and ER in tumors. However, EGF has been linked to tumor progression in a variety of model systems.

In mice that have a high incidence of spontaneous breast tumors, removal of the submandibular glands (a rich source of EGF) reduces the rate of tumor formation [115]. It is also possible that TGF-α is a paracrine factor secreted by surrounding stromal tissue to stimulate growth of the cancer. It is interesting to note that TGF-α and EGF have been isolated from human milk [148, 216]. It appears that TGF-α can regulate the growth of breast cancer cells in vivo, although the precise mechanisms remain to be defined.

Insulin-like Growth Factors

Insulin-like growth fctors (IGF-I and IGF-II) represent two members of a family that have similar biologic activities: stimulation of sulfate incorporation into cartilage, insulin-like activity, and mitogenic activity. They are closely related to insulin, with similar A and B domains, and have 47% identity with insulin [15, 20].

There is an analogous c domain, but this length is different in IGF-I and IGF-II and, unlike insulin, is not excised from the mature form found in the circulation. IGF-I and IGF-II share 60% amino acid homology [213]. IGF-I is expressed primarily in adult liver and fibroblasts, but immunoreactive IGF-I can be found in human milk and semen [18, 17, 47, 172]. In situ hybridization of human fetal tissues with oligonucleotide probes demonstrates hybridization in many tissues of mesenchymal origin. IGF-II is primarily expressed in fetal tissue and is thought to be the primary mediator of fetal growth; its role in the adult is not entirely clear [77]. In serum, both IGF-I and IGF-II are complexed with binding proteins that render them biologically inactive [139, 23].

IGF-I acts through a receptor analogous to the insulin receptor; that is, a heterotetramer with two extracellular α-chains and two β-chains that span the cell membrane. The β-chains have tyrosine kinase activity. Although IGF-I and IGF-II are homologous polypeptides, it is surprising that the putative IGF-II receptor is quite dissimilar. The IGF-II receptor is a single polypeptide chain and, unlke several other growth factor receptors, is not a tyrosine kinase. Either ligand can bind to either receptor, although the affinity for their own receptor is higher. IGF-I and IGF-II can also bind to insulin receptor, but with a much lower affinity [150, 195].

Both IGF-I and IGF-II have been cloned from liver libraries. The IGF-I cDNA probe hybridizes with as many as six different length mRNA species in both tumor and normal tissues. The IGF-II probe hybridizes weakly with a single 5.3 kb message in liver, but size differences have been reported in different tissues and tumors [20, 96, 161, 19].

Breast cancer cell lines have IGF-I receptor [71], and authentic IGF-I stimulates monolayer growth in these cells [87]. Immunoreactive IGF-I activity can be found in media conditioned by several breast cancer cell lines. The highest levels of activity are in the estrogen-unresponsive cell lines. Normal IGF-I is a 7.6 K dalton protein, but it is tightly associated with serum-binding proteins, increasing the size of the protein to 150 K–200 K dalton. After acid gel filtration of conditioned media, the size of the complex is 30 K–50 K dalton, and this is significantly larger than mature IGF-I. However, after acid/ethanol extraction, conditioned media contain a substance that comigrates within a fraction of authentic IGF-I on column chromatography. Immunoreactive IGF-I secretion in MCF-7 is induced 2- to 3-fold by estrogen [87, 16]. EGF, TGF-α, and insulin also stimulate immunoreactive IGF-I production in these cells. Cycloheximide will block estrogen-induced increases in immunoreactive IGF-I, suggesting that estrogen induces de novo synthesis of immunoreactive IGF-I [88, 89].

Poly-A-selected RNA hybridized to IGF-I cDNA probe yields a pattern that reveals multiple species of RNA, but a 300 base pairs message is similar to that seen in human liver [87]. Estrogen does not appear to increase the level of IGF-I message [89]. Other cancers that have been reported to produce IGF-I included colon, hemangiosarcoma, liposarcoma, and lung [132, 190]. Because of the multiple transcript sizes noted, it is not entirely clear if breast cancer, or any other cancers, secrete authentic IGF-I or a closely related polypeptide hormone.

The predominant form of IGF-II that exists in the serum is 7.6 K dalton, however, a 10 K dalton form also exists [78, 80]. The 10 K dalton form has been found in cerebrospinal fluid, amniotic fluid, pituitary, and brain. IGF-II cDNA hybridizes to mRNA form normal adult granulosa cells of the ovary, liver, and brain, while many fetal tissues seem to produce IGF-II. Some human cancers, including colon cancer, liposarcoma, rhabdomyosarcoma, Wilms' tumor, hepatoblastoma, and pheochromocytoma, have been reported to express IGF-II [190, 79, 151, 174].

There is some evidence that IGF-II may be expressed in human breast cancer. Some breast cancer cell lines bind IGF-II in a fashion suggesting that IGF-II receptor may be present on these cells, additionally IGF-II stimulates thymidine incorporation in these cells [85]. IGF-II stimulates the proliferation of T47D cells in culture and allows tumor formation in the athymic mouse. T47D also contains mRNA for IGF-II [85, 146]. It is possible that these effects are due to the ability of IGF-II to stimulate IGF-I receptor. Work from our laboratory suggests that authentic IGF-II is expressed in some breast cancer cell lines and tumors [212].

Therefore, hormone responsive and unresponsive cell lines secrete an IGF-I, and perhaps an IGF-II, like material. In hormone responsive cell lines, the IGF-I secretion can be increased by estrogen treatment. Recent evidence suggests that factors can be isolated from human platelets and uterine tissue by Bio-Gel P-10 chromatography and reverse phase HPLC that can stimulate cultured estrogen receptor positive MCF-7 cells. These factors have had their partial amino acid sequence determined, and found to share homology with IGF-I and IGF-II, yet appear to be truncated IGFs or fragments of unique polypeptides. They are also 10 to 100 times more potent than authentic IGF-I [102, 142]. Therefore the evidence suggests that IGFs are likely important factors in the growth regulation of breast cancer, however the exact species of IGF remains to be defined.

Platelet-Derived Growth Factor

PDGF was originally isolated from the α-granules of blood platelets, and is known to be a mitogen as well as a chemotactic factor for fibroblasts and smooth muscle cells [9]. PDGF exists as a dimer with two polypeptide subunits, PDGF-A and PDGF-B, and is active as a heterodimer or homodimer [203, 99, 8]. PDGF, in fibroblast systems, is a "competency factor" and allows density-arrested fibroblasts to enter a new wave of DNA synthesis. Once stimulated, the cell can become responsive to "progression factors," such as IGF-I and EGF, and can continue traversing the cell cycle [160, 162b]. PDGF-B chain is the cellular homolog of a viral oncogene, v-*sis* of simian sarcoma virus, which is transforming in fibroblasts [203, 98, 118]. PDGF expression has been noted in a variety of cultured tumors, most notably in sarcomas and gliomas [22, 82, 140]. PDGF acts through its receptor, which is a tyrosine kinase [64, 211]. However, in many human tumors, the number of receptors is lower than that in normal cells, suggesting that in those malignancies, there is a downregulation of PDGF receptor. Alternatively, PDGF receptors are internalized as the cell is stimulated [86, 83]. Since PDGF receptor cannot be found in some human tumors, PDGF may act primarily on the stroma as a paracrine factor. However, in fibroblast systems PDGF-specific antibody will inhibit proliferation and transformation. This suggests that PDGF can act as an autocrine growth factor [160]. However, in some instances PDGF is apparently not secreted by the cell, but remains associated with the membrane. This may suggest that PDGF can transform without release into the medium [153]. In these instances, PDGF-specific antibodies may not inhibit proliferation. Treatment of fibroblasts with PDGF can also stimulate the secretion of other growth factors, such as IGF-I [42].

Breast cancer cell lines secrete PDGF-related substance that can stimulate growth of mouse fibroblasts in platelet-poor plasma. Immunoprecipitation of metabolically labeled MCF-7 and MDA-MB-231 demonstrates a 28 K and 14 K dalton protein in both cellular extracts and conditioned media. When this protein is eluted from nonreducing gels, its activity is blocked with PDGF-specific antiserum. mRNA isolated from both cell lines detects PDGF-A and PDGF-B message, and estrogen treatment of MCF-7 increases both A- and B-chain mRNA [31, 81, 163, 21]. However, PDGF receptor has not been found in human breast cancer cells.

Although in several model systems PDGF is thought to represent an autocrine growth factor, it is not clear that PDGF acts this way in breast cancer. In breast cancer, the evidence suggests that PDGF may act as an estrogen-regulated paracrine growth factor. In this model, PDGF produced by breast cancer would stimulate surrounding fibroblasts and perhaps other stromal tissues. This would lead to proliferation, and possibly release of other growth factors by the stromal tissues that would stimulate growth of the cancer.

Transforming Growth Factor *β*

TGF-*β* was originally described as a factor stimulating the anchorage-independent growth of non-transformed AKR-2B and NRK cells; however, TGF-*α* or EGF must also be present to stimulate NRK cells [183, 135, 154]. TGF-*β* is distinguished from TGF-*α* because it does not compete with EGF for receptor binding, and later isolation of the cDNA showed different nucleotide sequences [55]. TGF-*β* is composed of two 12 K dalton chains linked by disulfide bonds, and recent evidence suggests that there may be two different porcine TGF-*β* chains that can form two homodimers or a heterodimer, giving rise to TGF-*β*1, TGF-*β*2, and TGF-*β* 1.2. There are likely three cell surface receptors for TGF-*β*, 280 K, 65 K, and 85 K dalton [40]. TGF-*β* is an unusual growth factor; in some systems it is stimulatory, but in other systems it appears to be growth-inhibitory [191, 156]. It has been suggested that these different properties relate to the type of TGF-*β* receptor–ligand interaction. Specifically, stimulation of the 280 K dalton receptor by TGF-*β*1 or TGF-*β*2 generates a growth-inhibitory signal. The function of the lower molecular weight receptors is uncertain [40, 128]. TGF-*β* has also been shown to be involved in the processes of normal development and wound healing, it seems likely that these effects may be mediated through more than one receptor–ligand interaction [128].

TGF-β is growth-inhibitory for breast cancer cells, and breast cancer cells secrete TGF-β into the media. Concentrated conditioned media obtained from MCF-7 breast cancer cells together with EGF cause anchorage-independent growth of NRK cells. Serial dilution of the conditioned media gave a response curve parallel to one obtained from authentic platelet-derived TGF-β. Radioreceptor assays show that material from conditioned media binds competitively with authentic TGF-β to the A549 lung carcinoma cell, and the displacement curve of conditioned media is similar to that of TGF-β. Immunoprecipitation of conditioned media shows that the material comigrates with authentic TGF-β. When this material is acid-dialyzed and fractionated by gel exclusion chromatography, a high and low molecular weight activity is seen that is identical in size to acid-dialyzed TGF-β. mRNA obtained from MCF-7 expresses an expected single-sized 2. 5 kb message. These data confirm that MCF-7 produces authentic TGF-β [55, 109].

In MCF-7 cells, the production of TGF-β is coupled to hormonally controlled growth regulation. Secretion of TGF-β is enhanced by growth-inhibitory antiestrogens and dexamethasone, while growth-stimulatory insulin and estradiol decrease secretion. In an antiestrogen-resistant MCF-7 variant, this increase in production of TGF-β can no longer be seen, suggesting that the level of TGF-β in conditioned media is coupled to growth regulation. Increased production of TGF-β by antiestrogens appears to be mediated via the ER. Increasing amounts of estrogen added to antiestrogen decrease the amount of TGF-β production, suggesting that competition for the ER by an agonist will reverse the antiestrogen binding and decrease TGF-β production. The mechanism of increased TGF-β production is likely to be posttranscriptional, as estrogen and antiestrogen treatment do not change the level of TGF-β mRNA in Northern or slot-blot analysis. The intracellular pools of TGF-β are not altered by hormone stimulation as the amount of immunofluorescent TGF-β does not change with hormonal treatment. Degradation of secreted TGF-β does not appear to be altered either, as radiolabeled TGF-β added to conditioned media is not digested after 6 h [109].

TGF-β can also regulate the growth of estrogen-unresponsive cell lines. Receptor for TGF-β can be detected on all cell lines. Monolayer growth of MDA-MB-231, an ER negative and highly tumorigenic cell line, can be inhibited by TGF-β or by conditioned media obtained from antiestrogen-treated MCF-7. Use of high density MCF-7 as a feeder layer for MDA-MB-231 inhibits anchorage-independent colony formation by 20%, and when antiestrogens are added, the inhibition is doubled. Antiestrogen treatment of MDA-MB-231 alone does not cause growth inhibition. These effects are primarily due to TGF-β, as antibody directed against TGF-β can restore normal growth in MDA-MB-231 treated with conditioned media from MCF-7 [109].

In summary, TGF-β secretion by an ER cell line is under hormonal control. A hormone-unresponsive cell line also has high affinity receptors for TGF-β. However, unlike TGF-α or IGF-related protein, TGF-β appears to be a negative growth regulator, and may act in an autocrine or paracrine fashion. The overall growth of breast cancer may therefore be under the control of both positive and negative autocrine/paracrine factors.

52 K Dalton Protein

Rochefort and colleagues have identified a 52 K dalton protein that is secreted into the culture media of ER+ cell lines [157]. This protein has been purified to homogeneity and is a cathepsin D-like protease bearing mannose-6-phosphate signals. The protein can be taken up by MCF-7 cells and processed into a 34 K dalton protein. Purified 52 K dalton protein is growth-stimulatory, and may account for 40% of the mitogenic effects of estrogen [36, 199]. It is increased by estrogen stimulation of the ER+ cell lines, and this is accompanied by an increase in its mRNA levels. It is constitutively synthesized by ER− cell lines. It appears to degrade proteoglycan and extracellular matrix. Clinical studies suggest that its expression correlates with poor patient outcome and with the presence of lymph node metastases [157].

However, the role of 52 K dalton protein in growth regulation is not entirely clear. In some antiestrogen-resistant cell variants, 52 K dalton protein is inducible by tamoxifen [49]. In other antiestrogen-resistant MCF-7 clones, decreased level of the protein is seen when treated with antiestrogens, yet cell growth is not inhibited [30, 33]. This suggests that the 52 K dalton protein is regulated by estrogen, but may not be important in the regulation of cell growth.

Mammary Tumor-Derived Growth Factor

Human mammary tumor-derived growth factor (h. MTGF) has been purified from human breast cancers and is a heat- and acid-labile 16 K dalton protein. It is mitogenic for human foreskin fibroblasts and some human breast cancer cell lines. It has been suggested that h. MTGF has an affinity for heparin, and it may act as a stimulant for both epithelial cells and stromal elements [162a]. Of note is that h. MTGF may belong to the family of fibroblast growth factors (FGF). These factors are of similar molecular size (16 K–18 K dalton) and bind heparin. FGF has been isolated from many tissues, particularly from the brain and from neural tissues. FGFs are mitogenic for fibroblasts and vascular endothelial cells and are thought to be angiogenic factors [67, 133]. Therefore, h.MTGF may be an angiogenic factor for breast cancer, allowing neovascularization of the solid breast cancer.

Autocrine Motility Factor

Other factors may act to increase the metastatic potential of breast cancer. Autocrine motility factor (AMF) is a 55 K dalton protein isolated from a human melanoma cell line. AMF is a chemotactic protein for tumor cells and is not an attractant for neutrophils. It stimulates the random motility of the producer cells and binds to the cell membrane. It is not known to be related to any other peptides, and its activity cannot be replaced or blocked by EGF or TGF-β. *ras*-transformed NIH3T3 cells produce large amounts of AMF and can also respond to the factor [120].

AMF has also been isolated from the human breast cancer cell line MDA-MB-435. AMF produced by MDA-MB-435 stimulates the random motility of the producer cells. This is accompanied by alterations in cell shape and pseudopodia extension. These pseudopodia express laminin and fibronectin recognition receptors at a 20-fold greater concentration than plasma membrane from unstimulated cells [76]. Therefore, besides growth-regulatory peptides, breast cancer cells produce autocrine factors that lead to increased motility and potentially increased invasiveness.

Other Factors

Mammary-derived growth factor (MDGF-I) is a 62 K dalton protein that has been purified from human milk. MDGF-I can also be found in conditioned media from human breast cancer cell lines and in extracts prepared from biopsies of breast cancer [10]. Its effect on NRK cells is to increase collagen synthesis. MDGF-I is mitogenic for mouse mammary cells, and also increases the synthesis of collagen and laminin. In ovariectomized mice, MDGF-I and estrogens act synergistically to increase growth in ductal and alveolar cells. MDGF-I may be important in causing deposition of collagen by stromal cells in the early development of breast cancer [166].

Growth factors mediate their effects through their receptors, so regulation of receptor is likely to be important in growth regulation. EGF receptor is expressed in greater numbers in ER—cell lines, and these lines are not responsive to estrogens. This increase in expression is in part due to increased transcription in these cell lines. There is no evidence for gene amplification. The significance of the inverse relationship between ER level and EGF receptor level is still unclear; however, it is possible that the two receptors interact in some fashion [50]. A homologous oncogene (*neu*, c-*erb*-B2, HER2) has been found in breast cancer, and amplification of this gene has been correlated with advanced disease and poor patient outcome in several studies [177,.198, 43]. It seems probable that c-*erb*-B2 codes for a growth factor receptor; however, the nature of its ligand has not yet been determined.

Other investigators have found that human serum is inhibitory to the growth of ER+ human breast cancer in culture. The cell lines T47–DA8 and C7MCF7–173 are dependent on estrogen to form tumors in athymic mice, yet estrogen added to serum-free conditioned media does not accelerate their growth. These cell lines are inhibited by addition of 10% charcoal–dextran-stripped human female serum. This serum inhibition is concentration dependent. Similar inhibitory activity is seen in charcoal–dextran-stripped fetal bovine serum. This inhibition can be overcome by adding estrogen to the culture media, and androgens, glucocorticoids, and progestins do not alter the inhibition. This inhibitory activity is reversed by very low (3×10^{-11}M) concentrations of estradiol, suggesting that the inhibitory activity is not simply due to estrogen-binding proteins [180, 28, 179]. It is possible that these effects are due to TGF-β, but further characterization of these inhibitory factors may yield new negative regulatory factors.

Establishment of Estrogen Independence

The preceding sections have dealt with growth factors that are secreted by the cell, and some of these factors (TGF-α, IGF-I-related peptide, TGF-β, 52 K dalton protein) have already been shown to be regulated by estrogen. It is clear that not all human breast cancers respond to estrogen, and many clinical samples do not have ER. As proposed in the introduction, estrogen may act as an important proximal step in the generation of cancer, however maintenance of the malignant phenotype may bypass estrogen-related events. Constitutive expression of previously estrogen-regulated growth factors could be one way to maintain malignancy.

Our laboratory has performed calcium phosphate transfection of v-Ha-*ras* into the estrogen-responsive cell line, MCF-7 to examine the events associated with estrogen-independent tumor growth [104]. The cellular homolog of v-Ha-*ras* is c-Ha-*ras* and is activated in a variety of human tumors [204, 186]. In breast cancer, however, there is not consistent evidence for c-Ha-*ras* activation or amplification. In the carcinosarcoma cell line Hs578T, c-Ha-*ras* has been found to be activated by point mutation (codon 12) while a cell line derived from the normal breast elements of the same patient did not display this mutation. However, other studies of DNA-extracted from tumor tissue have demonstrated an allelic loss of the c-Ha-*ras* locus without evidence of mutation, gene rearrangement, or amplification, and this is associated with *ras* expression at the mRNA level [113, 72, 187, 43]. In the rat, formation of tumors by nitrosomethylurea causes tumors with point mutations in the Ha-*ras* locus [214]. It seems possible that Ha-*ras* activation may be a common feature of breast cancer, but has not yet been detected. Recent work in other cancer systems suggests that in order to define point mutations in *ras*, techniques more sensitive than those applied thus far to breast cancer must be used [26, 68, 27].

The protein product of v-Ha-*ras* is p21, which is bound to the inner surface of the plasma membrane and is a weak GTPase. GTPases are important in signal transduction of receptor–ligand interactions, and it is thought that activated *ras* reduces the level of GTPase activity, thereby allowing continued stimulation by GTP [182]. The p21 *ras* protein has been detected in malignant and benign breast tissue [143].

MCF-7 cells stably transfected with v-Ha-*ras* lose much of their estrogen requirement for growth. MCF-7*ras* is tumorigenic in 85% of inoculated castrated female nude mice, while the parent MCF-7 has an absolute requirement for estrogen in this system [104]. MCF-7*ras* secretes 3 to 5-fold more TGF-α, immunoreactive IGF-I, and TGF-β than the nontransformed parent line. Conditioned medium from MCF-7*ras* was mitogenic for the parent MCF-7. There is no change in PDGF production. MCF-7*ras* still expresses ER, and quantities of EGF receptor and IGF-I receptor are not significantly changed. MCF-7*ras* also expresses laminin receptor at a level comparable to estrogen-stimulated cells, and is more invasive in vitro [6]. MCF-7 *ras* is less responsive to estrogen, TGF-α, or IGF-I [59].

These data suggest that introduction of an oncogene product into an estrogen-responsive cell line can stimulate tumorigenesis without further estrogen stimulation. This increase in tumorigenesis is accompanied by an increased constitutive production of several polypeptide growth factors. This suggests that agents other than estrogen can be growth-regulatory, and estrogen can be bypassed entirely in this model system. It is possible that establishment of estrogen independence in vivo may be due to further, as yet undefined, oncogene activation.

Therapeutic Implications

By understanding factors involved in the growth regulation of breast cancer, perhaps more rational therapeutic agents can be designed. The use of antiestrogens to exploit the estrogen dependence of some breast cancers is an example of designing treatment strategies based on observations of the biology of breast cancer. In this chapter several potential growth-promoting and growth-inhibiting factors have been outlined. It has been proposed that some of these factors act as autocrine or paracrine stimuli. Interruption of a potential autocrine loop could modulate breast cancer growth.

The most direct method of interrupting an autocrine loop would be to synthesize a pharmacologic agent that binds to, but does not stimulate, the receptor, as has been done with the antiestrogens. An "anti-IGF" or "anti-TGF-α" agent could compete with the authentic growth factor for the receptor to cause a decrease in receptor-stimulated second messages. However, synthesizing a polypeptide that could remain stable in serum may be difficult, owing to the many serum proteases. In addition, many normal cells express IGF or EGF receptor, and interference with normal receptor function may have unforeseen consequences.

By characterizing the growth factors involved in breast cancer, it may also be possible to synthesize a fusion protein consisting of a toxin coupled to a growth factor. Since many receptor–ligand complexes are internalized within the cell, this would allow the toxin a specific access to the cell which it would not have normally. Current in vitro work is proceeding with EGF and TGF-α coupled to *Pseudomonas* exotoxin or ricin A chain [5, 39]. Identifying specific breast cancer growth factors could lead to similar fusion proteins that would be directed against the tumor.

Interfering with receptor–ligand binding with an antibody is a strategy that has been employed with varying degrees of success in the treatment of human cancer. Anti-Tac in T-cell leukemia/lymphoma is an example of this strategy [201]. Antibodies directed against growth factors are also undergoing clinical testing (anti-bombesin in small cell lung cancer) [46]. Both of these therapies were designed to interfere with a putative autocrine loop, and it is still too early to evaluate therapeutic results. Similar anti-receptor antibodies could be employed in breast cancer; however, it is most clear if all human breast cancers express enough specific receptor to make this strategy successful. Many "specific" anti-tumor antibodies have been developed against cell surface antigens and then coupled with radioactive or toxic moieties [69, 112, 158]. Anti-receptor antibody could be coupled with these agents, just as the growth factors themselves can be made toxic, to deliver more specific radiotherapy or toxin therapy to the tumor. Again, the limiatations relate to the abundance and specificity of growth factor receptors expressed in breast cancer, although initial attempts at synthesizing immunotoxins directed against breast cancer cell surface antigens have been made [25, 117].

Most growth factor receptors (IGF receptor, EGF receptor) are tyrosine kinases, and it appears that tyrosine phosphorylation is the important first step in triggering the effects of growth factor–receptor interaction. Tyrosine kinase inhibitors are currently being tested in vitro [138, 194]. By interfering with generation of the second messenger, these inhibitors could also be growth-inhibitory in human breast cancer.

Since, by definition, autocrine growth factors are produced by the cancer, agents could be used to interfere with the transcription of these growth factors. Several systems utilizing anti-sense RNA (RNA introduced into the cell of opposite polarity to the coding sequence of interest) have shown that the protein product can be interfered with, and resultant phenotypic changes occur in the cell [93, 209, 51]. In experimental systems, this has usually been accomplished by introduction of either an entire anti-sense gene or a fragment of the gene, with resultant chromosomal integration of the foreign DNA. It would be extremely difficult to target tumor cells for gene introduction, but similar results could be obtained if the anti-sense RNA were given parenterally and then taken up by the cells. Stabilization of the anti-sense RNA can be partially accomplished by the production of RNA synthesized with methylphosphonates. These compounds resist ribonucleases in the serum or intracellular space, and experimentally have been shown to be active [178]. In this manner, specific genes and gene products could be targeted to decrease breast cancer growth.

Some of the growth factors implicated in growth regulation of breast cancer were originally described in systems investigating normal growth. The hypothalamic–pituitary control of IGF-I synthesis is well known. Growth hormone increases IGF-I secretion and growth hormone release is under the control of both positive and negative regulatory releasing hormones. Somatostatin inhibits growth hormone secretion, and can decrease IGF-I levels. If immunoreactive IGF-I derived from breast cancer cells is under hormonal control, then somatostatin may be able to inhibit its production and control tumor growth. somatostatin has been used in some sarcomas, with experimental evidence of tumor response [116, 134, 170].

Finally, a direct way of decreasing the growth of a cancer is to identify growth-inhibitory factors. As previously mentioned, TGF-β, and perhaps other unidentified serum components, are growth-inhibitory for breast cancer cells in culture. If these proteins are also active in vivo, then a simple way to arrest growth would be to supply these substances in pharmacologic doses. Another member of the TGF-β family is Mullerian inhibitory substance [128]. This compound may have some therapeutic activity against ovarian cancer [70]. In an analogous way, inhibitory substances could be given to breast cancer patients.

References

1. Adams DJ, McGuire WL (1985) Quantitative enzyme-linked immunosorbent assay for the estrogen-regulated Mr 24,000 protein in human tumors. Correlation with estrogen and progesterone receptors. Cancer Res 45: 2445-2449
2. Aitken SC, Lippman ME (1982) Hormonal regulation of net DNA synthesis in MCF-7 human breast cancer cells in culture. Cancer Res 42: 1727-1735
3. Aitken SC, Lippman ME (1983) Hormonal regulation of de novo pyrimidine synthesis and utilization in human breast cancer cells in tissue culture. Cancer Res 43: 4681-4690
4. Aitken SC, Lippman ME (1985) Effects of estrogens and antiestrogens on growth-regulatory enzymes in human breast cancer cells in tissue culture. Cancer Res 45: 1611-1620
5. Akiyama S, Seth P, Pirker R, Fitzgerald D, Gottesman MM, Pastan I (1985) Potentiation of cytotoxic activity of immunotoxins on cultured human cells. Cancer Res 45: 1005-1007
6. Albini A, Graf JO, Kitten T, Kleinman HK, Martin GR, Veillete A, Lippman ME (1986) Estrogen and v-*ras*^{H} transfection regulate the interactions of MCF-7 breast carcinoma cells to basement membrane. Proc Natl Acad Sci USA 83: 8182-8186
7. Allegra JC, Lippman ME (1978) Growth of a human breast cell line in serum-free hormone-supplemented medium. Cancer Res 38: 3823-3829
8. Antoniades HN (1981) Human platelet-derived growth factor (PDGF): purification of PDGF-I and PDGF-II and separation of their reduced subunits. Proc Natl Acad Sci USA 78: 7314-7317
9. Antoniades HN, Scher CD, Stiles CD (1979) Purification of the platelet-derived growth factor. Proc Natl Acad Sci USA 76: 1809-1813
10. Bano M, Salomon DA, Kidwell WR (1985) Purification of a mammary derived growth factor from human milk and human mammary tumors. J Biol Chem 260: 5745-5752
11. Barrack ER, Coffey DS (1980) The specific binding of estrogen and androgens to the nuclear matrix of sex hormone responsive tissues. J Biol Chem 255: 7265-7275
12. Bates SE, Davidson NE, Valverius E, Freter CE, Dickson RB, Kudlow JE, Tam JP, Lippman ME, Salomon DS (1988) Expression of transforming growth factor α and its messenger ribonucleic acid in human breast cancer: Its regulation by estrogen and its possible functional significance. Mol Endocrinology (In press)
13. Bates SE, McManaway ME, Lippman ME, Dickson RB (1986) Characterization of estrogen responsive transforming activity in human breast cancer cell lines. Cancer Res 46: 1707-1713
14. Bates SE, Valverius E, Salomon D, Stampfer M, Lippman ME, Dickson RB (1987) Expression and estrogen regulation of transforming growth factor (TGF) mRNA in human breast cancer. Proc Am Assoc Cancer Res 28: 233
15. Baxter RC (1986) The somatomedins: insulin like growth factors. Adv Clin Chem 25: 49-115
16. Baxter RC, Maitland JE, Raisur RL, Reddel R, Sutherland RL (1983) High molecular weight somatomedin-C (IGF-I) from T47D human mammary carcinoma cells: immunoreactivity and bioactivity. In: Spencer EM (ed) Insulin-like growth factors/somatomedins. DeGruyter, Berlin, pp 615-618
17. Baxter RC, Martin JL, Handelsman DJ (1984) Identification of human semen insulin-like growth factor-I/somatomedin C immunoreactive and binding protein. Acta Endocrinol (Copenh) 104: 420-427

18. Baxter RC, Zaltsman Z, Turtle JR (1984) Immunoreactive somatomedin C/insulin-like growth factor I and its binding protein in human milk. J Clin Endocrinol Metab 58: 955-959
19. Bell GI, Gerhard DS, Fong NM, Sanchez-Pescador R, Rall LB (1985) Isolation of the human insulin-like growth factor genes: insulin-like growth factor II and insulin genes are contiguous. Proc Natl Acad Sci USA 82: 6450-6454
20. Bell GI, Merryweather JP, Sanchez-Pescador R, Stempien MM, Priestly L, Scott J, Ball CB (1984) Sequence of a cDNA clone encoding human preproinsulin-like growth factor II. Nature 310: 775-777
21. Betsholtz C, Hohnsson A, Heldin CH, Westermark B, Lind P, Urdea MS, Eddy R, Shows TB, Philpott K, Mellor AL, Knott TJ, Scott J (1986) cDNA sequence and chromosomal localization of human platelet derived growth factor A chain and its expression in tumor cell lines. Nature 320: 695-700
22. Betsholtz C, Westermark B, Ek B, Heldin C-H (1984) Coexpression of a PDGF-like growth factor and PDGF receptors in a human osteosarcoma cell line: implications for autocrine receptor activation. Cell 39: 447-457
23. Binoux M, Hossenlopp P, Hardouin S, Sevrin D, Lassare C, Gourmelen M (1986) Somatomedin (insulin-like growth factors) binding proteins, molecular forms and regulation. Horm Res 24: 141-151
24. Bishop HM, Elston CW, Blamey RW (1979) Relationship of oestrogen-receptor status to survival in breast cancer. Lancet ii: 283-284
25. Bjorn MJ, Groetsema G, Scalapino L (1986) Antibody-*Pseudomonas* exotoxin A conjugates cytotoxic to human breast cancer cells in vitro. Cancer Res 46: 3262-3267
26. Bos JL, Fehran JL, Hamilton SR, Verlan-de Vries M, Van Boom JH, Van der Eb AJ, Vogelstein B (1987) Prevalence of *ras* gene mutations in human colorectal cancers. Nature 237: 293-297
27. Bos JL, Verlaan-deVries M, van der Eb HJ, Janssen JW, Delnel R, Lowenberg B, Lolly LP (1987) Mutations in N-*ras* predominant in acute myeloid leukemia. Blood 69: 1237-1241
28. Briand P, Lykkesfeldt AE (1987) The effect of estradiol on the growth of human breast cancer may depend on a growth inhibitor in serum. Proc Am Assoc Cancer Res 28: 246
29. Bringman TS, Lindquist PB, Derynck R (1987) Different transforming growth factor α species are derived from a glycosylated and palmitoylated transmembrane precursor. Cell 48: 429-440
30. Bronzert DA, Greene GL, Lippman ME (1985) Selection and characterization of breast cancer cell line resistant to the antiestrogen LY 17018. Endocrinology 117: 1409-1417
31. Bronzert DA, Pantazis P, Antoniades HN, Kasid A, Davidson N, Dickson RB, Lippman ME (1987) Synthesis and secretion of PDGF-like growth factor by human breast cancer cell lines. Proc Natl Acad Sci USA 84: 5763-5767
32. Bronzert DA, Silverman S, Lippman ME (1985) Induction of a secreted protein in human breast cancer cells. Proceedings of the 67th Annual Endocrine Society Meeting, Baltimore 1985 (abstr 1007)
33. Bronzert DA, Triche TJ, Gleason P, Lippman ME (1984) Isolation and characterization of an estrogen-inhibited variant derived from the MCF-7 breast cancer cell line. Cancer Res 44: 3942-3951
34. Butler WB, Kelsey WH, Goran N (1981) Effects of serum and insulin on the sensitivity of the human breast cancer cell line MCF-7 to estrogens and antiestrogens. Cancer Res 41: 82-88
35. Butler WB, Kirkland WL, Jorgensen TL (1979) Induction of plasminogen activator by estrogen in a human breast cancer cell line (MCF-7). Biochem Biophys Res commun 90: 1328-1334

36. Capony F, Morisset M, Barret AJ, Capony JP, Broquet P, Vignon F, Chambon M, Louisot P, Rochefort H (1987) Phosphorylation, glycosylation, and proteolytic activity of the 52-Kd estrogen-induced protein secreted by MCF-7 cells. J Cell Biol 104: 253-262
37. Chablos D, Vignon F, Keydar I, Rochefort H (1982) Estrogens stimulate cell proliferation and induce secretory proteins in a human breast cancer cell line (T47D). J Clin Endocrinol Metab 55: 276-283
38. Chambon P (1987) Structure of the human oestrogen responsive pS2. Nucleic Acids Res 15: 1401-1414
39. Chaudbary UK, Fitzgerald DJ, Adhya S, Pastan I (1987) Activity of a recombinant fusion protein between transforming growth factor type and *Pseudomon* as toxin. Proc Natl Acad Sci USA 84: 4538-4542
40. Cheifetz S, Wentherbee JA, Tsang MSS, Anderson JK, Mole JE, Lucas R, Massague J (1987) The transforming growth factor β system, a complex pattern of cross-reactive ligands and receptors. Cell 48: 409-415
41. Ciocca DR, Adams DJ, Edwards DP, Bjerke RJ, McGuire WL(1983) Distribution of an estrogen induced protein with a molecular weight of 24,000 in normal and malignant human tissues and cells. Cancer Res 43: 1204-1210
42. Clemmons DR, Shaw DS (1983) Variables controlling somatomedin production by cultured human fibroblasts. J Cell Physiol 115: 137-143
43. Clina MJ, Battifora H, Yokota J (1987) Proto-oncogene abnormalities in human breast cancer: correlations with anatomic features and clinical course of disease. J Clin Oncol 5: 999-1006
44. Cohen SJ, Ushiro H, Stoscheck C, Chiners N (1982) A native 170,000 epidermal growth factor receptor-kinase complex from shed membrane vesicles. J Biol chem 257: 1523-1531
45. Cowan K, Levine R, Aitken S, Goldsmith M, Douglass E, Clendeninn N, Nienhuis A, Lippman ME (1985) Dihydrofolate reductase gene amplification and possible rearrangement in estrogen-responsive methotrexate resistant human breast cancer cells. J Biol Chem 257: 15079-15086
46. Cuttita F, Carney DN, Mulshine J, Moody TW, Fedorko J, Fisher A, Minna J (1985) Bombesin-like peptides can function as autocrine growth factors in small cell lung cancer. Nature 316: 823-827
47. D'Ercole AJ, Applewhite GT, Underwood LE (1980) Evidence that somtomedin is synthesized by multiple tissues in the fetus. Dev Biol 75: 315-328
48. Darbe P, Yates J, Curtis S, King RJB (1983) Effect of estradiol on human breast cancer cells in culture. Cancer Res 43: 349-354
49. Davidson NE, Bronzert DA, Chambon P, Gelmann EP, Lippman ME (1986) Use of two MCF-7 cell variants to evaluate the growth regulatory potential of estrogen-induced products. Cancer Res 46: 1904-1908
50. Davidson NE, Gelmann EP, Lippman ME, Dickson RB (1987) EGF receptor gene expression in estrogen receptor positive and negative human breast cancer cell lines. Mol Endocrinology 1: 216-223
51. De Benedetti A, Pytel BA, Balioni C (1987) Loss of (2'-5') oligo adenylate synthetase activity by production of antisense RNA results in lack of protection by interferon from viral infections. Proc Natl Acad Sci USA 84: 658-662
52. De Larco JE, Todaro GJ (1978) Growth factors from murine sarcoma virus transformed cells. Proc Natl Acad Sci USA 75: 4001-4005
53. Derynck R (1987) Transforming growth factor-alpha: structure and biological activities. J Cell Biochem 32: 293-304
54. Derynck R, Goeddel DV, Ullrich A, Gutterman JU, Williams RD, Bringman TS, Berger WH (1987) Synthesis of messenger RNAs for transforming growth factors α and β and the epidermal growth factor receptor by human tumors. Cancer Res 47: 707-712

55. Derynck R, Jarret JA, Chen EY, Eaton DH, Bell JR, Assoian RK, Roberts AB, Sporn MB, Goeddel DV (1985) Human transforming growth factor β. Complementary DNA sequence and expression in normal and transformed cells. Nature 316: 701-705
56. Derynck R, Roberts AB, Eaton DH, Winkler MC, Goeddel DV (1985) Human transforming growth factor α precursor sequence, gene structure, and heterologous expression. In: Feramisco J, Ozanne B, Stiles C (eds) Cancer cells 3: growth factors and transformation. Cold Spring Harbor Laboratory, Cold Spring Harbor, pp 79-86
57. Derynck R, Roberts AB, Winkler ME, Chen Ey, Goeddel DV (1984) Human transforming growth factor -α (precursor structure and expression in *E. coli.* Cell 38: 287-297
58. Dickson RB, Huff KK, Spencer EM, Lippman ME (1986) Induction of epidermal growth factor-related polypeptides by 17β-estradiol in MCF-7 human breast cancer cells. Endocrinology 118: 138-142
59. Dickson RB, Kasid A, Huff KK, Bates S, Knabbe C, Bronzert D, Gelmann EP, Lippman ME (1987) Activation of growth factor secretion in tumorigenic states of breast cancer induced by 17β estradiol or v-*rasH* oncogene. Proc Natl Acad Sci USA 84: 837-841
60. Dickson RB, McManaway M, Lippman ME (1986) Estrogen induced factors of breast cancer cells partially replace estrogen to promote tumor growth. Science 232: 1540-1543
61. Edwards DP, Martin PM, Horwitz KB, Chamness GC, McGuire WL (1980) Subcellular compartmentalization of estrogen receptors in human breast cancer cells. Exp Cell Res 127: 197-213
62. Edwards DP, Murphy Sr, McGuire WL (1980) Effect of estrogen and antiestrogen on DNA polymerase in human breast cancer. Cancer Res 40: 1722-1726
63. Eisman JA, Martin TJ, MacIntyre I, Framptin RJ, Moseley JM, Whitehead R (1980) 1,25-Dihydroxyvitamin D_3 receptor in a cultured breast cancer cell line (MCF-7 cells). Biochem Biophys Res Commun 93: 9-18
64. Ek B, Heldin C-H (1982) Characterization of a tyrosine-specific kinase activity in human fibroblast membranes stimulated by platelet-derived growth factor. J Biol Chem 257: 10486-10492
65. Engle LW, Young NW (1978) Human breast carcinoma cells in continuous culture: a review. Cancer Res 38: 4327-4339
66. Fitzpatrick SL, La Chance MP, Schultz GS (1984) Characterization of epidermal growth factor receptor and action on human breast cancer cells in culture. Cancer Res 44: 3442-3447
67. Folkman J, Klagsburn M (1987) Angiogenic factors. Science 235: 442-447
68. Forrester K, Almoguera C, Han K, Grizzle WE, Perucho M (1987) Detection of high incidence of K-*ras* oncogenes during human colon tumorigenesis. Nature 327: 298-303
69. Frankel AE, Houston LL, Issel BF, Fatham G (1986) Prospects for immunotoxin therapy in cancer. Annu Rev Med 37: 125-142
70. Fuller AF Jr, Krane IM, Budzik GP, Donahoe PK (1985) Mullerian inhibiting substance reduction of colony growth of human gynecologic cancers in a stem cell assay. Gynecol Oncol 22: 135-148
71. Furlanetto RW, Di Carlo JN (1984) Somatomedin C receptors and growth effects in human breast cells maintained in long-term tissue culture. Cancer Res 44: 2122-2128
72. Graham KA, Richardson Cl, Minden MD, Trent JM, Buick RM (1985) Varying degrees of amplification of the N-*ras* oncogene in the human breast cancer cell line MCF-7. Cancer Res 45: 2201-2205

73. Green S, Walter P, Kumar V, Krust A, Bornertt J-M, Argos P, Chambon P (1986) Human oestrogen receptor cDNA: sequence, expression and homology to v-*erb* A. Nature 320: 134-139
74. Greene GL, Gilna P, Waterfield M, Baker H, Hort Y, Shine J (1986) Sequence and expression of human estrogen receptor complementary DNA. Science 231: 1150-1154
75. Greig RG, Trainer DC (1986) Shaping future strategies for the pharmacological control of tumor cell metastases. Cancer Metastasis Rev 5: 3-14
76. Guirguis R, Marguiles J, Taraboletti G, Schiffman E, Liotta L (1987) Cytokine induced pseudopodial protrusion coupled to tumor cell migration. Nature 329: 261-263
77. Han VK, D'Ercole AJ, Lund PK (1987) Cellular localization of somatomedin (insulin-like growth factor) messenger RNA in the human fetus. Science 236: 193-197
78. Hasselbacher G, Humbel R (1982) Evidence for two species of insulin-like growth factor II (IGF-II and 'big' IGF-II) in human spinal fluid. Endocrinology 110: 1822-1824
79. Hasselbacher GK, Irminger J-C, Zapf J, Ziegler WT, Humbel RE (1987) Insulin-like growth factor II in human adrenal pheochromocytomas and Wilms' tumors: expression at the mRNA and protein level. Proc Natl Acad Sci USA 84: 1104-1106
80. Hasselbacher GK, Schwab ME, Pasi A, Humbel RE (1985) Insulin-like growth factor II (IGF-II) in human brain: regional distribution of IGF-II and of higher molecular mass forms. Proc Natl Acad Sci USA 82: 2153-2157
81. Heldin C-H, Hammacher A, Betsholtz C, Westermark B Role of PDGF-like growth factors in autocrine stimulation of cell growth. J Cell Biochem 11A: [Suppl] 2
82. Heldin C-H, Johnsson A, Wennergen S, Wernstedt C, Betsholtz C, Westermark B (1986) A human osteosarcoma cell line secretes a growth factor structurally related to a homodimer of PDGF-A chain. Nature 319: 311-314
83. Heldin C-H, Westermark B, Wasteson A (1981) Specific receptors for platelet-derived growth factor on cells derived from connective tissue and glia. Proc Natl Acad Sci USA 78: 3664-3668
84. Hennekens CT, Speizer FE, Rosner B et al. (1979) Use of permanent hair dyes and cancer among registered nurses. Lancet i: 1390-1393
85. Hirsh KS, Sledge Jr GW, Roth BJ, Falcone JF (1897) In vitro interactions of IGF-II with human breast cancer (BC) cell lines grown in serum-free media. Proc Am Assoc Cancer Res 28: 240
86. Huang JS, Huang SS, Deuel TF (1984) Transforming protein of simian sarcoma virus stimulates autocrine growth of SSV-transformed cells through PDGF cell surface receptors. cell 39: 79-87
87. Huff KK, Kaufman D, Gabbay KH, Spencer EM, Lippman ME, Dickson RB (1986) Human breast cancer cells secrete an insulin-like growth factor-I-related polypeptide. Cancer Res 46: 4613-4619
88. Huff KK, Knabbe C, Kaufman D, Lippman ME, Dickson RB (1987) Hormonal regulation of insulin-like growth factor I (IGF-I) secretion from MCF-7 human breast cancer cells. J cell Biochem IIA: [Suppl] 28
89. Huff KK, Knabbe C, Lindsay R, Lippman ME, Dickson RB (1988) Multihormonal regulation of insulin-like growth factor-I related protein in MCF-7 human breast cancer cells. Mol Endocrinology X:X (mansuscript submitted)
90. Huseby RA, Maloney TM, McGrath CM (1984) Evidence for a direct growth-stimulating effect of estradiol on human MCF-7 cells in vivo. Cancer Res 44: 2654-2659
91. Ibbotson KJ, Harrod J, Gowen M, D'Souza S, Smith DD, Winkler ME, Derynck R, Mundy GR (1986) Human recombinant transforming growth factor alpha stimulates bone resorption and inhibits formation in vitro. Proc Natl Acad Sci USA 83: 2228-2232

92. Ikeda T, Danielpour D, Sirbasku BA (1984) Isolation and properties of endocrine and autocrine type mammary tumor cell growth factors (estromedins). In: Bresciani F, King RJB, Lippman ME, Namer M, Raynaud JP (eds) Progress in cancer research and therapy, vol 31. Raven, New York, pp 171-186
93. Izant JG, Weintraub H (1983) Constitutive and conditional suppression of exogenous and endogenous genes by anti-sense RNA. Science 229: 345-352
94. Jakesz R, Smith CA, Aitken S, Huff KK, Schuette W, Schackney S, Lippman ME (1984) Influence of cell proliferation and cell cycle phase on expression of estrogen receptor in MCF-7 breast cancer cells. Cancer Res 44: 619-625
95. Jakolew SB, Breathnack R, Jeltsch J, Chambon P (1984) Sequence of the pS2 mRNA induced estrogen in the human breast cancer cell line MCF-7. Nucleic Acids Res 12: 2861-2874
96. Jansen M, Van Schaik FMA, Ricker AT, Bullock B, Woods PE, Gabbay KH, Nussbaum AL, Sussenback JS, Vander Branch JR (1983) Sequence of cDNA encoding human insulin-like growth factor I precursor. Nature 306: 609-611
97. Jensen EV, Desombre ER (1972) Mechanism of action of the female sex hormones. Annu Rev Biochem 41: 203-230
98. Johnsson A, Heldin Ch, Wateson A, Westermark B, Devel TF, Huang JS, Seeburg PH, Gray A, Ullrich A, Scrace G, Stroobant P, Waterfield MS (1984) The *c-sis* gene encodes a precursor of the B chain of platelet-derived growth factor. EMBO J 3: 921-928
99. Johnsson A, Heldin Ch, Westermark B, Wasteson A (1982) Platelet-derived growth factor identification of constituent polypeptide chains. Biochem Biophys Res Commun 104: 66-74
100. Jordan VC (1987) Laboratory models of breast cancer to aid the elucidation of antiestrogen action. J Lab Clin Med 109: 269-277
101. Kao RT, Stern R (1986) Collagenases in human breast carcinoma cell lines. Cancer Res 46: 1349-1354
102. Karey KP, Marquardt H, Sirbasku DA (1987) Identification of platelet derived human mammary tumor cell growth factors as IGF-I and IGF-II by purification and partial amino acid sequencing. Proc Am Assoc Cancer Res 28: 54
103. Kasid A, Davidson N, Gelmann E, Lippman ME (1986) Transcriptional control of thymidine kinase gene expression by estrogens and antiestrogens in MCF-7 human breast cancer cells. J Biol Chem 261: 5562-5567
104. Kasid A, Lippman ME, Papageorge AG, Lowy DR, Gelmann EP (1985) Transfection of v-*ras*^{H} DNA into MCF-7 cells bypasses their dependence on estrogen for tumorigenicity. Science 228: 725-728
105. Katzenellenbogen B, Norman MJ, Eckert RL, Peltz SW, Mangel WF (1983) Bioactivities, estrogen receptor interactions, and plasminogen activator-inducing activities of tamoxifen and hydroxy-tamoxifen isomers in MCF-7 human breast cancer cells. Cancer Res 44: 112-119
106. Kim M, Warren TC, Kimball ES (1985) Purification and characterization of a low molecular weight transforming growth factor from the urine of melanoma patients. J Biol Chem 260: 9237-9243
107. Kimball ES, Bohn WH, Cockley KD, Warren TC, Sherwin SA (1984) Distinct high-performance liquid chromatography pattern of transforming growth factor activity in urine of cancer patients as compared with that of normal individuals. Cancer Res 44: 3613-3619
108. King WJ, Greene GL (1984) Monoclonal antibodies localize estrogen receptor in the nuclei of target cells. Nature 307: 747-749
109. Knabbe C, Lippman ME, Wakefield L, Flanders K, Kasid A, Derynck R, Dickson RB

(1987) Evidence that TGFβ is a hormonally regulated negative growth factor in human breast cancer. Cell 48: 417-428

110. Knight WA III, Livingston RB, Gregory RJ (1977) Estrogen receptor as an independent prognostic factor for early recurrence in breast cancer. Cancer Res 37: 4469-4471
111. Kobrin MS, Samosondar J, Kudlow JE (1986) α-Transforming growth factor secreted by untransformed bovine anterior pituitary cells in culture. J Biol Chem 261: 14414-14419
112. Kozak RW, Atcher RW, Gansow OA, Friedman AM, Hines JJ, Waldmann TA (1986) Bismuth-212-labelled anti-Tac monoclonal antibody: alpha-particle-emitting radionuclides as modalities for radioimmunotherapy. Proc Natl Acad Sci USA 83: 474-478
113. Kraus MH, Yuasa Y, Aaronson SA (1984) A position 12-activated H-*ras* oncogene in all Hs578T mammary carcinosarcoma cells but not normal mammary cells of the same patient. Proc Natl Acad Sci USA 81: 5384-5388
114. Kudlow JE, Khosraui MJ, Kobin MS, Mak W (1984) Inability of anti-epidermal growth factor receptor antibody to block "autocrine" growth stimulation in transforming growth factor alpha-secreting melanoma cells. J Biol Chem 259: 11895-11900
115. Kurachi H, Okamoto S, Oka T (1985) Evidence for the involvement of the submandibular gland epidermal growth factor in mouse mammary tumorigenesis. Proc Natl Acad Sci USA 81: 5940-5943
116. Lambert SW, Reubi JC (1986) The potential use of somatostatin analogs in the treatment of cancer. Fifth NCI-EORTC symposium on new drugs in cancer therapy, oct 22-24, 1986, Amsterdam, 7:4
117. Le Maistre CF, Edwards DP, Kvolick KA, McGuire WL (1987) An immunotoxin cytotoxin for breast cancer cells *in* vitro. Cancer Res 47: 730-734
118. Leof EB, Proper JA, Goustin AJ, Shipley GD, Dicorleto PE, Moses HL (1986) Induction of c-*sis* mRNA and activity similar to platelet-derived growth factor: a proposed model for indirect mitogenesis involving autocrine activity. Proc Natl Acad Sci USA 83: 2453-2457
119. Leung BS, Qureshi S, Leung JS (1982) Response to estrogen by the human mammary carcinoma cell line CAMA-1. Cancer Res 42: 5060-5066
120. Liotta LA, Mandler R, Murano G, Katz DA, Gordon RK, Chiang PK, Schiffman E (1986) Tumor cell autocrine motility factor. Proc Natl Acad Sci USA 83: 3302-3306
121. Lippman ME (1984) Definition of hormones and growth factors required for optimal proliferation and expression of phenotypic responses in human breast cancer cells. In: Barnes DW, Sirbasku DA, Sata GH (eds) cell culture methods for molecular and cell biology, vol 2. Liss, New York, pp 183-200
122. Lippman ME (1985) Endocrine responsive cancers of man. In: Williams RH (ed) Textbook of endocrinology. Saunders Philadelphia, pp 1309-1326
123. Lippman ME, Bolan G, Huff K (1976) The effects of estrogens and antiestrogens on hormone-responsive human breast cancer in long term culture. Cancer Res 36: 4595-4601
124. MacMahon B, Cole P, Brown J (1973) Etiology of human breast cancer: a review. JNCI 50: 21-42
125. Marquardt H, Hunkapiller MW, Hood LE, Todaro GJ (1984) Rat transforming growth factor. Structure and relation to epidermal growth factor. Science 223: 1079-1082
126. Marquardt H, Hunkapiller MW, Hood LE, Twardzik DR, DeLarco JE, Stephenson JR, Todaro GJ (1983) Transforming growth factors produced by retrovirus-transformed rodent fibroblasts and human melanoma cells: amino acid sequence homology with epidermal growth factor. Proc Natl Acad Sci USA 80: 4684-4688

127. Marquardt H, Todaro GJ (1982) Human transforming growth factor. Production by a melanoma cell line, purification and initial characterization. J Biol Chem 257: 5220-5225
128. Massaque J (1987) The TGFβ family of growth and differentiation factors. Cell 49: 430-438
129. Matrisian LM, Pathak M, Magun BE (1982) Identification of an epidermal growth-factor related transforming growth factor from rat fetuses. Biochem Biophys Res Commun 107: 1761
130. McGuire WL, Clark GM, Dressler LG, Owens MA (1986) Role of steroid hormone receptors as prognostic factors in primary breast cancer. NCI Monogr 1: 19-23
131. Miller AB, Bullbrook RD (1980) The epidemiology and etiology of breast cancer. N Engl J Med 303: 1246-1248
132. Minuto F, Del Monte PD, Baweca A, Fortini P, Cariola G, Catarambone G, Giordano G (1986) Evidence for an increased somatomedin C/insulin-like growth factor I content in primary human lung tumors. Cancer Res 46: 985-988
133. Mira-y-Lopez R, Joseph-silverstein J, Rifkin DB, Ossowski C (1986) Identification of a pituitary factor responsible for enhancement of plasminogen activator activity in breast tumor cells. Proc Natl Acad Sci USA 83: 7780-7784
134. Moreau JP, De Feudis FU (1987) Pharmacologic studies of somatostatin and somatostatin-analogues: therapeutic advances and perspectives. Life Sci 40: 419-437
135. Moses HL, Branum EL, Proper JA, Robinson JE (1981) Transforming growth factor production by chemically transformed cells. Cancer Res 41: 2842-2848
136. Myal Y, Shiu RPC, Bhawmick B, Bala M (1984) Receptor binding and growth promoting activity of insulin-like growth factors in human breast cancer cells (T47D) in culture. Cancer Res 44: 5486-5490
137. Naito S, Von Eschenbach AC, Fidler IJ (1987) Different growth pattern and biologic behavior of human renal cell carcinoma implanted into different organs of nude mice. JNCI 78: 377-385
138. Nakumura H, Iituka Y, Imoto M, Ishiki K, Naganana H, Takeuchi T, Umezawa H (1986) The structure of an epidermal growth factor-receptor kinase inhibitor, erbastatin. J Antibiot (Tokyo) 39: 314-315
139. Nissley SP, Rechler MM (1984) Insulin-like growth factor: biosynthesis receptors and carrier proteins. In: Li CH (ed) Hormonal proteins and peptides vol XII. Academic, New York, pp 128-203
140. Nister M, Heldin C-H, Wasteson A, Westermark B (1982) A platelet-derived growth factor analogue produced by a human clonal glioma line. Ann NY Acad Sci 397: 25-35
141. O'Connell DL, Hulka BS, Chambless LE, Wilkinson WE, Deubner DC (1987) Cigarette smoking, alcohol consumption and breast cancer risk. JNCI 78: 229-231
142. Ogaswara M, Marquardt H, Sirbasku DA (1987) Further purification of uterine derived growth factors for mammary tumor cells: partial amino acid sequence identification as a truncated form of IGF-I. Proc Am Assoc Cancer Res 28: 58
143. Oguchi N, Thor A, Page DL, Hard PH, Halter SA, Schlom J (1986) Expression of the 21,000 molecular weight *ras* protein in a spectrum of benign and malignant human mammary tissue. Cancer Res 46: 2511-2519
144. Osborne CK, Hamilton B, Titus G, Livingston RB (1980) Epidermal growth factor stimulation of human breast cancer cells in culture. Cancer Res 40: 2361-2366
145. Page MJ, Field JK, Everett NP, Green CD (1983) Serum regulation of the estrogen responsiveness of the human breast cancer cell line MCF-7. Cancer Res 43: 1244-1249
146. Peres R, Betsholtz C, Westermark B, Heldin C-H (1987) Frequent expression of growth factors for mesenchymal cells in human mammary carcinoma cell lines. Cancer Res 47: 3425-3429

147. Perroteau E, Salomon D, Debortali M, Kidwell W, Hazarika P, Pardue R, Dedman J, Tam J (1986) Immunological detection and quantitation of alpha transforming growth factors in human breast carcinoma cells. Breast Cancer Res Treat 7: 201-210
148. Petrids PE, Hosang M, Shooter E, Esch FS, Bohlen P (1985) Isolation and characterization of epidermal growth factor from human milk. FEBS Lett 187: 89-95
149. Puca GA, Sica V, Nola E (1974) Identification of a high affinity nuclear acceptor site for estrogen receptor of calf uterus. Proc Natl Acad Sci USA 171: 979-983
150. Rechler MM, Nissley SP (1986) Insulin-like growth factor (IGF)/somatomedin receptor subtypes: structure, function, and relationships to insulin receptor and IGF carrier proteins. Horm Res 24: 152-159
151. Reeve AE, Eccles MR, Wilkins RJ, Bell GI, Millon LJ (1985) Expression of insulin-like growth factor II transcripts in Wilms' tumor. Nature 317: 258-260
152. Reiner GCA, Katzenellenbogen BS (1986) Characterization of estrogen in MDA-MB-134 human breast cancer cells. Cancer Res 46: 1124-1131
153. Robbins KC, Leal F, Pierce JH, Aaronson SA (1985) Biosynthetic pathway of the *v-sis*/PDGF-2 gene product in SSV-transformed cells. EMBO J 4: 1783-1792
154. Robertz AB, Anzano MA, Lamb LC, Smith JM, Frolik CA, Marquardt H, Todaro GJ, Sporn MB (1982) Isolation from murine sarcoma cells of a new class of transforming growth factors potentiated by epidermal growth factor. Nature 295: 417-419
155. Roberts AB, Anzanio MA, Lamb LL, Smith JM, Sporn MB (1981) New class of transforming growth factors potentiated by epidermal growth factor: isolation from non-neoplastic tissues. Proc Natl Acad Sci USA 78: 5339-5343
156. Roberts AB, Anzano MA, Wakefield LM, Roche NS, Stern DF, Sporn MB (1985) Type β transforming growth factor: a bifunctional regulator of cellular growth. Proc Natl Acad Sci USA 82: 119-123
157. Rochefort H, Capony F, Cavialles V, Garcia M, Morisset M, Freiss G, Vigvon F (1987) An estrogen induced procathepsin secreted by breast cancer cells: role in breast cancer growth and invasion? Proc Am Assoc Cancer Res 28: 247 (abst 978)
158. Rosen ST, Zimmer AM, Goldman-Leikin R, Gordon LI, Kazikiewicz JM, Kaplan EH, Variakojis D, Marder RJ, Dyekewicz MS, Piergles A (1987) Radioimmunodetection and radioimmunotherapy of cutaneous T-cell lymphomas using an I131-labelled monoclonal antibody: an Illinois cancer council study. J Clin Oncol 5: 562-573
159. Rosenthal A, Lindquist PB, Bringman TS, Goeddel DV, Derynck R (1986) Expression in rat fibroblasts of a human transforming growth factor α and cDNA results in transformation. Cell 46: 301-309
160. Ross R, Raines EW, Bowel-Pope DF (1986) The biology of platelet-derived growth factor. Cell 46: 155-169
161. Rotwein P (1986) Two insulin-like growth factor I messenger RNAs are expressed in human liver. Proc Natl Acad Sci USA 83: 77-81
162a. Rowe JM, Kasper S, Shiu RP, Friesen HG (1986) Purification and characterization of a human mammary tumor-derived growth factor. Cancer Res 46: 1408-1412
162b. Rozengurt E (1986) Early signals in the mitogenic response. Science 234: 161-166
163. Rozengurt E, Sinnett-Smith J, Taylor-Papadimitriou J (1985) Production of PDGF-like growth factor by breast cancer lines. Int J Cancer 36: 247-252
164. Sakagami Y, Inaguma Y, Sakakura T, Nishizuka Y (1984) Intestine-like morphology of adult mouse glandular stomach by implanting of fetal intestinal mesenchyme. Cancer Res 44: 5845-5849
165. Sakum T, Sakagami Y, Nishizuka Y (1981) Accelerated mammary cancer development by fetal salivary mesenchyma isografted to adult mouse mammary epithelium. JNCI 66: 953-959

166. Salomon DS, Kidwell WR (1987) Tumor-associated growth factors in malignant rodent and human mammary epithelial cells. Proc Am Assoc Cancer Res 28: 248
167. Salomon DS, Zweibel JA, Bano M, Losonczy I, Felnel P, Kidwell WR (1984) Presence of transforming growth factors in human breast cancer cells. Cancer Res 44: 4069-4077
168. Sapino A, Peitribiasi F, Bussolati G, Marchiso PC (1986) Estrogen- and tamoxifen-induced rearrangement of cytoskeletal and adhesion structures in breast cancer MCF-7 cells. Cancer Res 46: 2526-2531
169. Satao M, Yoshida H, Hayashi Y, Miyakami K, Bundo T, Yanagowa T, Yura Y, Azuma M, Ueno A (1985) Expression of epidermal growth factor and transforming growth factor in a human salivary gland adenocarcinoma cell line. Cancer Res 45: 6160-6167
170. Schally AV, Comary-Schally AM, Redding TW (1984) Antitumor effects of analogs of hypothalamic hormones in endocrine dependent cancers. Proc Soc Exp Biol Med 175: 259-281
171. Schatzkin A, Jones DY et al. (1987) Alcohol consumption and breast cancer in the epidemiologic follow-up study of the first National Health and Nutritional Examination Survey. N Engl J Med 316: 1169-1174
172. Schimpff RM, Donnadieu M, Gautier M (1981) Somatomedin activity measured as sulphation factor in culture media from normal human liver and connective tissue explants. Effects of growth hormone. Acta Endocrinol (Copenh) 98: 24-28
173. Schreiber AB, Winkler ME, Derynk R (1986) Transforming growth factor α: a more potent angiogenic mediator than epidermal growth factor. Science 232: 1250-1253
174. Scott J, Cowell J, Robertson ME, Priestly LM, Wadey R, Hopkins B, Pritchard J, Bell GI, Rall LB, Graham CF, Knott TJ (1985) Insulin-like growth factor II nerve expression in Wilms' tumor and embryonic tissues. Nature 317: 260-262
175. Sherwin C, Twardzink PR, Bohn WH, Cockley KD, Todaro GJ (1983) High molecular weight transforming growth factor activIty in the urine of patients with disseminated cancer. Cancer Res 43: 403-407
176. Shiu RP, Dembinski TC, Dubik D (1987) Estrogen action in human breast cancer: its requirement of a pituitary derived growth factor and its activation of cellular genes. Proc Am Assoc Cancer Res 28: 237
177. Slamon DJ, Clark GM, Wong SG, Levin WJ, Ullrich A, McGuire WL (1987) Human breast cancer: correlation of relapse and survival with amplification of the HER-2/*neu* oncogene. Science 235: 177-182
178. Smith CC, Aurelian L, Reddy MP, Miller PS, Ts'o P (1986) Antiviral effect of an oligo nucleoside methyl phosphonate complementary to the splicejunction of herpes simplex type 1 immediate early pre-mRNAs 4 and 5. Proc Natl Acad Sci USA 83: 2787-2791
179. Soto AM, Sonnenschien C (1987a) Cell proliferation of estrogen-sensitive cells: the case of negative control. Endocr Rev 8: 44-52
180. Soto AM, Sonnenschien C (1987b) Negative controls for the proliferation of breast tumor cells. Proc Am Assoc Cancer Res 28: 248
181. Soule HD, McGrath CM (1980) Estrogen responsive proliferation of clonal human breast carcinoma cells in athymic mice. Cancer 10: 177-189
182. Spiegel AM (1987) Signal transduction by guanine nucleotide binding proteins. Mol Cell Endocrinol 49: 1-16
183. Sporn MB, Roberts AB, Wakefield LM, Assoian RK (1986) Transforming growth factor β: biological function and chemical structure. Science 233: 532-534
184. Strobl JS, Thompson EB (1985) Mechanism of steroid hormone action. In: Auricchio F (ed) Sex steroid receptors. Field Educational Halia Acta Medica, Rome, pp 9-36

185. Stromberg K, Pigott DA, Ranchalis JE, Twardzik DR (1982) Human term placenta contains transforming growth factors potentiated by epidermal growth factor: isolation from non-neoplastic tissues. Proc Natl Acad Sci USA 78: 5339-5343
186. Tanaka T, Slamon D, Battifora H, Cline MJ (1986) Expression of p21 *ras* oncoproteins in human cancers. Cancer Res 46: 1465-1470
187. Theillet C, Lidereau R, Escot C, Hutzell P, Brunet M, Gest J, Schlom J, Callahan R (1986) Loss of a C-H-ras^1 allele and aggressive human primary breast carcinomas. Cancer Res 46: 4776-4778
188. Todaro GJ, DeLarco JE, Cohen S (1976) Transformation by murine and feline sarcoma viruses specifically blocks binding of epidermal growth factor to cells. Nature 264: 26-31
189. Todaro GJ, Fryling C, DeLarco JE (1980) Transforming growth factors produced by certain human tumor cells: polypeptides that interact with epidermal growth factor receptors. Proc Natl Acad Sci USA 77: 5238
190. Tricoli JV, Rall LR, Zarakousis CP, Herrera L, Petrelli N, Bell GI, Shows TB (1986) Enhanced levels of insulin-like growth factor messenger RNA in human colon carcinomas and liposarcomas. Cancer Res 46: 6169-6173
191. Tucker RF, Shipley GD, Moses HL, Holley RW (1984) Growth inhibitor from BSC-1 cells closely related to platelet type β transforming growth factor. Science 226: 705-707
192. Twardzik DR, Kimball ES, Sherwin SA, Ranchalis JE, Todaro GS (1985) Comparison of growth factors functionally related to epidermal growth factor in the urine of normal and human tumor-bearing athymic nude mice. Cancer Res 45: 1934-1939
193. Twardzik DR, Ranchalis JE, Todaro GJ (1982) Mouse embryonic transforming growth factors related to those isolated from tumor cells. Cancer Res 42: 590-593
194. Uehara Y, Hori M, Takeuchi T, Umezawa H (1986) Phenotypic change from transformed to normal induced by benzoquinonoid ansamycins accompanies inactivation of $p60^{src}$ in rat kidney cells infected with Rous sarcoma virus. Mol Cell Biol 6: 2198-2206
195. Ullrich A, Gray A, Tam AW, Yang Feng T, Tsubokawa M, Collins C, Henzel W, Le Bon T, Kathuria S, Chen E, Jacobs S, Francke U, Ramachandran J, Fujita-Yamaguchi Y (1986) Insulin-like growth factor I receptor primary structure: comparison with insulin receptor suggests structural determinants that define functional specificity. EMBO J 5: 2503-2512
196. Ushiro H, Cohen SJ (1980) Identification of phosphotyrosine as a product of epidermal growth factor-activated protein kinase in A431 cell membranes. J Biol Chem 255: 8363-8365
197. Valverius E, Bates SE, Salomon DS, Stampfer M, Clark R, McCormick F, Lippman ME, Dickson RB (1987) Production of transforming growth factor alpha by human mammary epithelial cells and sublines. Proceedings of the annual meeting of the endocrine Society, Indianopolis (abstr 306)
198. van de Vijor M, van de Bersselaar R, Devilee P, Cornelisse C, Peterse J, Nusse R (1987) Amplification of the *neu* (c-*erb* B_2) oncogene in human mammary tumors is relatively frequent and is often accompanied by amplification of the linked c-*erb-A* oncogene. Mol Cell Biol 7: 2019-2023
199. Vignon F, Capony F, Chambon M, Freiss G, Garcia M, Rochefort H (1986) Autocrine growth stimulation of the MCF-7 breast cancer cells by the estrogen-regulated 52 Kd protein. Endocrinology 118: 1537-1545
200. Vignon F, Derocq DF, Chambon M, Rochefort H (1983) Estrogen induced proteins secreted by the MCF-7 human breast cancer cells stimulated their proliferation. CR Acad Sci Endocrinol (Paris) 296: 151-157

201. Waldmann TA (1986) The interleukin-2 receptor on malignant cells: a target for diagnosis and therapy. Cell Immunol 99: 53-60
202. Walter P, Green S, Greene G, Krust A, Bornert JM, Jeltsch J-M, Straub A, Jensen E, Scrace G, Waterfield M, Chambon P (1985) Cloning of the human estrogen receptor cDNA. Proc Natl Acad Sci USA 82: 889-893
203. Waterfield MD, Scrace GT, Whittle N, Stroobant P, Johnsson A, Waterson A, Westermark B, Heldin CH, Huang JS, Deuel TF (1983) Platelet-derived growth factor is structurally related to the putative transforming protein p28 *sis* of simian sarcoma virus. Nature 305: 35-39
204. Weinberg RA (1984) *Ras* oncogenes and the molecular mechanisms of carcinogenesis. Blood 64: 1143
205. Welsh CW (1985) Host factors affecting the growth of carcinogen-induced rat mammary carcinomas: a review and tribute to Charles Brenton Huggins. Cancer Res 45: 3415-3443
206. Welshons WV, Lieberman ME, Gorski J (1984) Nuclear localization of unoccupied estrogen receptors. Nature 307: 747-749
207. Westley B, Rochefort H (1980) A secreted glycoprotein induced by estrogen in human breast cancer cell lines. Cell 20: 353-362
208. Willett WC, Stampfer MJ, Colditz GA, Rosner BA, Hennekens CH, Speizer FE (1987) Moderate alcohol consumption and the risk of breast cancer. N Engl J Med 316: 1174-1180
209. Wold BJ, Kim SK (1985) Stable reduction of thymidine kinase activity in cells expressing high levels of anti sense RNA. Cell 42: 129-138
210. Wynder EL, Rose DP, Cohen CA (1986) Diet and breast cancer in causation and therapy. Cancer 58 [Suppl 8]: 1804-1813
211. Yarden Y, Escobedo JA, Kwang WJ, Yang-Feng TL, Daniel TO, Tremble PM, Chen EY, Ando ME, Harkins RN, Franks U, Fried VA, Ullrich A, Williams LT (1986) Structure of the receptor for platelet-derived growth factor helps define a family of closely related growth factors. Nature 323: 226-232
212. Yee D, Cullen KJ, Paik S, Perdue JF, Hampton B, Schwartz A, Lippman ME, Rosen N (1988) Insulin-like growth factor II mRNA expression in human breast cancer. Cancer Res 48: 6691-6697
213. Zapf J, Froesch ER (1986) Insulin-like growth factors/somatomedins: structure, secretion, biological actions, and physiologic role. Horm Res 24: 121-130
214. Zarbl H, Sukumar S, Arthur AU, Martin-Zuria D, Barbacid M (1985) Direct mutagenesis of Ha-*ras*-1 oncogenes by *N*-nitroso-*N*-methylurea during initiation of mammary carcinogenesis in rats. Nature 315: 382-385
215. Zava DT, McGuire WL (1977) Estrogen receptor: unoccupied sites in nuclei of a breast tumor cell line. J Biol Chem 252: 2703-3708
216. Zwiebel JA, Bano M, Nero E, Salomon DS, Kidwell WR (1986) Partial purification of transforming growth factors from human milk. Cancer Res 46: 933-939

In Vitro Predictive Sensitivity Testing in the Therapeutic Assessment of Breast Cancer

J.T. Emerman

Department of Anatomy, University of British Columbia, Vancouver, B. C., Canada

Introduction

The choice of endocrine therapy and chemotherapy used in the treatment of breast cancer is largely empirically derived, based on data obtained from clinical trials [32]. However, patients with the same tumor pathology may not respond to the same cytotoxic drugs. Steroid hormone receptors, used to predict hormone responsiveness of breast tumors, greatly improve the probability of response, but does not ensure that a patient will benefit from endocrine manipulations. Inappropriate treatments result in valuable time lost for alternative therapy and unnecessary suffering from side effects of antineoplastic agents. A major aspect of breast cancer biology responsible for therapeutic failures is tumor heterogeneity; tumors contain varying numbers of hormone- and drug-responsive and hormone- and drug-resistant cells [47].

It would be of obvious clinical value to develop an assay that would lead to selection of the most effective treatment for the individual patient. To be clinically applicable, the assay must be rapid, simple, and inexpensive. To be valid, the assay must correlate positively with patient response.

Much information has accrued from assays with human tumor cell lines, but this cannot be used to predict drug response in patients; it only indicates the potential effects of antineoplastic agents as each patient's tumor is unique. It has recently been reported that drug sensitivities of cells from tumors passaged several times correlate with clinical responses [2, 50]. However, these assays take 4-6 weeks to complete. Furthermore, cell lines developed from a given tumor may not respond to drugs in the same way as the original tumor cell population [6], just as drug sensitivities between primary tumors and metastases may vary [128].

To eliminate the potential problems associated with tumor cell lines, in vitro assays have been designed to identify the sensitivities of freshly obtained human tumor specimens to therapeutic agents. This chapter does not attempt to review the details of in vitro predictive sensitivity tests nor to present an extensive review of the literature [21, 103], but to give an overview of current assays, an to describe our model for predictive testing of human breast carcinomas.

Scientists have been developing in vitro assays to determine sensitivities of fresh tumor specimens to antineoplastic agents for the past 30 years. A variety of techniques have been utilized to measure drug-induced cytotoxicity of cells in

Ragaz/Ariel (Eds.), High-Risk Breast Cancer

explant culture or cell culture, including morphological criteria [140], inhibition of cellular metabolism [22], inhibition of radioactive precursor incorporation [8], and reduced ability of isolated cells to form colonies [15, 43]. Current assays can be divided into three broad groups based on the time required to complete the assay. Short-term assays measure cell responses to drugs immediately following drug exposure and are completed in a matter of hours [39, 79, 105]. Medium-term assays measure cell sensitivities to drugs following a recovery period after drug treatment and generally take a few days [63, 86, 139]. Long-term assays determine cell growth 14-21 days following drug treatment [15, 102, 112].

Short-Term Assays

In most short-term assays, cells in suspension [39, 105, 127] or tumor fragments [16] are incubated with a cytotoxic drug for 3 h. For the last hour, a radioactive precursor of DNA or RNA is added to determine drug interference with nucleic acid precursor incorporation. A variation of the short-term assay provides for a longer drug exposure time [145]. Cell suspensions are incubated with drugs for 24 h, followed by a 1-h exposure to [^{3}H] TdR (tritiated thymidine). Response to hormones has been determined by incubating tumor fragments with hormones for 48 h and measuring [^{3}H] TdR incorporation at different times throughout this period [94]. Although the inhibition of nucleic acid precursor incorporation during or immediately after drug exposure does not necessarily imply cell death, positive correlations with clinical responses have been reported [16, 39, 79, 94] and are similar to those reported for clonogenic assays (discussed later in this chapter).

Medium-Term Assays

Medium-term assays generally utilize monolayer cultures [86, 139]. An antitumor drug is added to the culture medium for 1-2 days. Following removal of the drug, the cells are allowed to recover for a period of 1-2 days before the effects of the drug are determined. Alternatively, isolated cells may be maintained in soft agar (discussed later in this chapter) and growth determined by labeled nucleoside incorporation following a recovery period after drug exposure. This takes advantage of the specificity of soft agar for tumor cells while permitting a shorter time for completion of the assay than colony counting [61, 119]. A medium-term assay in which cells are cultured over an agar base in a liquid top layer allows the cells to be harvested directly without having to be released from the gel [35, 125, 45]. Theoretically, the recovery period following exposure to cytotoxic agents allows for a more accurate measurement of cell viability than determining inhibition of nucleic acid precursor incorporation immediately after drug treatment. Several determinants of cytotoxicity are utilized in medium-term tests, such as cell counts [69, 49], dye exclusion tests [59, 134], inhibition of nucleic acid precursor incorporation [119, 98, 115, 125, 57], and inhibition of protein precursor incorporation [70, 20,

136, 6, 34, 63, 139]. Good correlations between these assays and clinical responses have been demonstrated [70, 49, 136, 17].

Some investigators use multicellular spheroids rather than monolayer cultures for in vitro assays as the former reproduce the three-dimensional architecture of solid tumors in vivo [10, 88, 64]. Spheroids are formed from single-cell suspensions in spinner flasks [118], or from cells seeded onto nonadhesive surfaces [144, 42]. Recently, boluses of tumor cells have been embedded in collagen gel matrices to preserve tumor architecture [83, 84]. This three-dimensional arrangement allows for different microenvironments and metabolic gradients to be established that likely approximate those in solid tumors in vivo [10, 125]. The cells in the inner regions of the spheroid are exposed to different concentrations of therapeutic agents and for different lengths of time from those in the outer regions. Not only is it more difficult for cytotoxic agents to penetrate cells in the center of the spheroid, but also the cells are more resistant to these agents, since there is a decrease in growth rate resulting from oxygen and nutrient deficiencies and an accumulation of catabolic products. This is similar to poorly vascularized areas in solid tumors. Hypoxic cells of inner cell layers have been shown to be radioresistant [106, 40]. They may also respond differently to chemotherapeutic agents compared with cells receiving sufficient oxygen [40].

Organ cultures or tumor fragments [94, 77, 16, 84, 111, 135] are utilized to preserve cell-matrix and cell-cell interactions in vivo. The use of pieces of tissue also eliminates the trauma of tissue dissociation. However, tumor pieces may contain a considerable amount of stroma, and are not necessarily representative of the entire tumor.

Long-Term Assays

The application of cell cloning [95] for in vitro predictive sensitivity assays was demonstrated with mouse myeloma cells [93]. Modifications of this technique have resulted in long-term clonogenic assays for human solid tumors with soft agar [15, 43, 102], agarose [65], or methylcellulose [12]. Following tumor dissociation, the cell suspension is incubated for 1 h in the presence of chemotherapeutic agents. The cells are then seeded as isolated cells in a semisolid medium. Cytotoxicity of drugs is determined by measuring the number of colonies that arise from the single cells after 14-21 days in culture.

The clonogenic assay is based on the assumption that only a small percentage of the total tumor cell population, the stem cells, maintain the growth of the tumor and it is the stem cells that have the ability to form colonies in a semisolid medium. Proponents of the clonogenic assay suggest that a predictive sensitivity test should measure the effects of therapeutic agents only on the stem cell population. Assessing drug effects on all cell types within a tumor is misleading since most of the tumor cell population has a limited number of potential divisions. Positive correlations between clonogenic assay results and clinical responses have been demonstrated, ranging from 56% to 84% for predicting patient response, and from 76% to 100% for predicting patient resistance [131].

Although the clonogenic assay has proven to be a very useful tool in predictive sensitivity testing, less than 50% of human tumors produce sufficient colonies for assessing responses to therapeutic agents [109, 7, 123]. Passaging of cells before assay has been shown to enhance the cloning efficiency [100]. However, this prolongs the assay, which already requires 2-3 weeks to complete, and increases the probability of cellular alterations in drug sensitivities. Additional methodological problems have been identified [109, 123]. Preparation of single-cell suspensions is difficult and clumps of cells may be mistaken for colonies. The definition of a colony is arbitrary, generally ranging from 30 to 50 cells. Counting colonies is subjective and will be difficult to automate. A variety of nonmalignant tissues can also grow in soft agar [115], including fibrocystic breast tissue [130, 104]. Therefore, the assay may not be measuring clonal growth of the stem cell population alone. Furthermore, the culture conditions are far removed from the in vivo situation, permitting the measurement of drug effects on only a small population of cells within a tumor that has the capacity to proliferate as isolated cells in a semisolid matrix. This may not be relevant to the treatment of solid tumors, most of which are heterogeneous. The presence of mixed populations of cells within a tumor has been shown to influence the sensitivities of cells to therapeutic agents [82].

The percentage of breast carcinomas that can grow in the soft agar clonogenic assay is low [110, 130, 104]. Furthermore, there is a poor correlation between responses to drugs in the clonogenic assay and risk factors for breast cancer and clinical responses to chemotherapy [104, 57, 23]. The responses of breast cancer cell lines to hormones suggest that the assay may be useful for predicting hormone sensitivities of fresh breast cancer specimens [37, 31]. However, under the present conditions, there appears to be little correlation between exposure to hormones of fresh specimens in vitro and hormone treatment in vivo [23, 90, 132]. There may be potential for the use of the clonogenic assay in predicting sensitivities of breast cancers as recent modifications of culture conditions have resulted in improved correlations with clinical disease [52, 55].

Smith et al. [112] have developed a clonogenic assay for human breast cancers that uses second-passage cells grown on irradiated fibroblast feeder layers in conditioned medium. This has greatly improved the plating efficiency of these tumors. Additionally, they have shown that cells from normal breast tissue grow in this system and their responses to therapeutic agents are similar to those of cells from tumor tissue from the same patient and suggest that a patient's normal cells may be cultured to determine drug sensitivities of their malignant counterparts [113]. However, correlations with clinical responses have yet to be determined.

Proposed Assay for Breast Carcinomas

Breast cancers are comprised of a heterogeneous population of cells, and tumor heterogeneity contributes to the growth kinetics [47] and drug sensitivities [82, 81] of tumors. Thus, a representative sample of the tumor cell population should be cultured in order to maintain heterogeneity. For this reason, we have concentrated on developing a monolayer culture system to measure hormone and drug sensitivities of breast cancers. As discussed already, monolayer cultures do not retain the three-dimensional architecture of tumors in vivo as do spheroids or tumor fragments; however, relatively high seeding densities permit cell-cell interactions and cell growth fractions that approximate conditions in vivo [33]. Interactions between subpopulations affecting drug sensitivities in monolayer culture have been described [82]. The importance of the seeding density is further demonstrated by studies showing that cells in monolayer culture in a logarithmic phase of growth respond to anticancer agents differently from those in a stationary growth phase [24].

Substrates

Conventional monolayer cultures maintained on plastic or glass substrates are not appropriate for drug sensitivity testing of both normal and malignant mammary epithelium since the cells do not grow well and the cultures are quickly overgrown with fibroblasts [18, 97]. Recently, a defined medium has been developed for the continuous growth of human breast epithelial cells in monolayer culture [44]. Also, it has been demonstrated that breast epithelium will grow continuously in medium containing low calcium levels [116]. These culture systems may prove useful for drug sensitivity assays. However, it must be considered that optimal conditions for growth of cells in culture are not necessarily those that permit the continuous growth of cells, nor those that encourage maximal growth, but conditions that are comparable to those experienced by the cells in vivo. Measuring the response of tumor cells to therapeutic agents in the absenc of factors present in vivo disregards the fact that tumor behavior is correlated with its environment [107, 82, 80].

Collagen gel matrices more closely simulate the in vivo situation than do artificial substrates. We [25, 26, 27, 28, 30] and others [41, 68, 137, 141, 143] have demonstrated that normal and malignant mammary epithelial cells can grow and express differentiated functions comparable to counterpart cells in vivo when maintained on or in hydrated collagen matrices. Furthermore, tumor cells can retain their states of malignant progression [66, 30]. For development of an in vitro sensitivity assay, we have utilized a collagen substrate, but it has been necessary to use a dehydrated collagen matrix for the assay to be clinically feasible [27]. Further modifications may also be required to minimize errors in chemosensitivity testing. However, this culture system should be applicable to studying the effects of hormones and drugs on breast cancer cell survival.

Medium Constituents

An appropriate nutrient environment is also required for chemosensitivity testing. Defined media containing hormones and growth factors and animal sera-supplemented media are used to stimulate cell growth [107, 4, 142, 92, 44]. However, these media may be inadequate for determining the effects of therapeutic agents on cells in culture if they are deficient in factors that influence cell-drug interactions in vivo. Therefore, we suggest the medium in which the cultured cells are grown should include the patient's serum since this serum may provide host factors that influence regulation of cell growth and interact with therapeutic agents.

Procedures and Results

Our procedure for preparing human mammary epithelial cells for culture is briefly outlined. Mammary tissue is dissociated in collagenase and hyaluronidase followed by differential centrifugation of the cell suspension to select for a highly enriched population of epithelial cells. Single cells or small cell aggregates are collected by filtration through a 150-μm Nitex filter. Autoradiographic analysis of [^{3}H] TdR incorporation into DNA has demonstrated that the epithelial cells grow on collagen gels while fibroblast growth is restricted, comparable to the growth properties of these cell types in vivo (Fig. 1) [27]. We have demonstrated that normal and malignant human breast epithelium have different growth properties when cultured (a) in a defined medium designed specifically for the growth of human mammary cells [44], (b) in medium containing fetal bovine serum, and (c) in medium containing human serum. Medium containing human serum is superior to

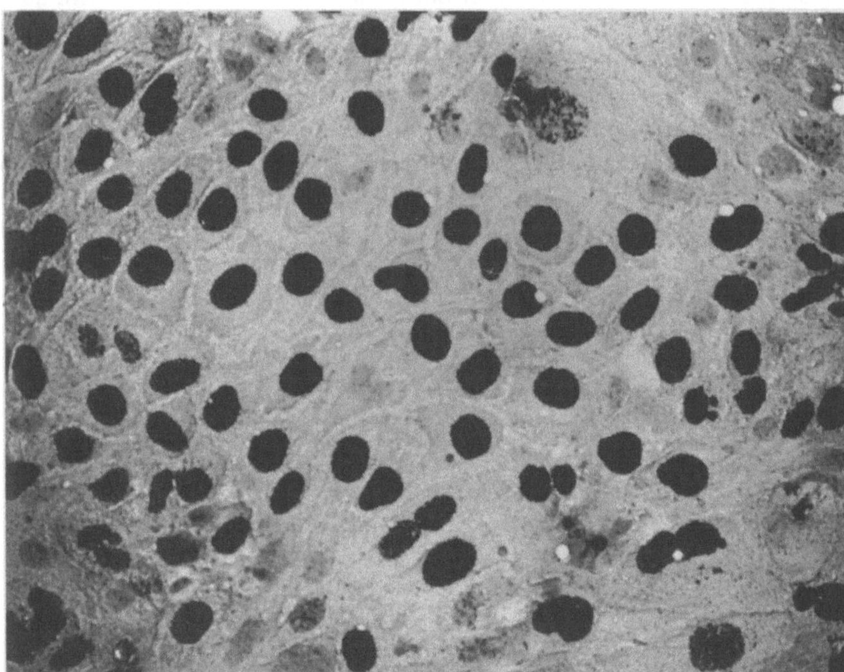

Fig. 1. Autoradiograph of human mammary tumor cells cultured on a collagen gel in the presence of 5% human serum. Following a 24-h exposure to 1 μCi/ml [^{3}H] TdR, the nuclei of cells forming the epithelial sheet are labeled [27]

the other media in supporting attachment and growth of these cells (Fig. 2) [27]. Human serum from all donors tested is superior to the other media in supporting growth, however, there is significant variation in the ability of different human serum samples to support the growth of cells from a given tumor [27], indicating the importance of using the serum of the patient from whom the tissue is excised. Similar results are obtained with dehydrated collagen substrates.

The experiments to be described demonstrate that cells cultured in different media show considerable variability in their response to the same cytotoxic agent. The protocol for testing the sensitivities of cells to chemotherapeutic agents is as follows [27]. Cells are seeded at a density of 2×10^5 cells/cm^2 onto dehydrated collagen-coated wells of a 96-well dish. Drugs at concentrations pharmacologically achievable in vivo and one-tenth of this level, are added to 1-day-old cultures. After drug exposure for 24 h, the cultures are allowed a recovery period in drug-free medium for 48 h, then incubated with [^{3}H] TdR for 24 h. Cytotoxicity is measured by inhibition of [^{3}H] TdR incorporation into DNA. The results are expressed as a percentage of untreated controls. The sensitivities to three chemotherapeutic agents, Adriamycin (AD), melphalan (MEL), and 5-fluorouracil (5-FU), of breast tumor cells cultured in different media is shown in Fig. 3 [27]. The cytotoxicity of all three drugs on cells from patients 1 and 2 was consistently greater in the presence of the patient's serum than fetal bovine serum (Fig. 3a-c). Cells from patient 3 cultured in the patient's serum varied in their sensitivities to the lower concentrations of AD and MEL from those cultured in defined medium (Fig. 3d, e). Precursor incorporation into DNA by AD of cells from patient 3 was inhibited by 5-FU in the patient's

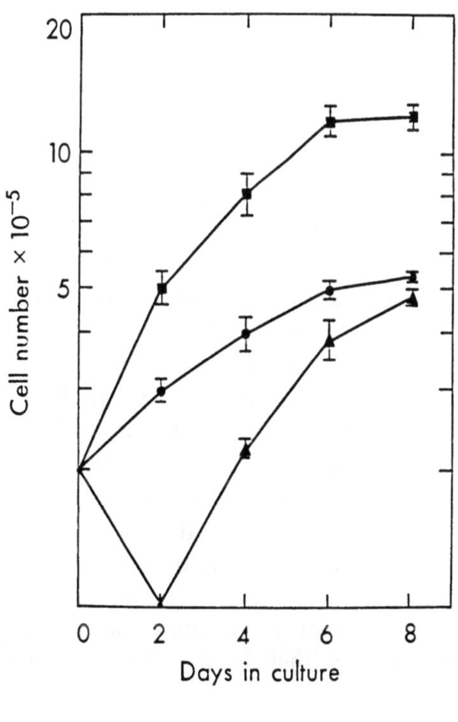

Fig. 2. Growth of human mammary tumor cells cultured on collagen gels in defined medium (*triangles*), medium supplemented with 5% fetal bovine serum (*circles*), or medium containing 5% human serum (*squares*). Medium containing human serum was superior to the other media in supporting growth of these cells [27]

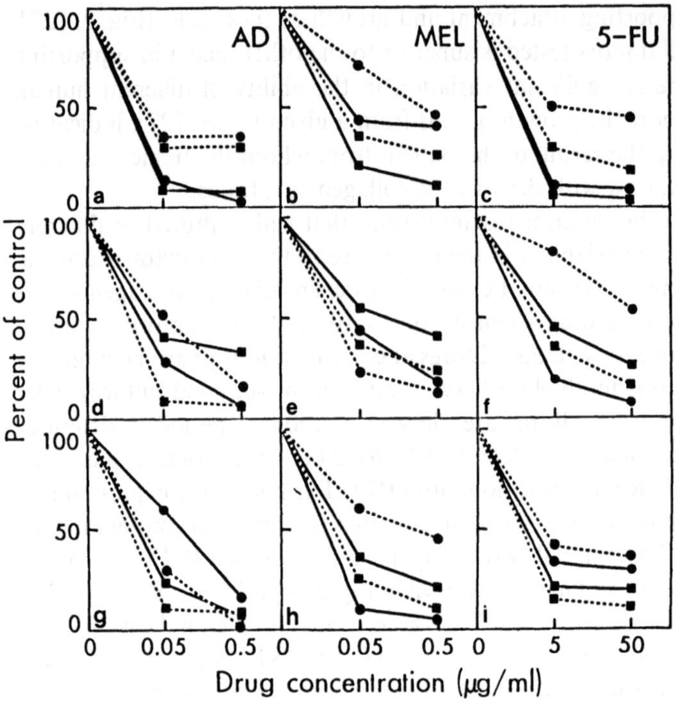

Fig. 3a–j. Variations in chemosensitivities of human mammary tumor cells cultured on dehydrated collagen matrices in different media. **a–c** cells from patients 1 (*circles*) and 2 (*squares*), maintained in serum from the patient (*full lines*) or fetal bovine serum (*broken lines*), **d–f** cells from patients 3 (*circles*) and 4 (*squares*), maintained in serum from the patient (*full lines*) or defined medium (*broken lines*), **g–i** cells from patients 5 (*circles*) and 6 (*squares*), maintained in serum from the patient (*full lines*) or serum from a normal human donor (*broken lines*). Cells were exposed to Adriamycin (**a, d, g**), melphalan (**b, e, h**), and 5-fluorouracil (**c, f, i**) [27]

serum, but not in defined medium (Fig. 3f). AD and MEL were more toxic to cells of patient 4 in defined medium than in the patient's serum (Fig. 3d,e). Inhibition of precursor incorporation into DNA of cells from patient 5 was greater in serum from a normal human donor than in the patient's serum (Fig. 3g), whereas the reverse was true for the effects of MEL (Fig. 3h). The variability in response of the same cells to the same chemotherapeutic agent cultured in different media illustrates the caution that must be exercised in extrapolating data obtained in vitro to the in vivo situation. Although the validity of using the patient's serum for predictive sensitivity tests must be confirmed by clinical correlations, this serum should provide optimal conditions for such assays since it provides an environment more closely simulating in vivo conditions than do other media.

We are also utilizing this in vitro assay to determine the effects of combination endocrine therapy and chemotherapy on breast carcinoma cells (J. T. Emerman and A. W. Tolcher 1988, unpublished work). Cortisol, known to influence human mammary epithelial cell growth in culture [120, 36, 62], is used in the experiments described later. Cultures are incubated with the hormone for the length of the assay in the presence of the patient's serum, which is treated with dextran-charcoal to remove endogenous steroids. Inhibition of cell growth by cortisol decreased cell sensitivity to the cytotoxic effects of AD (Fig. 4a). In contrast, if cortisol stimulated cell growth, the cells were more responsive to the inhibitory effects of AD (Fig. 4b). This supports other studies demonstrating that the growth-promoting effects of hormones enhance cell kill by chemotherapeutic agents [14, 67, 71, 54].

Problems with In Vitro Assays

Although there are positive correlations between in vitro sensitivity tests and clinical responses, one can still not predict with confidence the most appropriate form of treatment for individual cancer patients. There are several problems that plague in vitro assays in general that no doubt contribute to discrepancies between results in culture and in vivo. The appropriate drug concentrations and exposure times in culture that reflect those in vivo are not known. This is further complicated by the fact that drug concentrations within a tumor, although lower than those measured in plasma, are unknown and will vary in different regions of the tumor

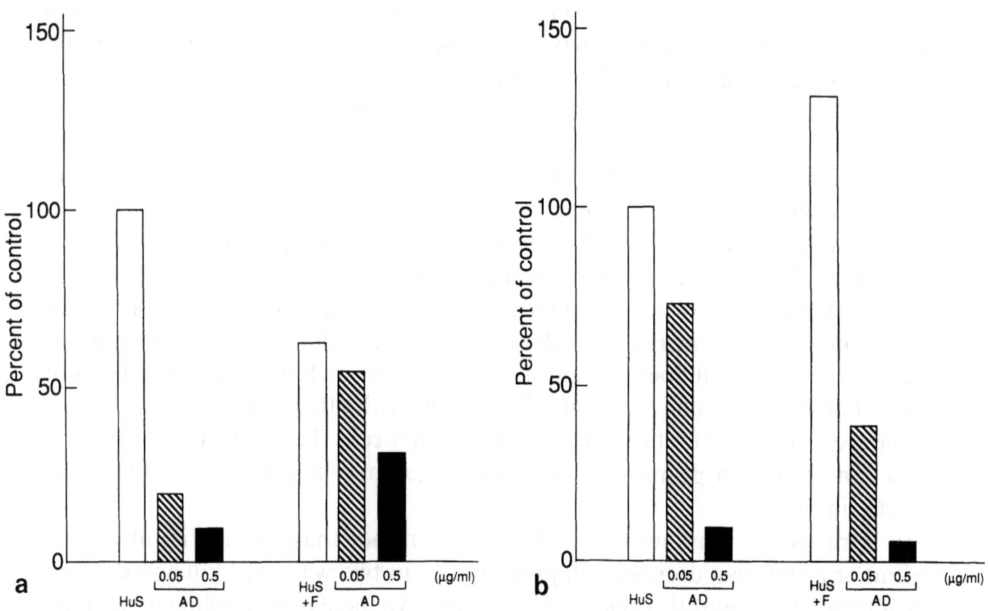

Fig. 4a,b. Effect of cortisol (F; 3 μg/ml) on the inhibition of [^{3}H] TdR incorporation into DNA by Adriamycin (AD) in human mammary tumor cells. Cells were grown on dehydrated collagen matrices in medium containing 5% dextran-charcoal-treated serum from the patient, plus or minus F. **a** decreased cell growth induced by F resulted in increased resistance to AD cytotoxicity, **b** stimulation of cell growth by F increased the sensitivity of the cells to AD and between tumors, depending on vascularization. Current data indicate that clinically relevant concentrations in vitro appear to be approximately one-tenth of the peak plasma concentration [1, 7, 98]. Higher concentrations may predict resistance, but may also produce false-positive responses [101, 85, 1]. The use of high drug concentrations in vitro, however, may identify those tumors that are not sensitive at low concentrations, but are sensitive at high concentrations. This could lead to selection of high dose drug treatment or regional administration of drugs [19, 91, 117, 129]. Ideally, a range of concentrations should be used to plot a dose-response curve, but this is usually not feasible, owing to an insufficient number of tumor cells for assay.

An accurate assessment of cytotoxic activity of cell-cycle-dependent drugs, drugs with a prolonged plasma half-life, and those administered daily may require a prolonged exposure time in culture of 24-48 h [1, 33, 86, 7, 78]. However, continuous exposure in vitro does not take into account host conversion, detoxification, and elimination [100].

Hormone and drug effects on metabolic processes may synchronize the cell population, producing false-negative or false-positive results [72, 5, 73, 89, 96]. On the other hand, the consequences of interference with a metabolic pathway may not be observed at the time of drug exposure [72, 86, 98, 138]. Therefore, it would appear that a recovery period is necessary following drug exposure. The length of the recovery period may vary, however, depending on the effect of the drug on the metabolic pathway in question. Good correlations with inhibition of protein precursors and clinical responses have been observed, with a recovery period of 24 h following drug treatment [34, 17, 86, 121]. For measuring inhibition of nucleic acid precursor incorporation, a recovery period of 48-96 h produces maximum effects [9, 51, 72, 119]. Owing to their mode of action, antimetabolites such as methotrexate and 5-FU initially increase [^{3}H] TdR incorporation into DNA. A decrease in [^{3}H] TdR is not observed until 72 h after exposure in vitro [34, 87, 76, 33, 119].

Certain drugs such as cyclophosphamide require activation to form cytotoxic metabolites [3]. Cytotoxic metabolites may be added directly to culture, or assays must be modified to activate compounds such as that described by Alley et al. [3], in which tumor cells are cocultured with rat hepatocytes. Although estrogen does not require bioactivation, it does not appear to act directly on human breast epithelium to stimulate proliferation [56, 80, 46]. It interacts with other factors present in vivo to produce growth-promoting agents for mammary cells. Therefore, the response of breast cancer cells in primary culture to estrogen may not accurately reflect the response in vivo.

In vitro assays must measure cell survival rather than metabolic inhibition. Antitumor agents can decrease cell proliferation in two ways: cell kill and delayed transit through the mitotic cycle [9, 51, 72, 119]. An increased doubling time of the population may produce results indistinguishable from those obtained by populations whose cells are actually killed. However, cell survival determinations such as counting viable cells or clones require large numbers of cells and are time and labor intensive. The procedures are, therefore, clinically unfeasible. Other tests that monitor the sensitivities of tumors to therapeutic agents and that are rapid and easily automated must be utilized. Precursor incorporation with [^{3}H] nucleosides and [^{3}H] amino acids has been shown to reflect changes in cell number and clonogenic survival [119, 86, 92, 98, 114, 138, 57] and correlate positively with clinical response [72, 94, 114, 122]. In contrast, other investigators have shown that changes in [^{3}H] TdR incorporation do not necessarily affect the proliferative potential of cells [126, 98, 58]. Colorimetric assays have been used to evaluate growth inhibition by antineoplastic agents. Intensity of hematoxylin-stained cells [75] or methylene blue-parafuchsin-stained cells [108] as well as dye exclusion tests [134] appear to give an accurate measure of cell number. Reduction of tetrazolium-based compounds by cell lines to a blue formazen product shows a good correlation with colony counts [11]. Other end points that may assess drug effects are being investigated, such as utilization of radiolabeled glucose [132] and flow cytometric analysis of cellular perturbations [48]. End points for in vitro assessment of cell death that reflect in vivo cell kill will ultimately be identified by correlating sensitiveities of cells in vitro with clinical responses. It is possible that using a single index of response may not give an accurate measure of cell death, and two or more parameters may be required.

Single-drug regimens are rarely used in clinical treatment. For most solid tumors, chemotherapeutic protocols generally involve 3-5 drugs. Drugs are selected for combination treatments based on their differences in mode of action, but this does not necessarily correlate with the biological responses of cells to drug combinations. In vitro sensitivity assays should be able to identify appropriate combination treatments for individual patients, but must be modified to accommodate multiple drug testing. To date, there have been few reports on the effects of drug combinations in vitro due to the requirement for large numbers of cells [1, 74, 60].

In addition to combination drug protocols, combination endocrine therapy and chemotherapy is used in breast cancer treatment, since the mechanism of action of hormones and cytotoxic drugs are different. Initially, it was assumed that endocrine treatment would eliminate the hormone-responsive cells while cytotoxic drugs would kill the cells not affected by the hormonal environment. However, it soon became apparent that if chemotherapy is most effective on cycling populations of cells and the hormone-responsive cells are the more rapidly growing cells in a heterogeneous tumor, there may be little benefit to combination therapy. Recent data have indicated that the modifying influences of hormones on tumor growth and metabolism may interfere with the cytotoxic effects of chemotherapeutic agents [133, 5, 29, 89, 13, 38, 53]. This is likely responsible for the conflicting results of hormone-drug combination therapy [99]. However, these studies have also demonstrated that the therapeutic efficacy of chemotherapeutic agents may be enhanced by utilizing the effects of hormones on tumor growth to increase the sensitivities of tumors to these agents. It has also recently been shown that the growth-stimulating effects of growth factors and hormones in vitro that result in an increase in the number of proliferating cells, increase cell sensitivity to chemotherapeutic agents ([67, 71, 54], J. T. Emerman and A.W. Tolcher 1988, unpublished work). These studies suggest that growth stimulation as well as growth inhibition by hormones should be incorporated into hormone-drug regimens. Much work remains to be done in this area to determine how combination endocrine therapy and chemotherapy can be used to its best advantage in clinical cancer treatment.

Concluding Remarks

Although it may be some time before the limitations of in vitro assays are overcome, research in this area is vital. An in vitro assay that can predict the sensitivities of tumor cells to hormones and drugs will permit a rapid assessment of the benefits of therapeutic agents for individual patients. It will also provide a greater insight into drug-drug and hormone-drug interactions for rational design of combination therapies. In addition, an in vitro assay can be used to determine the potency of new antitumor agents [124].

To be beneficial to the clinical management of cancer, an in vitro assay must ultimately result in improved survival rates. After the validity of an assay has been confirmed by retrospective studies, randomized, prospective clinical trials are needed to demonstrate the value of an assay compared with other assays and empirical derivations. We expect that an in vitro assay that most closely simulates in vivo conditions has the greatest chance for success in predictive sensitivity testing. However, in the final analysis, methodology is not important; clinical relevance is important. We must not give up the prospect of developing a clinically relevant assay that will contribute to improving the quality and quantity of life of cancer patients and to preventing the needless suffering caused by inappropriate therapies.

Acknowledgments The studies in the author's laboratory were supported by a grant from the National Cancer Institute of Canada and funds contributed by Mr. B.T. Wharton in memory of his wife, Nadia. J.T. Emerman is a research scholar of the National Cancer Institute of Canada.

References

1. Alberts DS, Salmon SE, Chen HSG, Moon TE, Young L, Surwit EA (1981) Pharmacologic studies of anticancer drugs with the human tumor stem cell assay. Cancer Chemother Pharmacol 6:253-264
2. Albrecht M, Simon WE, Hölzel F (1985) Individual chemosensitivity of in vitro proliferating mammary and ovarian carcinoma cells in comparison to clinical results of chemotherapy. J Cancer Res Clin Oncol 109: 210-216
3. Alley MC, Powis G, Appel PL, Kooistra KL, Lieber MM (1984) Activation and inactivation of cancer chemotherapeutic agents by rat hepatocytes cocultured with human tumor cell lines. Cancer Res 44: 549-556
4. Barnes D, Sato G (1980) Methods for growth of cultured cells in serum-free medium. Anal Biochem 102: 255-270
5. Benz C, Cadman E, Gwin J, Terrence W, Amara J, Eisenfeld A, Dannies P (1983) Tamoxifen and 5-fluorouracil in breast cancer: cytotoxic synergism in vitro. Cancer Res 43: 5298-5303
6. Berry RJ, Laing AH, Wills J (1975) Fresh explant culture of human tumours in vitro and the assessment of sensitivity to cytotoxic chemotherapy. Br J Cancer 31:218-227
7. Bertelsen CA, Sondak VK, Mann BD, Korn EL, Kern DH (1984) Chemosensitivity testing of human solid tumors: a review of 1582 assays with 258 clinical correlations. Cancer 53: 1240-1245

8. Bickis IJ, Henderson IWD, Quaster JH (1966) Biochemical studies of human tumors. II. In vitro estimation of individual tumor sensitivity to anticancer agents. Cancer 19: 103-113
9. Brereton HD, Bryant TL, Young RC (1975) Inhibition and recovery of DNA synthesis in host tissues and sensitive and resistant B16 melanoma after 1-2(2-chloroethyl)-3-(*trans*-4-methylcyclohexyl)-1-nitrosourea, a predictor of therapeutic efficacy. Cancer Res 35: 2420-2425
10. Carlsson J, Yuhas JM (1984) Liquid-overlay culture of cellular spheroids. In: Acker H, Carlsson J, Durand R, Sutherland R (eds) Spheroids in cancer research. Springer, Berlin Heidelberg NewYork, pp 1-23 (Recent results in cancer research, vol. 95)
11. Carmichael J, DeGraff WG, Gazdar AF, Minna JD, Mitchell JB (1987) Evaluation of a tetrazolium-based semiautomated colorimetric assay: assessment of chemosensitivity testing. Cancer Res 47: 936-942
12. Cillo C, Odartchenko N (1984) Cloning of human tumor cells in methylcellulose-containing medium. Hofmann V, Berens ME, Martz G (eds) Predictive drug testing on human tumor cells. Springer, Berlin Heidelbrg New York, pp 56-64 (Recent results in cancer research, vol. 94)
13. Clarke R, Van den Berg HW, Kennedy DG, Murphy RF (1985) Oestrogen receptor status and the response of human breast cancer cell lines to a combination of methotrexate and 17-β-oestradiol. Br J Cancer 51: 365-369
14. Conte PF, Fraschini G, Alama A, Nicolin A, Corsaro E, Conavese G, Rosso R, Drewinko B (1985) Chemotherapy following estrogen-induced expansion of the growth fraction of human breast cancer. Cancer Res 45: 5926-5930
15. Courtenay VD, Mills J (1978) In vitro colony assay for human tumours grown in immunesuppressed mice and treated in vivo with cytotoxic agents. Br J Cancer 37: 261-268
16. Daidone MG, Silvestrini R, Sanfilippo O, Zaffaroni N, Varini M, De Lena M (1985) Reliability of an in vitro short-term assay to predict the drug sensitivity of human breast cancer. Cancer 56: 450-456
17. Darling JL, Thomas DGT (1983) Results obtained using assays of intermediate duration and clinical correlations. In: Dendy PP, Hill BT (eds) Human tumour drug sensitivity testing in vitro. Academic, London, pp 269-280
18. Das NK, Hosick HL, Nandi S (1974) Influences of seeding density on multicellular organization and nuclear events in cultures of normal and neoplastic mouse mammary epithelium. J N C I 52: 849-861
19. Dedrick RL, Myers CE, Bungay PM, De Vita VT Jr (1978) Pharmacokinetic rationale for peritoneal drug administration in the treatment of ovarian cancer. Cancer Treat Rep 62: 1-11
20. Dendy PP, Bozman G, Wheeler TK (1970) In vitro screening test for human malignant tumours before chemotherapy. Lancet ii: 68
21. Dendy PP, Hill BT (eds) (1983) Human tumour drug sensitivity testing in vitro. Academic, London
22. Di Paolo JA, Dowd JE (1961) Evaluation of inhibition of human tumour tissue by cancer chemotherapeutic drugs with an in vitro test. J N C I 27: 807-815
23. Dittrich C, Jakesz R, Wrba F, Havelec L, Haas O, Spona J, Holzner H, Kolb R, Moser K (1985) The human tumour cloning assay in the management of breast cancer patients. Br J Cancer 52: 197-203
24. Drewinko B, Patchen M, Yang L-Y, Barlogie B (1981) Differential killing efficacy of twenty antitumor drugs on proliferating and nonproliferating human tumor cells. Cancer Res 41: 2328-2333

25. Emerman JT, Bartley JC, Bissel MJ (1981) Glucose metabolite patterns as markers of functional differentiation in freshly isolated and cultured mouse mammary epithelial cells. Exp Cell Res 134: 241-250
26. Emerman JT, Enami J, Pitelka DR, Nandi S (1977) Hormonal effects on intracellular and secreted casein in cultures of mouse mammary epithelial cells on floating collagen membranes. Proc Natl Acad Sci USA 74: 4466-4470
27. Emerman JT, Fiedler EE, Tolcher AW, Rebbeck PM (1987) Effects of defined medium, fetal bovine serum, and human serum on growth and chemosensitivities of human breast cancer cells in primary culture: inference for in vitro assays. In Vitro Cell Dev Biol 23: 134-140
28. Emerman JT, Pitelka DR (1977) Maintenance and induction of morphological differentiation in dissociated mammary epithelium on floating collagen membranes. In Vitro 13: 316-328
29. Emerman JT, Siemiatkowski J (1984) Effects of endocrine regulation of growth of a mouse mammary tumor on its sensitivity to chemotherapy. Cancer Res 44: 1327-1332
30. Emerman JT, Worth AJ (1985) Phenotypic stability of mouse mammary tumor cells cultured on collagen gels. In Vitro Cell Dev Biol 21: 49-56
31. Fan D, Schneider C, Fan S, Blank H, Gillen L, Morgan LR (1984) Effects of estrogen, tamoxifen and progesterone on a human breast cancer line in the soft-agar assay. In: Salmon SE, Trent JM (eds) Human tumor cloning. Grune and Stratton, Orlando, pp 477-486
32. Forrest APM (1986) Advances in management of carcinoma of breast. Surg Gynecol Obstet 163: 89-100
33. Freshney RI, Dendy PP (1983) Culture methods for assays of intermediate duration. In: Dendy PP, Hill BT (eds) Human tumour drug sensitivity testing in vitro. Academic, London, pp 69-89
34. Freshney RI, Paul J, Kane IM (1975) Assay of anticancer drugs in tissue culture: conditions affecting their ability to incorporate ^{3}H-leucine after drug treatment. Br J Cancer 31: 89-99
35. Friedman HM, Glaubiger DL (1982) Assessment of in vitro drug sensitivity of human tumor cells using [^{3}H] thymidine incorporation in a modified human tumor stem cell assay. Cancer Res 42: 4683-4689
36. Gaffney EV, Pigott D (1978) Hydrocortisone stimulation of human mammary epithelial cells. In Vitro 14: 621-624
37. Goldenberg GJ, Froese EK (1982) Drug and hormone sensitivity of estrogen receptor-positive and negative human breast cancer cells in vitro. Cancer Res 42: 5147-5151
38. Goldenberg GJ, Froese EK (1985) Antagonism of the cytocidal activity and uptake of melphalan by tamoxifen in human breast cancer cells in vitro. Biochem Pharmacol 34: 763-770
39. Group for Sensitivity Testing of Human Tumours (KSST) (1981) In vitro short-term test to determine the resistance of human tumours to chemotherapy. Cancer 48: 2127-2135
40. Gupta V, Costanzi JJ (1987) Role of hypoxia in anticancer drug-induced cytotoxicity for Ehrlich ascites cells. Cancer Res 47: 2407-2412
41. Haeuptle M, Suard YLM, Bogenmann E (1983) Effect of cell shape change on the function and differentiation of rabbit mammary cells in culture. J Cell Biol 96: 1425-1434
42. Haji-karim M, Carlsson J (1978) Proliferation and viability in cellular spheroids of human origin. Cancer Res 38: 1457-1464

43. Hamburger AW, Salmon SE (1977) Primary bioassay of human tumor stem cells. Science 197: 461-463
44. Hammond SL, Ham RG, Stampfer MR (1984) Serum-free growth of human mammary epithelial cells: rapid clonal growth in defined medium and extended serial passage with pituitary extract. Proc Natl Acad Sci USA 81: 5435-5439
45. Hanson JA, Bean EA, Coombs AM, Moore JL (1985) A comparison of two in vitro assays of cell response following in vitro drug and radiation exposures of human tumour xenograft cells. Br J Cancer 52: 637-640
46. Haslam SZ (1986) Mammary fibroblast influence on normal mouse mammary epithelial cell responses to estrogen in vitro. Cancer Res 46: 310-316
47. Heppner GH, Miller B, Cooper DN, Miller FR (1981) Growth interactions between mammary tumor cells. In: Brenner NJ, McGrath CM (eds) Cell biology of breast cancer. Academic, New York, pp 161-172
48. Hill BT, Whelan RDH, Rupniak HT, Dennis LY, Rosholt MA (1981) A comparative assessment of the in vitro effects of drugs on cells by means of colony assays or flow microfluorimetry. Cancer Chemother Pharmacol 7: 21-26
49. Holmes HL, Little JM (1974) Tissue-culture microtest for predicting response of human cancer to chemotherapy. Lancet ii: 985-987
50. Hölzel F, Albrecht M, Simon WE, Hänsel M, Metz R, Schweizer J, Dietel M (1985) Effectiveness of antineoplastic drugs on the proliferation of human mammary and ovarian carcinoma cells in monolayer culture. J Cancer Res Clin Oncol 109: 217-226
51. Houghton PJ, Taylor DN (1977) Fractional incorporation of [^{3}H] thymidine and DNA specific activity as assays of inhibition of tumour growth. Br J Cancer 35: 68-77
52. Hug V, Haynes M, Rashid R, Spitzer G, Blumenschen G, Hortobagyi G (1984) Improved culture conditons for clonogenic growth of primary human breast tumours. Br J Cancer 50: 207-213
53. Hug V, Hortobagyi G, Drewinko B, Finders M (1985) Tamoxifen-citrate counter-acts the antitumor effects of cytotoxic drugs in vitro. J Clin Oncol 3: 1672-1677
54. Hug V, Johnston D, Finders M, Hortobagyi G (1986) Use of growth-stimulating hormones to improve the in vitro therapeutic index of doxorubicin for human breast tumors. Cancer Res 46: 147-152
55. Hug V, Thames H, Hortobagyi G, Finders M (1986) Chemosensitivities of human clonogenic breast tumour cells. Eur J Cancer Clin Oncol 22: 971-981
56. Ikeda T, Liu Q, Danielpour D, Officer JB, Iio M, Leland FE, Sirbasku DA (1982) Identification of estrogen-inducible growth factors (estromedins) for rat and human mammary tumor cells in culture. In Vitro 18: 961-979
57. Jones CA, Tsukamoto T, O'Brien PC, Uhl CB, Alley MC (1985) Soft agarose culture human tumour colony forming assay for drug sensitivity testing: [^{3}H]-thymidine incorporation vs colony counting. Br J Cancer 52: 303-310
58. Jozan S, Gay G, Marques B, Mirouze A, David JF (1985) Oestradiol is effective in stimulating ^{3}H-thymidine incorporation, but not on proliferation of breast cancer cultured cells. Cell Tissue Kinet 18: 457-464
59. Kaltenbach JP, Kaltenbach MH, Lyons WB (1958) Nigrosin as a dye for differentiating live and dead ascites cells. Exp Cell Res 15: 112-117
60. Kennedy DG, Van den Berg HW, Clarke R, Murphy RF (1986) Enhancement of methotrexate cytotoxicity towards the MDA. MB. 436 human breast cancer cell line by dipyridamole. Biochem Pharmacol 35: 3053-3056
61. Kern DH, Drogemuller CR, Kennedy MC, Hildebrand-Zanki SU, Tanigawa N, Sondak VK (1985) Development of a miniaturized, improved nucleic acid precursor

incorporation assay for chemosensitivity testing of human solid tumors. Cancer Res 45: 5436-5441
62. Klevjer-Anderson P, Buehring GC (1980) Effect of hormones on growth rates of malignant and nonmalignant human mammary epithelia in culture. In Vitro 16: 491-501
63. Kornblith PL, Smith BH, Leonard LA (1981) Response of cultured human brain tumours to nitrosoureas: correlation with clinical data. Cancer 47: 255-261
64. Kwok TT, Twentyman PR (1985) The response to cytotoxic drugs of EMTG cells treated either as intact or disaggregated spheroids. Br J Cancer 51: 211-218
65. Laboisse CL, Augeron C, Potet F (1981) Growth and differentiation of human gastrointestinal adenocarcinoma stem cells in soft agarose. Cancer Res 41: 310-315
66. Lawler EM, Miller FR, Heppner GH (1983) Significance of three-dimensional growth patterns of mammary tissues in collagen gels. In Vitro 19: 600-610
67. Leclercq G, Devleeschouwer N, Danguy A, Verrijdt A, Heuson JC (1985) In vitro synergism between estrogens and cytotoxic agents. J Steroid Biochem 23: 1111-1113
68. Lee EYH, Lee WH, Kaetzel CS, Parry G, Bissell MJ (1985) Interaction of mouse mammary epithelial cells with collagenous substrata: regulation of casein gene expression and secretion. Proc Natl Acad Sci USA 82: 1419-1423
69. Lickiss JN, Cane KA, Baikie AG (1974) In vitro drug selection in antineoplastic chemotherapy. Eur J Cancer 10: 809-814
70. Limburg H, Heckmann C (1968) Chemotherapy in the treatment of advanced pelvic malignant disease with special reference to ovarian cancer. J Obstet Gynaecol 75: 1246-1250
71. Lippman ME, Cassidy J, Wesley M, Young RC (1985) Increasing the response rate to cytotoxic chemotherapy by endocrine means. J Steroid Biochem 23: 1173-1180
72. Livingstone RB, Titus GA, Heilbrun LK (1980) In vitro effects on DNA synthesis as a predictor of biological effect from chemotherapy. Cancer Res 40: 2209-2212
73. Lykkesfelt AE, Larsen JK, Christensen IJ, Briand P (1984) Effects of the antioestrogen tamoxifen on the cell cycle kinetics of the human breast cancer cell line, MCF-7. Br J Cancer 49: 717-722
74. MacKintosh FR, Evans TL, Sikic BI (1981) Methodologic problems in clonogenic assays of spontaneous human tumours. Cancer Chemother Pharmacol 6: 205-210
75. Madeddu L, Roy F, Leclercq G (1986) A new method for evaluating the inhibitory potency of antiestrogens on breast cancer cell lines. Anticancer Res 6: 11-16
76. Mann BD, Kern DH, Guiliano AE, Burk MW, Campbell MA, Morton DL (1982) Clinical correlations with drug sensitivities in the clonogenic assay: retrospective pilot study. Arch Surg 117: 33-36
77. Masters JRW (1983) An overview of the role of organ culture for human tumour biopsies. In: Dendy PP, Hill BT (ed) Human tumour drug sensitivity testing in vitro. Academic, London, pp 163-177
78. Matsushima Y, Kanzawa F, Hoshi A, Shimizu E, Nomori H, Sasaki Y, Saijo N (1985) Time-schedule dependency of the inhibiting activity of various anticancer drugs in the clonogenic assay. Cancer Chemother Pharmacol 14: 104-107
79. Mattern J, Volm M (1982) Clinical relevance of predictive tests for cancer chemotherapy. Cancer Treat Rev 9: 267-298
80. McGrath CM (1983) Augmentation of response of normal mammary epithelial cells to estradiol by mammary stroma. Cancer Res 43: 1355-1360
81. Miller BE, McInerney D, Jackson D, Miller FR (1986) Metabolic cooperation between mouse mammary tumor subpopulations in three-dimensional collagen gel cultures. Cancer Res 46: 89-93

82. Miller FR, Medina D, Heppner GH (1981) Preferential growth of mammary tumors in intact mammary fat pads. Cancer Res 41: 3863-3867
83. Miller BE, Miller FR, Heppner GH (1984) Assessing tumor drug sensitivity by a new in vitro assay which preserves tumor heterogeneity and subpopulation interactions. J Cell Physiol [Suppl] 3: 105-116
84. Miller BE, Miller FR, Heppner GH (1985) Factors affecting growth and drug sensitivity of mouse mammary tumor lines in collagen gel cultures. Cancer Res 45: 4200-4205
85. Moon TE (1980) Quantitative and statistical analysis of the association between in vitro and in vivo studies. In: Salmon SE (ed) Cloning of human tumor stem cells. Liss, New York, pp 209-221
86. Morgan D, Freshney RI, Darling JL, Thomas DGT, Celik F (1983) Assay of anticancer drugs in tissue culture: cell cultures of biopsies from human astrocytoma. Br J Cancer 47: 205-214
87. Myers CE, Young RC, Chabner BA (1976) Kinetic alterations induced by 5-fluorouracil in bone marrow, intestinal mucosa, and tumor. Cancer Res 36: 1653-1658
88. Nederman T, Twentyman P (1984) Spheroids for studies of drug effects. In: Acker H, Carlsson J, Durand R, Sutherland R (eds) Spheroids in cancer research. Springer, Berlin Heidelberg New York, pp 84-102 (Recent results cancer research, vol 95)
89. Osborne CK, Boldt DH, Estrada P (1984) Human breast cancer cell cycle synchronization by oestrogens and antioestrogens in culture. Cancer Res 44: 1433-1439
90. Osborne CK, Von Hoff DD, Mullins K (1985) Endocrine therapy testing of human breast cancers in the soft agar clonogenic assay. Breast Cancer Res Treat 6: 229-235
91. Ozols R, Gratzinger K, Myers C, Young RC (1979) Ovarian cancer (OC): intraperitoneal (IP) therapy with adriamycin (ADR). Proc Am Assoc Cancer Res 20: 978
92. Page MJ, Field JK, Everett NP, Green CD (1983) Serum regulation of the estrogen responsiveness of the human breast cancer cell line MCF-7. Cancer Res 43: 1244-1250
93. Park CH, Bergasgel DE, McCulloch EA (1971) Mouse myeloma tumor stem cells: a primary cell culture assay. J N C I 46: 411-422
94. Poulsen HS, Bichel P, Andersen J (1982) Short-term culture of human breast cancer: in vitro effects of hormones related to patient response. Br J Cancer 46: 67–74
95. Puck TT, Marcus PI (1955) A rapid method of viable cell titration and clone production with Hela cells in tissue culture: the use of X-irradiated cells to supply conditioning factors. Proc Natl Acad Sci USA 41: 432-437
96. Reddel RR, Murphy LC, Sutherland RL (1984) Factors affecting the sensitivity of T-47D human breast cancer cells to tamoxifen. Cancer Res 44: 2398-2405
97. Richards J, Pasco D, Yang J, Guzman R, Nandi S (1983) Comparison of the growth of normal and neoplastic mouse mammary cells on plastic, on collagen gels and in collagen gels. Exp Cell Res 146: 1-14
98. Roobol C, Sips HCM, Theunissen J, Atassi G, Bernheim JL (1984) In vitro assessment of cytotoxic agents in murine cancers: comparison between antiproliferative and antimetabolic assays. J N C I 72: 661-666
99. Rose C, Mouridsen HT (1984) Combined cytotoxic and endocrine therapy in breast cancer. In: Bresciani F, King RJB, Lippman ME, Namer M, Raynaud J-P (eds) Progress in cancer research and therapy vol 31. Raven, New York, pp 269-286
100. Rosenblum ML, Dougherty DV, Reese C, Wilson CB (1981) Potentials and possible pitfalls of human stem cell analysis. Cancer Chemother Pharmacol 6: 227-235
101. Salmon SE, Alberts DS, Durie BGM, Meyskens FL, Jones SE, Soehnlen B, Chen WS, Moon T (1980) Clinical correlations of drug sensitivity in the human tumor stem cell assay. In: Mathe G, Muggia FM (eds) Cancer chemo- and immunopharmacology I.

Springer, Berlin Heidelberg New York, pp. 300-305 (Recent results in cancer research, vol 74)
102. Salmon SE, Hamburger AW, Soehnlen B, Durie BG, Alberts DS, Moon TE (1978) Quantitation of differential sensitivity of human tumor stem cells to anticancer drugs. N Engl J Med 298: 1321-1327
103. Salmon SE, Trent JM (eds) (1984) Human tumor cloning. Grune and Stratton, Orlando
104. Sandbach J, Von Hoff DD, Clark G, Cruz AB, O' Brien M (1982) Direct cloning of human breast cancer in soft agar culture. Cancer 50: 1315-1321
105. Sanfilippo O, Daidone MG, Costa A, Canetta R, Silvestrini R (1981) Estimation of differential in vitro sensitivity of non-Hodgkin lymphomas to anticancer drugs. Eur J Cancer 17: 217-226
106. Sasaki T, Yamamoto M, Kuwahara K (1984) Lethal effect of bleomycin and peplomycin on Hela cells in multicell tumor spheroids. Cancer Res 44: 1374-1379
107. Sato G (1975) The role of serum in culture. In: Litwak G (ed) Biochemical action of hormones, vol 3. Academic, New York, pp 391-396
108. Sauter C, Cogoli M, Arrenbrecht S (1986) Interactions of cytotoxic and other drugs: rapid cell culture assay. Oncology 43: 46-49
109. Selby P, Buick RN, Tannock I (1983) A critical appraisal of the "Human tumour stem-cell assay". N. Engl J Med 308: 129-134
110. Sikic BI, Taber RL (1981) Human tumor clonogenic assays. Cancer Chemother Pharmacol 6: 201-203
111. Silvestrini R, Daidone MG, Costa A, Sanfilippo O (1985) Cell kinetics and in vitro chemosensitivity as a tool for improved management of patients. Eur J Cancer Clin Oncol 21: 371-378
112. Smith HS, Lan S, Ceriani R, Hackett AJ, Stampfer MR (1981) Clonal proliferation of cultured nonmalignant and malignant human breast epithelia. Cancer Res 41: 4637-4643
113. Smith HS, Lippman ME, Hiller AJ, Stampfer MR, Hackett AJ (1985) Response to doxorubicin of cultured normal and cancerous human mammary epithelial cells. J N C I 74: 341-347
114. Sondak VK, Bertelsen CA, Tanigawa N, Hildebrand-Zanki SU, Morton DL, Korn EL, Kern DH (1984) Clinical correlations with chemosensitivities measured in a rapid thymidine incorporation assay. Cancer Res 44: 1725-1728
115. Sondak VK, Giuliano AE, Kern DH (1984) Outcome of "non-malignant" specimens submitted for soft-agar clonogenic assay. In: Salmon SE, Trent JM (eds) Human tumor cloning. Grune and Stratton, Orlando, pp 327-341
116. Soule HD, McGrath CM (1986) A simplified method for passage and long-term growth of human mammary epithelial cells. In Vitro Cell Dev Biol 22: 6-12
117. Speyer JL, Collins JM, Dedrick RL, Brennan MF, Londer H, DeVita VT Jr, Myers CE (1979) Phase I and pharmacological studies of intraperitoneal (IP) 5-fluorouracil (5-FU). Proc Am Soc Clin Oncol 20: C-251
118. Sutherland RM, Durand RE (1976) Radiation response of multicell spheroids: an in vitro tumour model. Curr Top Radiat Res 11: 87-139
119. Tanigawa N, Kern DH, Hikasa Y, Morton DL (1982) Rapid assay for evaluating the chemosensitivity of human tumors in soft agar culture. Cancer Res 42: 2159-2164
120. Taylor-Papadimitriou J, Sheares M, Stoker MGP (1977) Growth requirements of human mammary epithelial cells in culture. Int J Cancer 20: 903-908
121. Thomas DGT, Darling JL, Paul EA, Mott TJ, Godlee JN, Tobias JS, Capra LG, Collins CD, Mooney C, Bozek T, Finn GP, Arigbabu SO, Bullard DE, Shannon N, Freshney RI (1985) Assay of anti-cancer drugs in tissue culture: relationship of relapse

free interval (RFI) and in vitro chemosensitivity in patients with malignant cerebral glioma. Br J Cancer 51: 525-532
122. Tubiana M, Pejovic MH, Chavaudra N, Contesso G, Malaise EP (1984) The long-term prognostic significance of the thymidine labelling index of breast cancer. Int J Cancer 33: 441-445
123. Twentyman PR (1985) Predictive chemosensitivity testing. Br J Cancer 51: 295-299
124. Twentyman PR, Fox NE, Wright KA, Workman P, Broadhurst MJ, Martin JA, Bleehen NM (1986) The in vitro effects and cross-resistance patterns of some novel anthracyclines. Br J Cancer 53: 585-594
125. Twentyman PR, Walls GA, Wright KA (1984) The response of tumour cells to radiation and cytotoxic drugs—a comparison of clonogenic and isotope uptake assays. Br J Cancer 50: 625-631
126. Van den Berg HW, Clarke R, Murphy RF (1981) Failure of 5-fluorouracil and methotrexate to destroy the reproductive integrity of a human breast cancer cell line (MCF-7) growing in vitro. Eur J Cancer Clin Oncol 17: 1275-1281
127. Volm M, Wayss K, Kaufmann M, Mattern J (1979) Pretherapeutic detection of tumour resistance and the results of tumour chemotherapy. Eur J Cancer 15: 983-993
128. Von Hoff DD, Clark GM, Forseth BJ, Cowan JD (1986) Simultaneous in vitro drug sensitivity testing on tumours from different sites in the same patient. Cancer 58: 1007-1013
129. Von Hoff DD, Clark GM, Weiss GR, Marshall MH, Buchok JB, Knight III WA, LeMaistre CF (1986) Use of in vitro dose response effects to select antineoplastics for high-dose or regional administration regimens. J Clin Oncol 4: 1827-1834
130. Von Hoff DD, Cowan J, Harris G, Reisdorf G (1981) Human tumor cloning: feasibility and clinical correlations. Cancer Chemother Pharmacol 6: 265-271
131. Von Hoff DD, Forseth B, Gonzales L (1986) Culture and sensitivity of tumors. Tex Med 82: 32-35
132. Von Hoff DD, Forseth B, Warfel LE (1985) Use of a radiometric system to screen for antineoplastic agents: correlation with a human tumor cloning system. Cancer Res 45: 4032-4038
133. Weichselbaum RR, Nove J, Hellman S, Piro AJ, Little JB (1979) Combination hormonal, chemotherapy and radiotherapy in vitro: implications for therapy in vivo. Int J Radiat Oncol Biol Phys 5: 1657-1661
134. Weisenthal LM, Marsden JA, Dill PL, Macaluso CK (1983) A novel dye exclusion method for testing in vitro chemosensitivity of human tumors. Cancer Res 43: 749-757
135. Wei-Zen W, Massey RJ, Heppner GH (1985) A 3-dimensional tumour growth inhibition assay for testing monoclonal antibody cytotoxicity. Cancer Immunol Immunother 20: 137-144
136. Wheeler TK, Dendy PP, Dawson A (1974) Assessment of an in vitro screening test of cytotoxic agents in the treatment of advanced malignant disease. Oncology 30: 362-376
137. Wilde CJ, Hasan HR, Mayer RJ (1984) Comparison of collagen gels and mammary extracellular matrix as substrata for study of terminal differentiation in rabbit mammary epithelial cells. Exp Cell Res 151: 519-532
138. Wilson AP, Ford CHJ, Newman CE, Howell A (1984) A comparison of three assays used for the in vitro chemosensitivity testing of human tumours. Br J Cancer 49: 57-63
139. Wilson AP, Neal FE (1981) In vitro sensitivity of human ovarin tumours to chemotherapeutic agents. Br J Cancer 44: 189-200
140. Wright JC, Cobb JP, Gumport SL, Golomb FM, Safodi D (1957) Investigation of the relation between clinical and tissue culture response to chemotherapeutic agents of human cancer. New Engl J Med 257: 1207-1211

141. Yang J, Elias JJ, Petrakis NL, Wellings SR, Nandi S (1982) Effects of hormones and growth factors on human mammary epithelial cells in collagen gel culture. Cancer Res 41: 1021-1027
142. Yang J, Larson L, Flynn D, Elias J, Nandi S (1982) Serum-free primary culture of human normal mammary epithelial cells in collagen gel matrix. Cell Biol Int Rep 6: 965-975
143. Yang N, Kube D, Park C, Furmanski P (1981) Growth of human mammary epithelial cells on collagen gel surfaces. Cancer Res 41: 4093-4100
144. Yuhas JM, Li AP, Martinez AO, Ladman AJ (1977) A simplified method for production and growth of multicellular tumour spheroids. Cancer Res 37: 3639-3643
145. Zirvi KA, Hill GJ, Hill HZ (1986) Comparative studies of chemotherapy of human tumor cells in vitro by tritiated thymidine uptake inhibition and soft agar clonogenic assay. J Surg Oncol 31: 123-126

The Role of Chromosome Analysis in the Investigation of Breast Cancer

D.E. Horsman

Cytogenetics Laboratory, Cancer Control Agency of British Columbia,
Vancouver, B.C., Canada

Introduction

Cancer cytogenetics is a rapidly growing field that has made significant contributions to our understanding of the genetic mechanisms of neoplasia. It has confirmed the clonal nature of malignant disease and has demonstrated that most if not all cancers are characterized by alterations in chromosome number and structure. The knowledge that there is concordance between the common sites of cancer-specific chromosomal changes and the location of normal genes and oncogenes involved in the control of cell proliferative activities has contributed to our current understanding of the chromosomal basis of neoplasia [50].

The major application of chromosome analysis has been in the investigation of hematopoietic malignancies. The majority of acute and chronic leukemias have been shown to have clonal chromosomal abnormalities, many of which are specific for certain subtypes of disease. Similar findings have been recently demonstrated in the non-Hodgkin's lymphomas. The identification of these "non random" chromosomal abnormalities has provided important diagnostic and prognostic information to the pathologist and clinician, as well as a focus for current research.

The valuable information arising from the chromosomal investigation of the leukemias and lymphomas has kindled new interest in the cytogenetics of solid tumors. These cancers have not received the same amount of attention, primarily owing to technical difficulties associated with obtaining metaphases from solid tumor tissue. Recent improvements in methodology, however, have permitted successful analysis of numerous types of solid tumor. This effort holds promise to provide the same kind of diagnostic and prognostic information that has accrued with the hematopoietic malignancies. With regards to breast cancer, there is a strong potential that chromosome investigation may be of value in defining different subtypes of disease and in predicting patient outcome.

Before discussing in detail the role of cancer cytogenetics in relation to solid tumors and breast cancer in particular, a perspective on the general field of cytogenetics will be provided, including a brief outline of chromosome morphology and nomenclature and a review of the established findings in leukemia and lymphoma.

Ragaz/Ariel (Eds.), High-Risk Breast Cancer

Chromosome Morphology and Nomenclature

The human chromosome complement can be analyzed during the metaphase stage of cell division with a photomicroscope. The normal structure of human chromosomes is determined by their DNA and protein composition and its interaction with the methods of cell fixation and staining used in the laboratory. Each chromosome is composed of two sister chromatids, consisting of identical molecules of DNA. The chromatids are held together at a localized constriction called the centromere. The location of the centromere varies along the length of each chromosome and serves as an identifying feature. For identification purposes, each chromosome can be divided into the short or p arm and a longer q arm, determined by the position of the centomere. A variety of special staining techniques are used to produce an alternating dark and light stain pattern along the length of the chromosome arms [36]. This banding pattern is constant for each normal chromosome and from one person to the next. The number of bands visible on each chromosome is dependent on the stage of metaphase at which the cell was fixed, with more bands being evident in late prophase and early metaphase than in late metaphase. The techniques utilized to reveal a greater number of chromosome bands are called high resolution banding [49]. A numbering system has been devised to identify each band on all of the chromosomes [18]. An individual chromosome can therefore be identified by its size, the location of the centromere, and the length and the characteristic banding pattern of the p and q arms. These features can also be utilized to interpret the makeup of structurally rearranged chromosomes. A normal human karyotype and a pictorial representation of the banding pattern of chromosome 1 are provided in Figs. 1 and 2.

The normal chromosome complement, or diploid number, in humans is 46, consisting of 22 pairs of autosomes and one pair of sex chromosomes. In cytogenetic nomenclature this is designated 46,XY and 46,XX for males and females, respectively. In cancer cells, change from the normal chromosome complement can result from a variety of mechanisms involving gain or loss of chromosomes or alterations in chromosome structure. Such alterations are not compatible with normal cell function and are only viable in neoplastic cells.

An abnormal, or aneuploid, chromosome number in a cell may arise from chromosome loss or duplication, usually the consequence of mitotic errors such as nondisjunction, endoreduplication, or cell fusion. If the resultant total chromosome number is less than 46, it is termed hypodiploidy, and if more than 46, hyperdiploidy. Structural changes result from multiple chromosome breaks with rejoining of the broken segments into abnormal chromosome configurations, thereby producing an alteration in the banding pattern of the affected chromosomes. With good quality chromosome preparations and high resolution banding, precise identification of the sites of breakage, or breakpoints, on the involved chromosomes is possible. If the new chromosome cannot be identified by its band pattern, it is called a marker.

In cytogenetic nomenclature, an abnormality is described following the total chromosome number and sex designation, with chromosome gains or losses noted with either a + or a − sign, i.e., 47, XX, +8. Rearrangements are designated by an

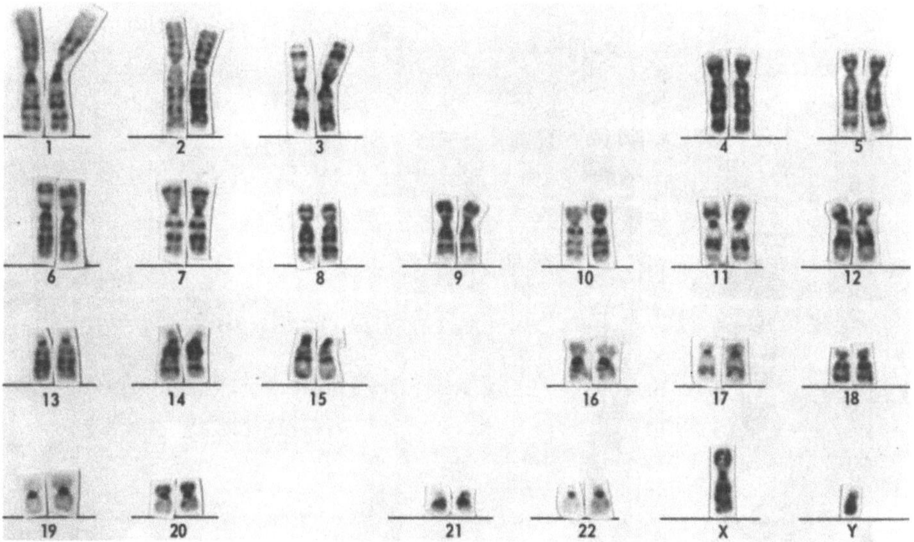

Fig. 1. A normal G-banded human karyotype: 250-band stage

abbreviation for the particular type of change found, with the affected chromosomes designated within brackets and separated by a semicolon. The breakpoint sites are then defined, i.e. 46,XY,t(9;22)(q34;q11) describes a translocation between chromosome 9 and 22, involving breakpoint sites 9q34 and 22q11, respectively.

During chromosome analysis of bone marrow or tumor tissue, the chromosomes of 25 or more metaphases are fully counted and analyzed to identify any cell line with a numerical or structural deviation from normal. A consistent alteration, defined as two or more cells with the same change, identifies the presence of a malignant clone.

Cancer Cytogenetics: History

The belief that chromosomes play an important role in the etiology of neoplasia was established in the early years of this century. This was most eloquently expressed in the 1914 monograph of Theodor Boveri [5]. His observations were consistent with the more recently proposed theories that cancer is a clonal disorder and that alteration in the genetic material, such as by chromosomal rearrangement, is a basic underlying mechanism in the genesis of cancer. The profound nature of his hypotheses, however, were not to be fully appreciated for another 50 years.

The development of cancer cytogenetics during the first half of this century was hampered by technical problems which precluded reliable chromosome counts or analysis of chromosome morphology. The development of tissue culture techniques

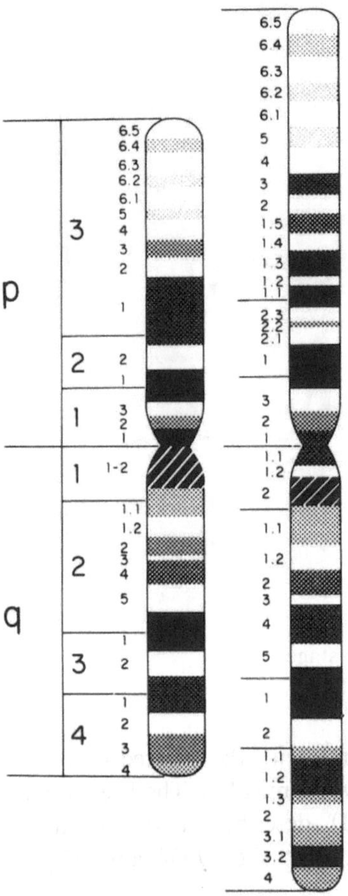

Fig. 2. A pictorial representation (idiogram) of high resolution banding of chromosome 1 showing the relationship between subbands at different stages of chromosome condensation

and improved cell fixation methods in the 1950s contributed greatly to improved chromosome preparations. Until the late 1960s, however chromosomes were stained by a solid staining method which permitted counting and grouping according to size and shape, but the detection of the most structural chromosomal rearrangements was not possible. Many of the early cancer investigations, therefore, revealed numerical abnormalities, but failed to identify the individual chromosomes involved or any recurrent rearrangements.

In 1960, Nowell and Hungerford identified in the bone marrow of seven patients with chronic myelogenous leukemia (CML) the presence of a common structural abnormality, initially thought to be a deleted G group chromosome [26]. In 1972, with the use of banding techniques this so-called Philadelphia (Ph^1) chromosome was shown to be the result of a reciprocal translocation between chromosomes 9 and 22 [30]. This was the first demonstration of a "non random" chromosomal abnormality associated with a specific disease and gave new impetus to the field of cancer cytogenetics.

Cancer Cytogenetics: General

The chromosomal changes encountered in human cancer consist of primary karyotypic changes that are related to the basic etiology of the disease and secondary changes that arise subsequently as the disease progresses [34]. Primary chromosomal changes are associated with early neoplastic events and are specific for a particular subtype of cancer, while secondary changes are nonspecifically associated with disease progression. Both are considered to play a crucial role in the behavior of the malignant cells.

Primary karyotypic changes are usually structural alterations such as translocations, inversions, and deletions. These are intra- and interchromosomal alterations resulting from chromosomal breakage and reunion. The net effect is the relocation of genes into abnormal chromosomal positions. There is a growing body of evidence that implicates one of the breakpoints in a rearrangement as the site of a proto-oncogene [19] which becomes abnormally activated when relocated into the vicinity of a transcriptionally active gene involved in the control of cell proliferation or differentiaion [20].

Secondary changes are usually additional numerical or structural changes that are superimposed upon primary structural rearrangements and arise sequentially as the malignant clone evolves. This occurs in all types of malignancies in a nonspecific manner, with greater degrees of karyotypic complexity being characteristic of advanced cancer. The progressive acquisition of secondary cytogenetic abnormalities, termed clonal evolution, produces an alteration of chromosomal dosage which may confer selective growth advantages. This is modulated by selection pressures and paralleled by biological alterations in the malignant clone such as increased invasiveness, development of drug resistance, or transformation to more aggressive disease.

Two other types of chromosomal abnormalities of importance in cancer cytogenetics are the chromosomal sites of gene amplification and fragile sites. Gene amplification is manifested as additional chromosomal material in the form of small acentric fragments, called double minutes (DM), or an expanded area within a chromosome region which stains in a homogeneous manner, termed homogeneously stained regions (HSR) [8]. These are often seen in advanced and aggressive neoplasms and are a reflection of selection pressures on individual genes. In a number of instances the amplified sequences have been shown to involve either oncogenes or genes for drug resistance. Fragile sites are chromosomal regions that are prone to breakage and rearrangement [23]. They are inherited in a mendelian fashion and may be cytogenetic windows onto transcriptionally active genes or sites of viral DNA insertion. A number of fragile sites have been mapped to the location of common cancer-associated breakpoints. Under the appropriate conditions, they may predispose the carrier of the fragile site to a structural rearrangement that plays a role in the initiation of cancer. Confirmation of an instrumental role in carcinogenesis, however, has yet to be proven.

The accumulation of a large amount of cytogenetic data from the hematopoietic malignancies and some solid tumors has led to the appreciation that there is a limited number of chromosomal breakpoint sites involved in cancer [25]. It is suspected that many of these sites harbor genes important in the development of a malignancy. The recent demonstration of concordance between the common cancer-related breakpoints and the loci of cell growth control genes, oncogenes, and fragile sites has provided the basis for the present theory of the chromosomal basis of neoplasia [50].

Chromosomes in Leukemia and Lymphoma

A brief review of the chromosomal findings in the leukemias and lymphomas will highlight some of the principles of the chromosomal involvement in cancer, including primary and secondary changes, clonal evolution, diagnostic and prognostic correlations, and the interaction of oncogenes with cell-type-specific functional genes.

Chronic myelogenous leukemia (CML) has been most extensively studied and the patterns of chromosomal involvement are well characterized [32]. In the chronic phase of CML, 95% of patients have a translocation involving chromosomes 9 and 22: t(9;22) (q34;q11). Some patients have additional changes during the chronic phase, but this becomes more prevalent as the disease transforms into the acute phase, when most patients develop additional chromosomal changes within the t(9;22) clone, i.e., +8, +19, duplication of the Ph^1 or of 17q. The detection of t(9;22) and the presence or absence of clonal evolution is of value in confirming the diagnosis and predicting disease stage and patient prognosis.

Molecular DNA investigation has demonstrated that in all cases of true CML the c-*abl* oncogene located at band 9q 34 is translocated onto chromosome 22 at band q11 into the midst of a gene called the bcr gene, the function of which is not yet known [9]. This produces a functional chimeric gene on the Ph^1 chromosome that is transcibed and translated into a novel protein with protein kinase activity. This abnormal protein has homology with the transforming protein product of the v-*abl* oncogene, and is believed to play a crucial role in the initiation and progression of CML.

The chromosomal investigation of the acute leukemias has proven of value for confirmation of diagnosis, provision of prognostic information, and for monitoring of remission and relapse. In acute lymphoblastic leukemia (ALL), up to 90% of patients can be shown to have a chromosomal abnormality at disease presentation and the karyotype is an independent prognostic indicator, regardless of other clinical parameters [45, 4]. The two most important types of abnormality are:

1. Hyperdiploidy, associated with the best prognosis within the entire group of ALL subtypes (and is an exception to the rule that a complex abnormal karyotype is associated with aggressive disease);
2. Translocation, conferring an especially poor prognosis. The translocations involve either a primitive stem cell (t(9;22), t(4;11)) or a highly proliferative cell (t(8;14)) which does not respond to standard chemotherapy [46] (Table 1).

The majority of patients with acute myelogenous leukemia (AML) have chromosomal abnormalities [51], most commonly nonspecific alterations such as +8, −7,

Table 1. Chromosomal abnormalities associated with acute lymphoblastic leukemia

Clonal abnormality	Fab morphology	Prognosis
Hyperdiploidy (50-70 chromosomes)	ALL-L1, L2	Good
Normal or near diploid	ALL-L1, L2	Medium
Hypodiploidy	ALL-L1, L2	Poor
Translocations		Poor
t(4;11)	ALL-L1, L2	
t(9;22)	ALL-L1, L2	
t(8;14)	ALL-L3	
t(1;19)	pre-B ALL	

Table 2. Chromosome abnormalities associated with acute myelogenous leukemia

Clonal abnormality	Fab morphology	Prognosis
+8 or other simple alterations	all subtypes	Medium
Translocations		
t(8;21)	AML-M2 (20%)	Good
t(15;17)	AML-M3 (100%)	Good
inv(16)	AML-M4 (25%)	Good
t(9;11)	AML-M5	Poor
t(6;9)	AML-M2, M4	Poor
t(9;22)	CML-BC	Poor
inv(3) or		
t(3;3)	AML and thrombocytosis	Poor?
Complex or multiple abnormalities	All subtypes	Poor

or complex karyotypic changes. A number of specific rearrangements associated with a specific morphological subtype of disease have also been defined which have important prognostic correlations (Table 2). With the recent availability of different types of treatment for acute leukemia, chromosome analysis has become an essential tool to identify subgroups of patients who may require different therapeutic protocols or alternative treatment such as bone marrow transplantation.

In malignant lymphoma, the prognosis may be influenced by the type of specific chromosomal rearrangement as well as by the presence or absence of clonal evolution [24]. A translocation (14; 18) is found in the majority of cases of follicular lymphomas, while other translocations (t(11;14), t(8;14)) are associated with diffuse lymphomas. These rearrangements characteristically involve the loci of the B-cell immunoglobulin genes or the T-cell receptor genes which become recombined with known or suspected oncogenes [38]. These genetic recombinations are believed to play an important role in the biology of these malignancies.

Chromosomes in Solid Tumors

In contrast to the large amount of information available on the chromosomal abnormalities in the hematopoietic malignancies, similar information for solid tumors has been slow to accumulate. Great difficulty has been experienced in obtaining good quality metaphases from cells of most solid tumors, and the complexity of the karyotypic changes encountered usually renders detailed analysis impossible.

To avoid these difficulties, attention was initially directed toward the analysis of malignant effusions and of permanent cell lines which provide a ready source of metaphases in fluid suspension. Effusions, however, represent metastatic disease from advanced and invasive carcinomas which have established complex karyotypes and are of limited value in the detection of primary chromosomal changes. Permanent cell lines, although convenient for cytogenetic analysis, are not easily established, especially from tumors that have not already metastasized. There has been limited success in establishing cell lines from some of the commoner cancers, including breast, prostate, and pancreatic cancer. The significance of the chromosome abnormalities identified in permanent cell lines, in relation to whether acquired in vivo or in vitro, provides an additional element of confusion.

Significant improvements in the processing of solid tumor tissue for chromosome analysis have been developed in the last few years [41]. These include mechanical and enzymatic disaggregation techniques which reduce the solid tissue to single cells or cell clusters which provide more numerous metaphases; the use of slides or plastic dishes coated with collagen or extracellular matrix to promote cell adherence and growth; and the use of improved media with growth factors and hormones. These improvements in cell culture have contributed to an improved success rate in solid tumor chromosome analysis.

The common solid tumors of childhood are the most intensively studied to date. Retinoblastoma, which occurs in both sporadic and hereditary form, is occasionally associated with a small interstitial deletion on chromosome 13 (13q14). This may be evident only in the tumor cells of sporadic cases, or may be found in both tumor and normal somatic cells of some patients with the familial form of this cancer [3, 7]. Similarly, Wilms' tumor arising in patients with congenital defects of the iris (aniridia), is often associated with a deletion of the short arm of chromosome 11 (11p13) [28]. Additional chromosomal changes, if present, provide evidence of aggressive disease that may not be apparent from the histologic features [10].

The chromosomal deletions associated with retinoblastoma and Wilms' tumor have demonstrated that loss or inactivation of normal genes on one chromosome, by a variety of potential mechanisms, may allow the expression of a malignant recessive allele present on the homologous chromosome [21, 6]. This is consistent with the "two-hit" theory of carcinogenesis developed by Knudson [22], and with the autosomal dominant pattern of inheritance of these hereditary cancers.

Neuroblastoma, which also occurs in familial and sporadic form, is also frequently found to have chromosome rearrangements. These usually involve structural alterations of the distal p arm of chromosome 1 [17]. The rearrangements of 1p involve breakage at a variety of different regions, and therefore may represent secondary changes involved in tumor progression. Multiple karyotypic abnormalities and DMs and HSRs are common in the more advanced and aggressive forms of neuroblastoma [14]. An oncogene similar to c-*myc* has been demonstrated to be amplified in neuroblastoma [35]. These n-*myc* amplified sequences can be identified within the HSRs [12]. From a prognostic standpoint, the demonstration of a normal karyotype or minor abnormalities has been correlated with early or treatment-responsive disease, while the presence of complex changes, DMs and HSRs, and molecular evidence of n-*myc* amplification, is predictive of an unresponsive and aggressive form of the disease [37].

Two other childhood tumors, Ewing's sarcoma and alveolar rhabdomyosarcoma, have been shown to have nonrandom chromosomal abnormalities [2, 42]. The identification of these respective rearrangements is of practical value in the differential diagnosis of these tumors from others with similar morphological features.

A number of adult tumors have been found to have specific chromosomal changes. The first identified was meningioma, being characterized by partial or complete loss of chromosome 22 [52]. The majority of cases have this abnormality, alone or with additional karyotypic changes. Simple monosomy 22 usually predicts a benign disease course, whereas those patients with more complex changes have a poorer prognosis.

Bladder cancer has been extensively investigated. The specific involvement of chromosome 1 and 11 is suspected, owing to recurrent observations of their association with this type of cancer [33]. Superficial, noninvasive lesions usually have a normal karyotype, but those with a chromosomal abnormality have a higher propensity to recurrence and more aggressive behavior. Bulky, invasive disease is always associated with complex abnormal karyotypes.

A number of other tumors have been shown to have specific chromosome involvement, at least in certain subtypes of the disease. In small cell carcinoma of lung, a 3p deletion or translocation is commonly found [44]. In a familial form of renal cell cancer, the site of the karyotypic changes may be on chromosome 3 [27]. Synovial sarcoma has recently been found associated with a translocation involving chromosomes X and 18 [43]. Other tumors have been extensively studied, including melanoma, colonic, ovarian, and endometrial carcinoma. An in-depth discussion of the cytogenetics of solid tumors can be found in more comprehensive reviews [31, 34].

Chromosomes in Breast Cancer

Of the many types of human solid tumors, breast carcinoma has received the most attention in an effort to identify any specific chromosomal changes that may be associated with disease etiology, with specific subtypes of disease, or with clinical behavior. Owing to the inherently low mitotic rate of breast cancer cells in vivo, it has proven very difficult to obtain metaphases from primary tumors. Many of the initial studies were performed on cell effusions or cell lines prior to the use of chromosome banding, and therefore the results are mainly of historical interest. The accumulated data from these prebanding studies have been reviewed by Sandberg [31]. It was established that almost all primary or metastatic lesions had complex karyotypes with chromosome counts in the 60-90 range, including numerous marker chromosomes. A small percentage had karyotypes in the near diploid range. Follow-up studies demonstrated that those patients with a near diploid karyotype had a survival advantage over patients with more complex karyotypic changes [1]. Information with regards to the identification of specific changes or breakpoint sites was not provided.

The more recent studies of breast cancer, utilizing a variety of preparative techniques on primary lesions, malignant effusions, and cell lines with chromosome banding methods have confirmed these general findings and permitted the identification of the extra and rearranged chromosomes involved. It was determined that certain chromosomes and breakpoint regions are over-represented and may be specifically associated with breast cancer. The results of these studies have been reviewed by Trent [40]. The possible nonrandom involvement of chromosomes 1, 6, 7, and 11 has been implicated. Chromosome 1 appears to be consistently abnormal in all cases, owing to either duplication or structural rearrangement affecting the q arm. It must be stated, however, that chromosome 1 is also commonly abnormal in other solid tumors and that such changes may be associated nonspecifically with tumor progression. Also, chromosomes 6, 7, and 11 were frequently abnormal, as a result of duplication, loss, deletion, translocation, or other rearrangement. There is, however, no consistency in involvement of any chromosome from one study to another, and the breakage sites on each suspect chromosome were scattered widely with no consistency from one case to another. Although these results have provided interesting and promising information, clearly a much larger number of cases will have to be thoroughly studied before any disease-specific breakpoint sites can be confirmed.

A number of interesting reports have appeared since the review by Trent in 1985 [40]. These are larger studies which have utilized direct analysis or short-term cultures applied to primary lesions or cell effusions. Smith et al. have utilized a special culture system with disaggregation techniques and specifically designed media including insulin, triiodothyrronine, epidermal growth factor, and conditioned media [39]. Successful culture of both benign and malignant breast epithelial cells has been confirmed by phenotypic markers. As these markers do not differentiate benign from malignant cells, an "invasion assay" was devised based on the ability of malignant cells to penetrate and invade a denuded amnion basement membrane layer. When this assay is used to confirm the malignant nature of the cultured cells, a majority of cases with "invasive" cells were shown to have diploid karyotypes. This confirmed the findings of their previous study in which the majority of cells in short-term cultures of breast carcinomas were diploid [48]. These results raise the question as to whether the acquisition of an abnormal karyotype is necessarily a primary tumorigenic event, and suggest that it may be indicative of malignant progression only. The authors admit that some unknown selection process, either within the culture system or in vivo, may be influencing their culture results. This method has shown, however, that diploid cells present in breast tumors may be capable of invasive growth.

Wolman et al. have also determined that chromosome aberrations in breast cancer cells evolve over time in culture, thereby questioning the relevance of cultured preparations to the in vivo situation [47]. In contrast, Gebhart et al., with the use of parallel investigation of fresh tissue from the patient and of specimens kept in culture, have demonstrated that the chromosomal changes follow predictable and parallel patterns of evolution in each situation [16]. Their short-term cultures of primary lesions and of cell effusions also detected near diploid and hyperdiploid karyotypes and confirmed the nonrandom involvement of previously implicated chromosomes. A novel approach of seeking the cytogenetic equivalents of gene amplification was also employed. Previous studies had correlated the presence of DMs with disease aggressiveness and patient outcome [15]. The authors were able to detect DMs in almost half of their cases and were able to correlate this with clinical behavior.

Until recently very few studies had been conducted with direct analysis of in vivo metaphases to avoid the problems of cultured specimens. Rodgers et al. [29] investigated 51 primary lesions by direct harvest of in vivo metaphases. Their technique yielded a 37% success rate in obtaining analyzable metaphases, with an additional 13% of cultures providing only countable metaphases. Nine cases in the near diploid range could be analyzed in detail. This revealed that all had a duplication of the terminal portion of the 1q arm arising by a variety of mechanisms. There was also frequent loss of chromosome 16 in both the near diploid and more aneuploid cases. The cases with the simplest karyotypes contained only a 1q marker and monosomy 16. The authors speculate that chromosome 1 may be involved in tumor initiation or progression by increased gene dosage effect, i.e., of oncogenes, and that chromosome 16 may also be implicated as a primary tumorigenic event in breast cancer. Ferti-Passantonopoulou et al. have also used a direct technique to investigate five cases of breast cancer. They found recurrent involvement of chromosome 1 and 11, but did not detect monosomy 16 in any of their cases [13].

The cytogenetics laboratory of the Cancer Control Agency of British Columbia has been involved in a developmental study of the cytogenetic aspects of breast cancer, utilizing a culture technique for benign and malignant breast epithelial cells developed by Emerman et al. [11]. This culture system uses mechanical and enzymatic disaggregation to produce single cells and cell clusters that are cultured on collagen-coated slides or in semisolid suspension. An important feature of the defined culture media is the inclusion of normal human serum and the omission of fetal calf serum. This provides the option of utilizing the patient's own serum for individual cultures. The cells can also be frozen for reculturing at a later date. The growing cells obtained by this technique have been confirmed to be breast epithelial cells by phenotypic marker studies. This culture system has provided high quality metaphases for cytogenetic analysis using in situ harvest of cultures on collagen-coated slides. We have obtained consistently analyzable metaphases from both benign and malignant specimens. A trypsinized harvest or harvest of metaphases from the semisolid suspension cultures would also be feasible.

The further development of these short-term culture methods for chromosome analysis of breast cancer will permit the prospective investigation of a series of breast cancer patients with correlation of results with histology and clinical staging. In addition, a high yield of chromosome abnormalities may permit a search for breast cancer-specific breakpoint sites or for specific karyotypic changes such as DMs which may correlate with disease subtype and prognosis. Of great interest will be the possibility of examining specific disease stages, such as preinvasive lesions and atypias to detect the presence of chromosomal changes for the purpose of screening and diagnosis. The renewable source of cells provides an important advantage to this system, allowing comparative studies using different methodologies with correlation over time by in vivo and in vitro analysis. It may be possible to correlate the chromosomal findings with the results from DNA flow cytometry and DNA studies performed on both the original and cultured specimen.

Despite these recent developments with direct analysis and short-term culture of breast cancer specimens, a number of questions remain unresolved. Will further experience with the direct technique be rewarded with a higher success rate? The high failure rate associated with direct metaphase preparation results in the loss of potentially important information that might be obtained through utilization of additional techniques such as short-term culture. There may be a biologic reason for the high failure rates and for the present lack of correlation of the chromosome results with the outcome of breast cancer; however, the growing experience with other solid tumors would suggest that these are primarily technical problems that will be overcome as more specimens are analyzed with improved methodology. With regards to short-term cultures, will a significant proportion of patients prove to have diploid or near diploid karyotypes, and will this correlate with early disease or a subtype of disease with different clinical behavior? Will the addition of growth factors and hormones to the culture media result in selective growth of certain cell lines or subclones within the malignant population which may bias the cytogenetic results? These questions will serve to stimulate additional investigation in this field, most likely by a combination of direct analysis and short-term culture. The experience with the hematopoietic malignancies has shown that the identification of the disease-specific chromosome abnormalities that we now recognize resulted from the improved success rate obtained with the combination of direct, short-term cultures and high resolution banding techniques. This should also prove to be the case with solid tumors.

Conclusions

The value of chromosome analysis in breast cancer has yet to be determined. A primary chromosomal lesion characterized as typical and selectively specific for breast cancer has not been found. This will require the investigation of a larger number of specimens by a combination of methods. Even primary changes associated with breast cancer are not detected, valuable information will be obtained of importance in patient prognosis and management, as it has with the hematopoietic malignancies. The use of standard chromosome analysis, in combination with DNA analysis for oncogene involvement and DNA flow cytometry will provide new insights into the basic biology of breast cancer in the near future.

Acknowledgment. The author gratefully acknowledges the encouragement and helpful criticism provided by Dr. Dagmar Kalousek in the preparation of this manuscript.

References

1. Atkin NB (1976) Cytogenetic aspects of malignant transformation. Karger, Basel, pp 71-72
2. Aurias A, Rimbaut C, Buffe D, Zucker JM, Mazabraud A (1984) Translocation involving chromosome 22 in Ewing's sarcoma. A cytogenetic study of four fresh tumors. Cancer Genet Cytogenet 12:21-25
3. Balaban G, Gilbert F, Nichols W, Meadows AT, Shields J (1982) Abnormalities of chromosome #13 in retinoblastomas from individuals with normal constitutional karyotypes. Cancer Genet Cytogenet 6: 213-221
4. Bloomfield CD, Goldman AI, Alimena G, Berger R, Borgström GH, Brandt L, Catovsky D, de la Chapelle A, Dewald GW, Garson OM, Garwicz S, Golomb HM, Hossfeld DK, Lawler SD, Mitelman F, Nilsson P, Pierre RV, Philip P, Prigogina E, Rowley JD, Sakurai M, Sandberg AA, Secker Walker LM, Tricot G, Van Den Berghe H, Van Orshoven A, Vuopio P, Whang-Peng J (1986) Chromosomal abnormalities identify high-risk and low-risk patients with acute lymphoblastic leukemia. Blood 67: 415-420
5. Boveri T (1914) Zur Frage der Entstehung maligner Tumoren. Fischer, Jena
6. Cavanee WK, Dryja TP, Phillips RA, Benedict WF, Godbout R, Gallie BL, Murphree AL, Strong LC, White RL (1983) Expression of recessive alleles by chromosomal mechanisms in retinoblastoma. Nature 305: 779-784
7. Chaum E, Ellsworth RM, Abramson DH, Haik BG, Kitchin FD, Changati RSK (1984) Cytogenetic analysis of retinoblastoma: evidence for multifocal origin and in vivo gene amplification. Cytogenet Cell Genet 38: 82-91
8. Cowell JK (1982) Double minutes and homogeneously stained regions: gene amplification in mammalian cells. Annu Rev Genet 16: 21-59
9. De Klein A, Hermans A, Bootsma D, Grosveld F, Heisterkamp N, Stam K, Groffen J (1986) The role of the Philadelphia translocation in chronic myelocytic leukemia. Ann Clin Res 18: 278-283
10. Douglass EC, Look AT, Webber B, Parham D, Wilimas JA, Green AA, Roberson PK (1986) Hyperdiploidy and chromosomal rearrangements define the anaplastic variant of Wilms' tumor. J Clin Oncol 4: 975-981
11. Emerman JT, Bissell MJ (in press) Cultures of mammary epithelial cells: extracellular matrix and functional differentiation. In: Maramorosch K (ed) Advances in cell culture. Academic, Orlando
12. Emmanuel BS, Balaban G, Boyd JP, Grossman A, Negishi M, Parmiter A, Glickman MC (1985) N-*myc* amplification in multiple homogeneously staining regions in two human neuroblastomas. Proc Natl Acad Sci USA 82: 3736-3740
13. Ferti-Passantonopoulu AD, Panami AD (1987) Common cytogenetic findings in primary breast cancer. Cancer Genet Cytogenet 27: 289-298
14. Franke F, Rudolph B, Christiansen H, Harbott J, Lampert F (1986) Tumour karyotype may be important in the prognosis of human neuroblastoma. J Cancer Res Clin Oncol 111: 266-272
15. Gebhart E, Brüderlein S, Tulusan AH, von Maillot K, Birkman J (1984) Incidence of double minutes, the cytogenetic equivalents of gene amplification in human carcinoma cells. Int J Cancer 34: 369-373

16. Gebhart E, Brüderlein S, Augustus M, Siebert E, Feldner J, Schmidt W (1986) Cytogenetic studies on human breast carcinomas. Breast Cancer Res Treat 8: 125-138
17. Gilbert F, Feder M, Balaban G, Brangman D, Lurie DK, Podolsky R, Rinaldt V, Vinikoor N, Weisband J (1984) Human neuroblastomas and abnormalities of chromosomes 1 and 17. Cancer Res 44: 5444-5449
18. Harnden DG, Klinger HP (eds) (1985) ISCN. An international system for human cytogenetic nomenclature. Karger, Basel
19. Heim S, Mitelman F (1987) Nineteen of 26 cellular oncogenes precisely localized in the human genome map to one of the 83 bands involved in primary cancer-specific rearrangements. Hum Genet 75: 70-72
20. Heim S, Mitelman F (1986) Proliferation-specific and differentiation-associated chromosomal breakpoints in human neoplasia—a unifying model. Hereditas 104: 307-312
21. Koufos A, Hansen MF, Lampkin BC, Workman ML, Copeland NG, Jenkins NA, Cavanee WK (1984) Loss of alleles at loci on chromosome 11 during genesis of Wilms' tumor. Nature 309: 170-172
22. Knudson AG (1971) Mutation and cancer: statistical study of retinoblastoma. Proc Natl Acad Sci USA 68: 820-823
23. Le Beau MM (1986) Chromosomal fragile sites and cancer-specific rearrangements. Blood 67: 849-858
24. Levine EG, Arthur DC, Frizzera G, Peterson BA, Hurd DD, Bloomfield CD (1985) There are differences in cytogenetic abnormalities among histologic subtypes of the non-Hodgkin's lymphomas. Blood 66: 1414-1422
25. Mitelman F (1984) Restricted number of chromosomal regions implicated in aetiology of human cancer and leukaemia. Nature 310: 325-327
26. Nowell PC, Hungerford DA (1960) A minute chromosome in human chronic granulocytic leukemia. Science 132: 1497
27. Pathak S, Strong LC, Ferrell RE, Trindade A (1982) Familial renal cell carcinoma with a 3;11 chromosome translocation limited to tumor cells. Science 217: 939-941
28. Riccardi VM, Hittner HM, Francke U, Yunis JJ, Ledbetter D, Borges W (1980) The aniridia-Wilms' tumor association: the critical role of chromosome band 11p13. Cancer Genet Cytogenet 2: 131-137
29. Rodgers CS, Hill SM, Hultén MA (1984) Cytogenetic analysis in human breast carcinoma. I. Nine cases in the diploid range investigated using direct preparations. Cancer Genet Cytogenet 13: 95-119
30. Rowley JD (1973) A new consistent chromosomal abnormality in chronic myelogenous leukaemia identified by quinacrine fluorescence and Giemsa staining. Nature 243: 290-293
31. Sandberg AA (1980) The chromosomes of human cancer and leukemia. Elsevier, New York, pp 485-490
32. Sandberg AA, Gemmill RM, Hecht BK, Hecht F (1986) The Philadelphia chromosome: a model of cancer and molecular cytogenetics. Cancer Genet Cytogenet 21: 129-146
33. Sandberg AA (1986) Chromosome changes in bladder cancer: clinical and other correlations. Cancer Genet Cytogenet 19: 163-175
34. Sandberg AA, Turc-Carel C (1987) The cytogenetics of solid tumors: relation to diagnosis, classification and pathology. Cancer 59: 387-395
35. Schwab M, Varmu HE, Bishop JM, Grzeschik K-H, Naylor SL, Sakaguchi AY, Brodeur G, Trent J (1984) Chromosome localization in normal human cells and neuroblastomas of a gene related to c-*myc*. Nature 308: 288-291
36. Seabright M (1971) A rapid banding method for human chromosomes. Lancet ii: 971-972
37. Seeger RC, Brodeur GM, Sather H, Dalton A, Siegel SE, Wong KY, Hammond D (1985)

Association of multiple copies of the N-*myc* oncogene with rapid progression of neuroblastomas. New Engl J Med 313: 1111-1116
38. Showe LC, Croce CM (1987) The role of chromosomal translocations in B- and T-cell neoplasia. Annu Rev Immunol 5: 253-277
39. Smith HS, Liotta LA, Hancock MC, Wolman SR, Hackett AJ (1985) Invasiveness and ploidy of human mammary carcinomas in short-term culture. Proc Natl Acad Sci USA 82: 1805-1809
40. Trent JM (1985) Cytogenetic and molecular biologic alterations in human breast cancer: a review. Breast Cancer Res Treat 5: 221-229
41. Trent J, Crickard K, Gibas Z et al. (1986) Methodologic advances in the cytogenetic analysis of human solid tumors. Cancer Genet Cytogenet 19: 57-66
42. Turc-Carel C, Lizard-Nacol S, Justrabo E, Favrot M, Philip T, Tabone E (1986) Consistent chromosomal translocation in alveolar rhabdomyosarcoma. Cancer Genet Cytogenet 19: 361-362
43. Turc-Carel C, Dal Cin P, Limon J, Li F, Sandberg AA (1986) Translocation X;18 in synovial sarcoma. Cancer Genet Cytogenet 23: 93
44. Whang-Peng J, Bunn PA Jr, Kao-Shan CS, Lee EC, Carney DN, Gazdar A, Minna JD (1982) A nonrandom chromosomal abnormality, del 3p (14-23), in human small cell lung cancer (SCLC). Cancer Genet Cytogenet 6: 119-134
45. Williams DL, Raimondi S, Rivera G, George S, Berard CW, Murphy SB (1985) Presence of clonal chromosome abnormalities in virtually all cases of acute lymphoblastic leukemia. New Engl J Med 313: 640-641
46. Williams DL, Harber J, Murphy SB, Look T, Kalwinsky DK, Rivera G, Melvin SL, Stass S, Dahl GV (1986) Chromosomal translocations play a unique role in influencing prognosis in childhood acute lymphoblastic leukemia. Blood 68: 205-212
47. Wolman SR (1983) Karyotypic progression in human tumors. Cancer Metastasis Rev 2: 257-293
48. Wolman SR, Smith HS, Stampfer M, Hackett AJ (1985) Growth of diploid cells from breast cancers. Cancer Genet Cytogenet 16: 49-64
49. Yunis JJ (1976) High resolution of human chromosomes. Science 191: 1268-1270
50. Yunis JJ (1983) The chromosomal basis of neoplasia. Science 221: 227-236
51. Yunis JJ, Brunning R, Howe RB, Lobell M (1984) High resolution chromosomes as an independent prognostic indicator of acute non-lymphocytic leukemia. New Engl J Med 311: 812-818
52. Zang DK (1982) Cytological and cytogenetic studies on human meningioma. Cancer Genet Cytogenet 6: 249-274

Subject Index

MIX
Papier aus verantwortungsvollen Quellen
Paper from responsible sources
FSC® C105338

If you have any concerns about our products,
you can contact us on
ProductSafety@springernature.com

In case Publisher is established outside the EU,
the EU authorized representative is:
Springer Nature Customer Service Center GmbH
Europaplatz 3, 69115 Heidelberg, Germany

Printed by Libri Plureos GmbH
in Hamburg, Germany